The Unofficial Guide™ to Women's Health

Carol A. Turkington
with Susan J. Probst, M.D.

IDG Books Worldwide, Inc.
An International Data Group Company
Foster City, CA • Chicago, IL • Indianapolis, IN
• New York, NY

IDG Books Worldwide, Inc.
An International Data Group Company
919 E. Hillsdale Boulevard
Suite 400
Foster City, CA 94404

Copyright © 2000 by Carol A. Turkington

All rights reserved, including the right of reproduction in whole or in part in any form.

This publication contains the opinions and ideas of its author[s] and is designed to provide useful advice to the reader on the subject matter covered. Any references to any products or services do not constitute or imply an endorsement or recommendation. The publisher and the author[s] specifically disclaim any responsibility for any liability, loss or risk (financial, personal or otherwise) which may be claimed or incurred as a consequence, directly or indirectly, of the use and/or application of any of the contents of this publication. The author and publisher are not engaged in rendering medical or other professional services in this publication. Circumstances vary for practitioners of the activities covered herein, and this publication should not be used without prior consultation from a competent medical professional.

Certain terms mentioned in this book which are known or claimed to be trademarks or service marks have been capitalized.

IDG Books Worldwide, Inc. does not attest to the validity, accuracy or completeness of this information. Use of a term in this book should not be regarded as affecting the validity of any trademark or service mark.

Unofficial Guides are a [registered] trademark of Macmillan General Reference USA, Inc., a wholly owned subsidiary of IDG Books Worldwide, Inc.

For general information on IDG Books Worldwide's books in the U.S., please call our Consumer Customer Service department at 800-762-2974. For reseller information, including discounts and previous sales, please call our Reseller Customer Service department at 800-434-3422.

ISBN: 0-02863666-X

Manufactured in the United States of America

10 9 8 7 6 5 4 3 2 1

First edition

For our daughter, Kara Kennedy

Acknowledgments

Thanks to all the experts who helped with advice, support, and information, especially the staff at Foxchase Cancer Center (including Susan Montgomery, Kathy Gillespie, and Josephine Costalas), the staffs at the institutes at the National Institutes of Health, and the American Psychological Association.

Thanks also to Dr. Susie Probst, to my editors, Randy Ladenheim-Gil and Sandra Birnbaum Wagman, for their skill and encouragement, and, as always, to my agent, Bert Holtje. And finally, special thanks to Kara and Michael for enduring my 18-hour days without complaint.

The *Unofficial Guide* Reader's Bill of Rights.............xxv
The *Unofficial Guide* Panel of Experts.....................xxxi
Introduction..xxxv

I Living a Longer, Healthier Life 1

1 Making Savvy Health Care Choices 3

How to Find a Good Health Care Provider 4
  How Available Will Your New Health Care Provider Be? 6
  "I Don't Want to Be a Partner!" 6

Be a Patient Your Health Care Provider Loves 7
  Before Your Office Visit 8
  During Your Office Visit 9

Do You Have a Good Partnership? 10
  Working Together as a Team 11
  If You're Unhappy with Your Health Care Provider... 13

If You Need a Specialist 13

"What's This Test Designed to Do?" 14
  You Can Say No! 15
  If You Agree to a Test 16

Home Medical Tests 16
  Urinalysis 16
  Blood Glucose 17
  Blood Pressure 17
  Blood in Stool 18
  Home Pregnancy Tests 18
  In-Home Ovulation Predictor Kit 18

Take Two Pills and Call Me in the Morning 19

Bogus Cures 20

If You Need Surgery... 20
Managed Care: Working the System 22
    The Downside of HMOs *23*
    Before You Join an HMO... ....*24*
    Are You Satisfied? *26*
    Understanding Your HMO Coverage *26*
    How to Get the Best HMO Care *27*
    If You've Got a Problem Getting Care... ......*29*
    External Review Boards *32*
Emergency! The Ins and Outs of the ER Visit 32
Choosing the Best Place for Your Treatment and Recovery 34
    Community Hospital or Specialty Center? *34*
    When Being at Home is the Right Choice *36*
Getting the Care You Need While in the Hospital 36
Patient's Bill of Rights 37
A Living Will 39
Just the Facts 41

2 Body Image 43

When Your Mirror Lies: Negative Body Image 43
    "I Hate My Body" *44*
    Body Dysmorphic Disorder *45*
Exploding the Diet Myths 46
    Why Weight Loss Diets Don't Work *46*
    Eat Out and Lose Weight *47*
    For Women Only: Special Nutritional Needs *48*
    Obesity *51*
Get Physical 53
    Designing Your Own Plan *53*
    See Your Doctor If... ....*55*
    Got Kids? *55*
    Exercise for Seniors *56*
Eating Disorders: Are You at Risk? 57
    Anorexia Nervosa *60*
    Bulimia Nervosa *62*

- Binge Eating 64
- Like Mother, Like Daughter 65
- For More Information... 65

Plastic Surgery 66
Cosmetic Breast Surgery 66
- Are They Too Small? 66
- Are They Too Big? 68

Nose Job (Rhinoplasty) 70
Suck the Fat Away 73
Tummy Tucks 76
Just the Facts 77

3 Checking Up Through All Stages of Life 79

How to Choose a Specialist 80
Birth to 11 Years 83
- Vaccinate! 83
- Chicken Pox: Is It Safe? 83
- Polio Vaccines: Give It a Shot 85
- DTP Versus DTaP 85
- Goodbye, Ear Infections! 86
- Sniff Away the Flu 86

The Teenage Years (12 to 19) 87
- Vaccinations 87
- What to Expect in a Physical 87
- Choosing a Gynecologist 89
- Your First Pap Smear 89
- Your First Pelvic Exam 91
- Eat Healthy, Stay Healthy 95

Young Adulthood (20 to 39) 96
- What to Expect in Your 20s 96
- What to Expect in Your 30s 97
- What You Can Do to Stay Healthy 97
- Do You Need a Special Doctor? 98
- Types of Specialists 99
- Locating a Doctor 99
- Test You Should Have 100
- Vaccines for Your 20s and 30s 100
- Contraception: What's Your Choice? 102
- Ask Your Doctor About... 103

Your Mature Years (40 to 64) 103
- What to Expect 103
- What You Can Do to Stay Healthy 104

Menopause: How to Choose a Specialist ...104
Tests 104
Bone Density Tests 104
Vaccinations 106
Ask Your Doctor About... 107
Your Older Years (Over 65) 107
What You Can Expect 108
Tests You Need 108
Get Your Shots! 108
What You Can Do to Stay Healthy 110
Ask Your Doctor About... 110
Special Vaccinations 110
Just the Facts 112

II Reproductive Health........................113

4 Keeping Your Reproductive System Healthy 115

Menstrual Problems 115
Absent Periods 116
Painful Periods 118
Heavy Flow 119
Abnormal Bleeding 121
Premenstrual Syndrome 123
PMS or Bad Temper? 124
What Is It? 125
Diagnosing the Problem 126
What You Can Do 127
Do Drugs Work? 128
Uterine Fibroids 129
Is It a Fibroid? 130
Tests Your Doctor May Do 130
To Treat or Not to Treat? 130
On the Horizon... 133
Can You Prevent Fibroids? 134
Endometriosis 134
How to Tell If It's Endometriosis 135
Complications 136
Tests Your Doctor Should Perform 137
Surgery: Yes or No? 138
Ovarian Problems 139
Ovarian Infections 141

Ovarian Cysts 141
   Tests Your Doctor Might Perform 142
   Treating Ovarian Cysts 142

Polycystic Ovarian Syndrome 143
   What Causes PCOS? 144
   Current PCOS Treatments 145
   On the Horizon... 146

Just the Facts 147

5 Fertility and Infertility 149

Birth Control 149
   Methods You Can Count On 150
   Methods That Don't Work 150

Natural Birth Control Methods 151

Barrier Methods 152
   Spermicide 153
   Condom: His and Hers 153
   Diaphragm 155
   Cervical Cap 156
   The Sponge: It's Back! 156

Intrauterine Device 158

Hormonal Contraception 159
   The Pill 160
   Contraceptive Implants 162
   Birth control Injections 163
   Birth control Interactions 165

Sterilization 165
   Female Sterilization 166
   Male Sterilization 167

Emergency Contraception:
The "Morning After" Pill 167

When Birth Control Fails... 168
   RU-486 (Mifepristone) 169
   Surgical Abortion 170

Infertility: Cause and Effect 170
   Is It Him... 171
   ...Or Is It Her? 172
   Factors Other Than Physical 172
   Are You Infertile? 174

Finding a Fertility Specialist 174
   Choosing a Good Doctor 176

What to Ask Your Doctor *177*
What to Expect on Your First Visit *177*
Infertility Tests 178
Getting a Second Opinion
(or Changing Doctors) 179
Unexplained Infertility 179
Fertility Drugs 180
Surgery 181
Artificial Insemination 181
Sperm Banks 181
  The Process... ....*182*
  Selecting a Donor *183*
  Confidentiality *183*
  Offspring Limits *184*
Assistive Reproductive Technology:
The Latest 184
  In Vitro Fertilization (IVF) *185*
  Gamete Intrafallopian Transfer *186*
  Zygote Intrafallopian Transfer *186*
  Donor Egg IVF *186*
  Frozen Embryos *187*
Just the Facts 187

6 Pregnancy **189**
Pregnancy Tests: Are They Reliable? 189
Choosing a Practitioner Who's Right
for You 190
  Obstetrician/Gynecologist *190*
  Perinatologist *191*
  Family Physician *191*
  Other Care Providers *192*
  So Many Choices... ....*193*
  Where to Find a Practitioner *193*
  Interviewing a Health Practitioner *194*
The Birth Site: The Inside Scoop 196
  The Hospital *197*
  The Birthing Center *198*
  Home Births *200*
Your First Prenatal Visit 200
Screening Tests: Do You Need Them? 201
  Basic Tests *201*

Ultrasound: How Many, How Often 202
　　Alpha-Fetoprotein (AFP) Test 203
　　Triple Screening 204
　　Amniocentesis: Not for Everyone 205
　　Chorionic Villus Sampling (CVS) 206
　　CVS Versus Amniocentesis 206
How You'll Look, What You'll Feel 207
First Trimester 207
　　What Your Baby Looks Like 208
　　How You May Feel 208
Second Trimester 208
　　What Your Baby Looks Like 210
　　How You May Feel 210
Third Trimester 211
　　What Your Baby Looks Like 211
　　How You May Feel 212
How to Have a Healthy Baby 213
　　Eat a Good Diet 213
　　Drink Up! 215
　　Vitamin Supplements 215
　　Exercise During Pregnancy 216
What to Avoid During Pregnancy 218
　　Alcohol 218
　　Cigarettes 220
　　Recreational Drugs 220
　　Caffeine 220
　　Artificial Sweeteners 221
　　Prescription and Over-the-Counter
　　　　Medicines 221
　　Hot Tubs and Saunas..............................222
　　Travel 222
　　Chemical Exposure 223
Problems: Not Likely, but Possible 223
　　Pre-term Labor 224
　　Preeclampsia: Can You Avoid It? 225
　　Abruptio Placentae 225
　　Bleeding 226
　　Placenta Previa 227
　　Ectopic Pregnancy 228
　　Infections 229
Are All Birthing Classes Equal? 232
Just the Facts 233

7 Childbirth 235

Labor: A Woman's Fears 235
Pain Control: The Real Deal 237
  Tranquilizers, Sedatives, and Narcotics *237*
  Local Anesthetics *237*
  Regionals: Epidurals and Spinal Blocks *238*
Get the Answers to Your Questions
Before Your Labor Begins 240
Labor: Is This the Real Thing? 240
  Signs of Labor *241*
  Contractions *243*
When to Call the Doctor 244
What to Take with You to the Hospital 245
What to Expect at the Hospital 246
Hospital Prep 246
The Next Step... 247
If Your Labor Is Induced 247
Latent Phase of First Stage of Labor 249
Active Phase of First Stage of Labor 249
Second Stage of Labor 250
Pushing 251
At Last—A Baby! 252
What Happens Now? 252
The Afterbirth 253
Cesarean Birth 254
  Is a C-Section Necessary? *254*
  What to Expect *255*
  After a Cesarean Birth *256*
  Vaginal Birth After C-Section *257*
If There's a Problem 257
  Miscarriage *258*
  Stillbirth *259*
  Birth Defects *261*
  Intrauterine Growth Restriction *262*
An Orange with Hair... 264
Holding Your Baby 265
Feeding Your Baby 266
Your Hospital Stay 266

Taking Your Baby Home 267
Postpartum 267
   If You Feel Depressed... 269
   What Your Baby Might Do 270
Wrapping It Up 270
Just the Facts 271

III Not All in Your Head: Mental Health Issues 273

8 Depression 275

Depression Quiz 276
   Why Are Women So Depressed? 276
   Serotonin Story 277
   Wintertime Blues: The Inside Scoop 278
   Hormones: The Female Difference 280
   Depression After Delivery 281
   Drugs and Depression 283

Are You at Risk? 283

Counseling: What the Experts Say 285
   Finding a Therapist 285
   Therapists: Heroes or Healers? 286
   Analysis or Talk Therapy? 287
   Paying for Treatment 288
   Is Your Therapist Really Helping? 289
   Squeezing Out Sexism 290
   If Your Therapist Acts Inappropriately... ..290

Do Antidepressants Work? 292
   What to Ask Your Doctor 293
   Hot Off the Lab Table: The Newest Drugs 294
   Cyclics: Do They Still Work? 296
   MAO Inhibitors: Are They Safe? 297
   Lithium: What You Need to Know 299

Electroconvulsive Treatment 300
   Pros and Cons 300
   ECT and Your Pregnancy 301

Alternatives 301
   St. John's Wort: Does It Work? 302
   Ins and Outs of Acupuncture 304
   Seeking Support 304
   Can You Relax Depression Away? 305

  Vitamins *305*
  Getting Better with Gingko *306*
  Banish Depression with a Cuppa Joe *306*
  Exercise—Is It Enough? *306*
 Down the Road: What You Can Expect 307
 Just the Facts 307

9 Stress, Anxiety, and Violence **309**
 How Stress Affects You 310
 How Stressed Are You? 311
  Stress Test *312*
  Keep a Stress Log *313*
 Dealing with Stress 314
  Breathing Can Help *315*
  Just Relax... ....*319*
  Meditate *320*
  Visualization *321*
  Exercise Stress Away *323*
  Diet and Stress *325*
  Anti-Stress Vitamins/Herbs *328*
  Social Support—Does It Work? *329*
  Stress Can Be Good *329*
 Anxiety: What's Normal? 330
  Anxiety Disorders: Are You at Risk? *330*
  Panic Disorder *331*
  Phobias *332*
  Generalized Anxiety Disorder *333*
  Do You Have an Anxiety Disorder? *333*
 Treatment 334
  Combining Counseling and Drugs *334*
  Kava *335*
 Dealing with Violent Relationships 335
  Is Your Partner an Abuser? *336*
  Are You at Risk? *337*
  What's Normal and What Isn't *337*
  Symptoms of Abuse *339*
  Getting Help: Where to Turn *340*
 Just the Facts 341

10 Substance Abuse **343**
 What Constitutes Abuse? 343
  Who's at Risk? *344*
  The Addictive Personality *345*

Smoking 345
   How to Quit *347*
   Patches and Gum *349*
   Acupuncture and Smoking *351*

Alcohol Abuse 351
   What's Your Risk? *353*
   Do You Have a Problem? *354*
   Getting Help for Someone Else *357*
   Support Groups—Working the Steps ...*359*

Legal and Illegal Drug Abuse 359
   Who's at Risk? *360*
   Prescription Drugs *361*
   Illicit Drugs *362*

Treatment 362
   Where to Get Help... ....*363*

Just the Facts 364

IV Symptoms, Diagnoses, and Treatments 365

11 Keeping Your Skin Healthy 367

How to Find a Great Skin Care Specialist 367
   Choosing a Dermatologist *368*
   What to Expect from a Good
     Dermatologist *369*

Acne 370
   Myths: Chocolate, French Fries,
     and More... ....*371*
   So What Does Cause Acne? *371*
   The Over-20 Acne Myths *373*
   Can You Prevent Acne? *373*
   Treat Yourself or See a Dermatologist? *374*
   Hot Off the Press: Newest Treatments *375*
   Don't Give Up! *377*
   Help for Acne Scars *378*

Is It Acne or Rosacea? 378
   Who Gets It? *379*
   Is It in Your Genes? *380*
   Treatment: The Newest Info *380*

Skin Cancer 381
   Check Your Skin Monthly *381*
   Mole or Cancer—Can You Tell the
     Difference? *383*

What to Expect with Skin Cancer 383
   Basal Cell Carcinoma *383*
   Squamous Cell Carcinoma *385*
   Malignant Melanoma *386*
   Skin Cancer Quiz *387*
Sun Safety: Help Keep Skin Cancer
at Bay 388
   Screening the Sun *389*
   Sunscreen Tips *390*
   Protect Your Eyes, Too! *392*
   Drugs and the Sun—Which Ones
      Don't Mix *392*
Indoor Tans 394
Just the Facts 396

12 Reducing the Risk for Cancers 397
Early Detection 398
Leading a Low-Risk Life 399
   You Are What You Eat *399*
   Alcohol *400*
   Hormones *400*
   Tobacco *401*
   Heredity *401*
Breast Cancer 402
   Charting Your True Risk *402*
      If You Have a Family History *403*
      Genetic Risk: What You Can Do *406*
      Take the Test: BRCA1 and BRCA2 ......*407*
      On the Horizon... ....*408*
   Warning Signs... ....*408*
   Getting a Good Mammogram *409*
   Things to Know Before Scheduling
      a Mammogram *410*
   Your Mammogram Rights *410*
   Ultrasounds Versus Mammograms *411*
   Needle And Tissue Biopsies: What to
      Ask *411*
      If Your Tests Are Positive... ....*413*
      What About a Clinical Trial? *414*
   Finding the Best Treatment *415*
   After Surgery *416*
   Surviving Breast Cancer *417*

    Prevention: From Tamoxifen to
       Mastectomy 418
    For More Information... 420

  Ovarian Cancer 420
    Charting Your Risk 421
    Screening Breakthroughs 423
    Hereditary Cancer Syndrome 423
    Treatment 424
    In the Future: New Treatments 424

  Endometrial Cancer 425
    Risk Factors 425
    Do You Have Endometrial Cancer? 426
    Tests Your Doctor May Do 426
    Treatment 427

  Cervical Cancer 427
    HPV and Genital Warts 428
    Early Warning Signs 429
    What Does Your Pap Smear Mean? 430
    New Treatments: What You
       Should Know 431

  Coping with Cancer 431
  Just the Facts 432

13 Cardiovascular Disease 433

  Symptoms to Take Seriously 435
  Types of Heart Problems 436
    Atherosclerosis 436
    Coronary Heart Disease 437
    Predicting a Stroke 437
    Are You at Risk for Stroke? 438
    Did You Have a Stroke? 439
    Mitral Valve Prolapse 440
    Congestive Heart Failure 440
    Heart Rhythm Disturbances 441

  Risk Factors for Heart Disease 442
  Why Are Women at Higher Risk? 443
  Questions to Ask Your Cardiologist 445
  High Blood Pressure 447
  Tips for Taking Blood Pressure 448
  Measuring Cholesterol 448

Triglycerides 450
General Heart-Smart Strategies 451
Checking Out Your Heart 453
Just the Facts 456

14 Osteoporosis 457

The Hard Truth About Weak Bones 458
What Causes Osteoporosis? 459
Got Milk? 460
Are You at Risk? 461
Symptoms of Osteoporosis 462
Diagnosis and Monitoring 462
Bone Density Tests: All You Need
to Know 464
   Ultrasound Densitometry 465
   Urine Tests 466
   Do You Need to Be Tested? 466
Treating Osteoporosis the Natural Way 467
   Is Your Diet Calcium-Friendly? 468
   Calcium Supplements: If You
      Need More 469
   It's Never Too Late... 470
   Can Vitamins Help? 470
   Magnesium: Slowing and
      Preventing Loss 471
   Exercise 472
Drug Treatments 473
   Alendronate 475
   Hormone Replacement Therapy 476
   Raloxifene (Evista) 478
   Calcitonin: The Nose Has It 480
Prevention Is Worth a Pound of Cure 480
   Start Young 481
   Soybeans: The Latest Preventative 481
   Parathyroid Hormone 482
In the Future... 482
Just the Facts 483

15 Infectious Diseases 485

Preventing Colds and Flu 486

Preventing Urinary Tract Infections 488
  UTIs During Pregnancy 489
  Do You Have a UTI? 489
  Tests Your Doctor Will Order 490
  How to Avoid UTIs 490
Preventing Vaginal Infections 491
  Yeast Infections 492
  Bacterial Vaginosis 493
  Trichomoniasis 494
Preventing Pelvic Inflammatory Disease 494
  Are You at Risk? 495
  PID Symptoms 495
  Treating PID 496
Preventing Toxic Shock Syndrome 496
Preventing Sexually Transmitted Diseases ...497
  If You Have Multiple Partners 498
  If You've Been Diagnosed 498
  Treatment Outlook 499
  Chlamydia 499
  Genital Warts 500
  Genital Herpes 502
  Gonorrhea 504
  Hepatitis B 505
  Syphilis 507
  HIV and AIDS 508
    Practicing Safe Sex 509
    Treatment 510
Still a Possibility: Preventing
Tuberculosis 510
  Latent Versus Active TB 511
  Who's at Risk? 511
  How Do You Know It's TB? 512
  Diagnosis: When to Get a TB Skin Test 512
  Can TB Be Treated? 512
Preventing Mononucleosis 513
  How Do You Know It's Mono? 513
  Diagnosing the Problem 514
  Complications 514
  Treatment Tips 515
Preventing Lyme Disease 515
Just the Facts 517

16 Autoimmune Diseases 519
What Causes Autoimmune Disease? 520
Is It My Hormones? 521
Do Autoimmune Diseases Run in Families? 523
Can You Catch an Autoimmune Disease? 524
Getting a Good Diagnosis 524
Treating Autoimmune Diseases 526
Connective Tissue Diseases 527
Lupus 527
Rheumatoid Arthritis 529
Systemic Sclerosis (Scleroderma) 530
Sjogren's Syndrome (Sjogren's Disease) ...531
Neuromuscular Diseases 531
Multiple Sclerosis (MS) 531
Myasthenia Gravis 532
Endocrine Diseases 533
Hashimoto's Thyroiditis 534
Graves' Disease 534
Insulin-Dependent (Type 1) Diabetes Mellitus (IDDM) 535
Inflammatory Bowel Disease 537
Crohn's Disease 537
Ulcerative Colitis 538
Autoimmune Skin Diseases 538
Psoriasis 538
Vitiligo 539
Other Autoimmune Diseases 539
Chronic Fatigue Syndrome 539
Sarcoidosis 540
Vasculitis Syndromes 541
Hematologic Autoimmune Diseases 542
Autoimmunity and Infertility 542
Tips for Managing Autoimmune Disease 543
What's New on the Research Horizon? 544
Just the Facts 545

V The Ticking Clock: Women and Aging 547

17 What to Expect as You Age 549

Younger-Looking Skin: The Eternal Quest 549
   Laser Resurfacing 550
      How It Works *551*
      The Pros and Cons *552*
      Finding the Best Doctor *553*
      Questions to Ask *553*
   Collagen Treatments 554
   Botox Injections 555
   Dermabrasion 556
   Skin Peels 557
   When the Chemical Peel Isn't for You... 558
      Vitamin A Derivatives *558*
      Vitamin A-Like Products *559*
      Do-It-Yourself Peels: Fruit Acids *560*
      AHAs Versus Retin-A *563*
      Risks of AHAs *563*
      Do Your Cosmetics Have AHAs? *566*
      Vitamin C: Just a Fad? *567*
      Should You Combine Skin Products? *568*
   Coping with Dry Skin 569
   Plastic or Cosmetic Surgery 571
      Finding a Plastic Surgeon *572*
      Face-Lifts *573*
      Eyelid-Lifts *575*
      Brow-Lifts *575*
   Hair—Too Much or Too Little? 575
      Treating Hair Loss *576*
      Gray Hair *577*
      Hair Dye: Does It Cause Cancer? *578*
      Hair Removal *579*
   Memory Loss 582
      A Simple Memory Test *583*
      Menopause-Related "Fuzzy Thinking" *583*
      Is It Alzheimer's? *584*
      Other Causes *585*
      Preventing Memory Problems *586*
      You Can Improve Memory *588*
   Just the Facts 589

18 **Menopause** **591**
   Ovulation 591
   When Will You Enter Menopause? 593

Is It Me or Is It Hot in Here? 595
Menstrual Period Changes 595
Hot Flashes 597
If You Can't Sleep... 599
Irritability and Mood Swings 599
Thinking and Memory Problems 600
Vaginal Dryness 601
Breast Changes 601
Headaches 601
Heart Palpitations 602
Loss of Sexual Interest 602
Urinary Changes 602
Facial Hair 603
Depression 604

How to Cope with Menopause Symptoms 604
Hot Flashes 604
Heavy Bleeding 606
Insomnia 607
Mood Swings and Irritability 607
Memory Problems 608
Vaginal Dryness 608
Headaches 610
Loss of Libido 610
Urinary Problems 610

Is It PMS or the Beginning of Menopause? 611

Finding the Right Health Care Provider 613
Consulting an Expert 614
10 Questions to Ask 615

Hormone Tests: Do They Work? 616

Hormone Replacement Therapy: Yes or No? 618
What Kind of HRT? 618
Progestins 620
Alphabet SERMs 621
Low-Dose Estrogen 622
A Little More, a Little Less... 623
Testosterone: Yes or No? 623
Birth Control Pills as HRT 625

HRT: What Method Should You Use? 626
Hormone Pills 626
Skin Patch 626
Vaginal Cream 627

     Injections *628*
     Vaginal Rings *628*
     On the Drawing Board... ....*628*
  Pros and Cons of HRT *629*
     HRT Risk and Heart Attacks ...*631*
     What the Experts Agree On *632*
  Is HRT Right for You? *632*
     You're a Good Candidate *633*
     Women at Risk *633*
     You're a Bad Risk *634*
     Who Should Absolutely Avoid HRT *634*
  What to Ask Your Health Care Provider *634*
  Side Effects of HRT *635*
  HRT Dosage Regimens *635*
     Continuous Estrogen and Cyclic
        Progestin *636*
     Cyclic Estrogen and Progestin *637*
     Continuous Estrogen and Progestin *637*
     Continuous Estrogen *637*
     Cyclic Estrogen *638*
     Continuous Progestin *638*
  Knowing When to Stop *638*
  Natural Hormone Replacement *638*
     Bioflavonoids *642*
     Cenestin *642*
  Just the Facts *643*

A Resource Directory *645*

B Further Readings *681*

  Index *683*

The *Unofficial Guide* Reader's Bill of Rights

We Give You More Than the Official Line

Welcome to the *Unofficial Guide* series of Lifestyles titles—books that deliver critical, unbiased information that other books can't or won't reveal—the inside scoop. Our goal is to provide you with the most accessible, useful information and advice possible. The recommendations we offer in these pages are not influenced by the corporate line of any organization or industry; we give you the hard facts, whether those institutions like them or not. If something is ill-advised or will cause a loss of time and/or money, we'll give you ample warning. And if it a worthwhile option, we'll let you know that, too.

Armed and Ready

Our hand-picked authors confidently and critically report on a wide range of topics that matter to smart readers like you. Our authors are passionate about their subjects, but have distanced themselves enough from them to help you be armed and protected, and help make you educated decisions as you go through the process. It is our intent that, from having read this book, you will avoid the pitfalls everyone else falls into and get it right the first time.

Don't be fooled by cheap imitations; this is the genuine article *Unofficial Guide* series from IDG Books. You may be familiar with our proven track record of the travel *Unofficial Guides,* which have more than three million copies in print. Each year thousands of travelers—new and old—are armed with a brand new, fully updated edition of the flagship *Unofficial Guide to Walt Disney World,* by Bob Sehlinger. It is our intention here to provide you with the same level of objective authority that Mr. Sehlinger does in his brainchild.

The Unofficial Panel of Experts

Every work in the Lifestyle *Unofficial Guides* is intensively inspected by a team of three top professionals in their fields. These experts review the manuscript for factual accuracy, comprehensiveness, and an insider's determination as to whether the manuscript fulfills the credo in this Reader's Bill of Rights. In other words, our Panel ensures that you are, in fact, getting "the inside scoop."

Our Pledge

The authors, the editorial staff, and he Unofficial Panel of Experts assembled for *Unofficial Guides* are determined to lay out the most valuable alternatives available for our readers. This dictum means that our writers must be explicit, prescriptive, and above all, direct. We strive to be thorough and complete, but our goal is not necessarily to have the "most" or "all" of the information on a topic; this is not, after all, an encyclopedia. Our objective is to help you narrow down your options to the best of what is available, unbiased by affiliation with any industry or organization.

In each *Unofficial Guide* we give you:

- Comprehensive coverage of necessary and vital information
- Authoritative, rigidly fact-checked data
- The most up-to-date insights into trends
- Savvy, sophisticated writing that's also readable.
- Sensible, applicable facts and secrets that only an insider knows

Special Features

Every book in our series offers the following six special sidebars in the margins that are devised to help you get things done cheaply, efficiently, and smartly.

1. "Timesaver"—tips and shortcuts that save you time
2. "Moneysaver"—tips and shortcuts that save you money
3. "Watch Out!"—more serious cautions and warnings
4. "Bright Idea"—general tips and shortcuts to help you find and easier or smarter way to do something
5. "Quote"—statements from real people that are intended to be prescriptive and valuable to you
6. "Unofficially..."—an insider's fact or anecdote

We also recognize your need to have quick information at your fingertips, and have thus provided the following comprehensive sections at the back of the book:

1. Resource Guide—lists of relevant agencies, associations, institutions, web sites, etc.
2. Further Readings—suggested titles that can help you get more in-depth information on related topics
3. Index

Letters, Comments, and Questions from Readers

We strive to continually improve the *Unofficial* series, and input from our readers is a valuable way for us to do that.

Many of those who have used the *Unofficial Guide* travel books write to the authors to ask questions, make comments, or share their own discoveries and lessons. For Lifestyle *Unofficial Guides,* we would also appreciate all such correspondence—both positive and critical—and we will make best efforts to incorporate appropriate readers' feedback and comments in revised editions of this work.

How to write us:

Unofficial Guides
Lifestyle Guides
IDG Books
1633 Broadway
New York, NY 10019

Attention: Reader's Comments

About the Authors

Carol A. Turkington is a medical writer with 25 years of professional experience. A former journalist and editor, she has worked as a medical writer and editor for Duke University Medical Center and as a senior writer in biobehavioral medicine for the American Psychological Association in Washington, D.C. Her books have included *The Perimenopause Sourcebook* (Contemporary Books), *Making the Prozac Decision: A Guide to Antidepressants* (Lowell House); *Hepatitis C: The Silent Epidemic* (Contemporary); and *Stress Management for Busy People* (McGraw-Hill). She lives in southern Pennsylvania with her husband Michael Kennedy and 9-year-old daughter Kara.

Susan J. Probst, M.D., is a board certified obstetrician/gynecologist with more than 20 years of experience in women's health care and related issues. A graduate of Temple University School of Medicine, she practices outside of Philadelphia, where she lives with her husband and two children.

The *Unofficial Guide* Panel of Experts

The *Unofficial* editorial team recognizes that you've purchased this book with the expectation of getting the most authoritative, carefully inspected information currently available. Toward that end, on each and every title in this series, we have selected a minimum of two "official" experts comprising the *Unofficial* panel who painstakingly review the manuscripts to ensure the following: factual accuracy of all data; inclusion of the most up-to-date and relevant information; and that, from an insider's perspective, the authors have armed you with all the necessary facts you need—but that the institutions don't want you to know.

For *The Unofficial Guide to Women's Health,* we are proud to introduce the following panel of experts:

Larry Glazerman, M.D. Dr. Glazerman has been practicing obstetrics and gynecology since 1980. He is a Clinical Assistant Professor of Obstetrics and Gynecology at the Pennsylvania State University School of Medicine and is actively involved in teaching residents, medical students, and practicing physicians. He is board certified in obstetrics and gynecology and a Fellow of the American College of Obstetricians and Gynecologists, as well as active in the American Association of Gynecologic Laparoscopists. In addition, he has received certification in endoscopic surgery by the Accreditation Council for Gynecologic Endoscopy.

He serves on the advisory boards of Planned Parenthood and the Allentown Women's Center and was selected as a national faculty member by Health Learning Systems and the University of Minnesota to teach other health care providers about evidence-based medicine. He is also the Pennsylvania state representative to ObGyn.net, one of the premier Internet sites for women's health care. Dr. Glazerman received a B.S. degree *cum laude* from Muhlenberg College and an M.D. degree from Jefferson Medical College.

R. Daniel Braun, M.D., FACOG Dr. Braun is Clinical Professor of Obstetrics and Gynecology at Indiana University School of Medicine in Indianapolis, IN. Dr. Braun is a graduate of the University of Toledo (B.S. 1960) and Baylor University College of Medicine (M.D. 1964). He served a one-year rotating internship at Marion County General Hospital, Indianapolis, and a four-year residency in obstetrics and gynecology at the Indiana University School of Medicine. He served at the U.S. Naval Hospital, Portsmouth, VA, in 1969 and 1970. He previously served on the staff of the Scott and White Clinic in Temple, TX. He was Professor and Chairman of Obstetrics and Gynecology at the

Chattanooga campus of the University of Tennessee. He has also served on the faculty at the University of North Dakota and Texas Tech University Health Sciences Center, Odessa.

M. Kelly Shanahan, M.D. Dr. Shanahan is a board certified obstetrician-gynecologist practicing in South Lake Tahoe, CA. Dr. Shanahan is also a Fellow of the American College of Obstetricians and Gynecologists and a member of the American Medical Women's Association. In addition to her private practice duties, Dr. Shanahan is an advisor for OBGYN.net (www.obgyn.net) and is the Women's Health Expert for ivillage's better health site (www.betterhealth.com). She writes an "ask the expert" column for Blue Cross (www.mylifepath.com), as well. A graduate of Bryn Mawr College and the University of Virginia School of Medicine, Dr. Shanahan completed her residency in ob/gyn at Temple University in Philadelphia in 1991. She had a daughter in 1998, a feat of which she is most proud.

Deborah Wage, MSN, FNP, CNM Ms. Wage is director of Nashville Women's Health Associates in Nashville, TN, a private midwifery practice. She delivers babies at Centennial Women's Hospital and Baptist Hospital in Nashville. Ms. Wage received her master's degree from Vanderbilt University School of Nursing. She is dual board certified as a family nurse practitioner and a nurse midwife. Ms. Wage has been providing health care to the Nashville community for eight years. She is co-president of Middle Tennessee Advance Practice Nurses and a member of the American College of Nurse Midwives and the American Academy of Nurse Practitioners. She is active at the local, state, and national levels in various activities to improve the quality of maternity services.

Introduction

In this past decade, there have been more medical advances for women than our grandmothers ever dreamed possible. It has been a long time coming. For far too long, science and federal agencies have ignored women's health needs and issues. That's all beginning to change.

Today, we're teetering on the brink of a new millennium, the dawn of an age when our daughters and granddaughters will enjoy a level of health care so attuned to their needs that they'll be able to live active and vigorous lives well into their 80s and beyond.

We owe it to ourselves to claim the responsibility for our own health care and move forward, so that we can live our lives to the best of our ability, unburdened by disability and poor health. We owe it to ourselves, and to our daughters, and to our daughters' daughters.

Make no mistake: Information *is* power. You cannot hope to make the most sensible health care decisions if you don't have all the facts, and that is certainly no more true than it is today—with so many sweeping changes in our health care system, the woman who roars gets the best health care.

Yet, the finest medical tests, diagnosticians, and medical specialists in the world are never going to be enough if we don't make sensible choices about using those resources. In these days of managed care, cost-cutting, and no-frills treatment, if you want good medical care you have to work for it. You need to use your common sense to help find the care that's right for you and avoid services (and costs) that you don't need. This book can help you do that.

If you work hard, you can be on your way to becoming a wiser medical consumer. The best way to protect yourself is to ask questions and be observant. If you don't like what you see, ask more questions. If your health care provider doesn't appreciate your questions, find another one who does. Become a working member of your health care team, be honest, and share responsibility for your care. In *The Unofficial Guide to Women's Health,* we'll help you cut through the confusion and bring you the very latest information on doing just that.

Research has shown quite clearly that when a woman visits a health care provider, the two most important factors are the amount of information she gets and how actively she can participate in her care. But with today's streamlined efforts to "manage" care, when time is money and communication gets lost in the shuffle, too many women don't get the answers they need.

The Unofficial Guide to Women's Health tries to answer the kinds of questions you'd like to ask—and those that you didn't even know you should be asking, including: How do you get good care in an HMO? What can you do if you aren't getting the care you think you should be? How do you choose a particular specialist? What are the newest, most recent tests and procedures? How can you join a clinical trial?

You'll learn which screening tests you need to have at each stage of your life and how to prepare for them. We'll tell you the newest research on plant estrogens and bring you the latest data on the pros and cons of hormone replacement therapy. We'll let you peek into the laboratory to find out what new drugs and treatments will be arriving within the next 10 years—such as the new blood test that may help reveal how you'll respond to treatment for breast cancer. We'll disclose some of the very newest infertility treatments for those who want to get pregnant, and the newest contraceptive devices for those who don't.

We'll show you why breast cancer is not inevitable (as a group, women are far more likely to die of heart disease than of breast cancer)—and we'll explain what those scary cancer statistics really mean. (For example, the fact that one out of every eight women of average risk will one day develop breast cancer also means that you have an 88 percent risk of not ever getting the disease.)

The belated recognition that women aren't just shorter, slighter versions of men ushers in a whole new generation of exciting innovations in medical practice, patient information, and health care testing and treatments. Best of all, the revolution in women's health has given women more choices and more control. At last, a recognition of a woman's right to be heard—and not to be patronized and dismissed—is becoming a reality in hospitals, medical centers, and health care professionals' offices across the country.

But with this newfound power comes an awareness that if we demand to be treated like intelligent adults, we can no longer turn over the reins of responsibility for our health care to others. We have choices to make in our own best interests, and it's time to make them.

Those choices may be simple: Knowing the importance of exercise, of eating fresh fruits and vegetables, of taking vitamin supplements. Or, they may be as incredible as knowing how a once-barren woman can become a mother, or having the ability to read in a woman's blood or her bones the diseases she is destined to develop.

It's just the beginning of an extraordinarily exciting time for women's health, as the Women's Health Initiative—the largest clinical study ever devised—tracks more than 160,000 of us in an effort to deepen our understanding of disease. Gender-based biology is the knowledge that we are first and foremost profoundly different from men: Women are three times more likely to develop autoimmune diseases, such as lupus and multiple sclerosis. We are twice as likely to get a sexually transmitted disease. Twice as likely to be depressed. Ten times more likely to contract HIV from unprotected sex. And significantly more likely to get lung cancer, osteoporosis, and heart attacks.

Did you know:

- After drinking the same amount of alcohol, women have higher blood alcohol levels than men, even after accounting for size differences.

- Women who smoke are more likely to get lung cancer than men who smoke the same amount.
- Women tend to wake up from anesthesia more quickly than men.
- Some pain medications are far more effective in relieving pain in women.
- Women are more likely to die from a heart attack in the hospital.
- A woman's stronger immune system protects her better from disease, but also makes her more susceptible to autoimmune disorders.
- Depression is twice as common in women, in part because our brains produce less serotonin.

New research is also discovering the very different ways that men and women process medication—in general, when a woman takes a pill, more of the medication is available in her bloodstream for use by her body and the medication tends to remain in her body for a longer period of time. These gender-related differences suggest that a "standard dose" for some medications (probably based on studies of men anyway) may be too high for women, especially elderly women.

In *The Unofficial Guide to Women's Health,* we acknowledge that many of you already understand a lot about the basics of good health care—you know all about the government food pyramid, that vegetables and fruits are good, and that saturated fats are bad. Most women know they should exercise, stop smoking, watch their alcohol intake. These are the health basics that we hear about every day—and we know very well what we *should* be doing, thank you very much. But an awful lot of us just don't do it.

We should be taking our vitamins and getting more calcium (especially as we approach menopause). We should be getting lots of exercise and plenty of sleep, and we shouldn't drink too much—or smoke at all. We should be cutting way down on animal protein, eliminating excess fat and eating lots of fruits and vegetables. But are we? Most of the women you know probably fall far short of the goal of "healthy living."

One of the problems is that Americans tend to have an "all or nothing" attitude. Deep down inside, we believe if we can't spend an hour a day, four days a week exercising like a runner training for a marathon, we shouldn't waste time doing it at all. We think we should cut out all fatty foods, but when we break down and have a Big Mac, we give up on our diet completely. We think if we can't spend an hour a day doing yoga, it doesn't do any good to try it for just 20 minutes.

This philosophy is related to the idea that if we can't win the game, we don't want to play.

Most of us don't have the time to live the sort of healthy life we "think" we should be living, and not being able to achieve the incredibly lofty goals we set for ourselves, we choose to do nothing. But it doesn't have to be that way.

In fact, a few halting small steps along that healthy trail are far, far better than sitting down by the side of the path in sullen sloth and giving up. Studies have shown that even the most moderate exercise—a walk around the block, for example—can pay real health benefits. You start out small, you do what you can do, and you build on that. You may not be ready to make drastic changes, but that doesn't mean that you can't take the first tiny steps toward living a more healthy lifestyle.

This book will show you that, in all aspects of your life, you can begin to use some of the newest information to live a healthy life. We've combed the most recent scientific journals in mental health, pediatric care, obstetrics and gynecology, cardiology, dermatology, cosmetic surgery, gastroenterology, sociology, infectious diseases, infertility, and oncology, surfed a wide range of Web sites, and interviewed lots of experts and consumers to find the hottest and most intriguing topics and information.

If you've ever wished for a helpful, knowledgeable health "insider" to stand by your side as you make your way through the medical establishment, you'll find the help you've been looking for in *The Unofficial Guide to Women's Health*.

So, if you've ever wondered if you have the right to look at your own hospital chart—or appeal the decision of your HMO—or demand a copy of your mammogram report on the spot—or find out what Pap test is the best—read on. You have a right to know. Your health depends on it.

PART I

Living a Longer, Healthier Life

GET THE SCOOP ON...
Finding a good health care provider ▪ Making your HMO work for you ▪ What to ask about your medications, tests you need, and upcoming surgery ▪ How to be a patient your health care provider loves ▪ The patient's bill of rights

Making Savvy Health Care Choices

The best medical tests, diagnosticians, and medical specialists in the world aren't enough if we don't make sensible choices about using those resources. In these days of managed care, cost cutting, and no-frills treatment, if you want good medical care you have to work for it. Use your common sense to help find the care that's right for you and avoid services (and costs) that you don't need. If you trust your common sense, you're on your way to becoming a wiser medical consumer.

The best way to protect yourself is to ask questions and be observant. If you don't like what you see, ask more questions. If your health care provider doesn't appreciate your questions, find another one. Become a working partner—be honest and share responsibility for your care—and the two of you will make a great team. This chapter will help you learn how to do just that.

How to find a good health care provider

If you don't have a primary health care provider, now is the time to get one. If you spend your time hopping from gynecologist to pulmonary specialist to dermatologist, you'll get good individualized care for specific problems—but a host of specialists working on separate health issues won't really get the whole picture of your health care situation. Many women also use a gynecologist as their only doctor, and if you find that works well, fine. Other women may want to find a health care provider who is a board certified family practitioner doctor or internist. These doctors have broad knowledge about a whole range of medical problems. To find a good family doctor, start by asking friends and family for recommendations. You also could call your local hospital for a list of affiliated physicians.

Another way to find a quality health care provider is to call the nearest training program in the field in which you are looking and ask to speak to the chief resident. Ask him or her to give you a list of three physicians. The local medical society is another good choice.

Check your local library for the *Compendium of Certified Medical Specialists* or the *Directory of Medical Specialists*. These sources list physicians' credentials and whether or not they are board certified. (Board certified means a doctor has undergone extra training in the field and has passed written and oral exams.) Most physicians are board certified, but not all specialists are—it is important to make sure that the specialist you choose is credentialed in the specialty he or she is advertising.

Once you've gathered all this information, narrow your choice to the health care providers who

Timesaver
Visit the Web site of the American Medical Association (www.ama-assn.org) to consult a list of every doctor in the U.S. Search by name or state to find a doctor's address, medical school, residency, year of graduation, and special awards.

have the most convenient locations, whose office hours are most convenient, who accept your type of insurance, who are affiliated with a good hospital, and whose office staff seems pleasant and well informed.

Take into consideration the type of practice you want—a single health care provider, partner, or group practice. Where is the office and how long does it take you to get there?

Once you've answered these questions, it's time to interview the finalists. Arrange a get acquainted visit. (You may have to pay for this visit, but it'll be worth it.) When you get to the health care provider's office, take a look around. Does the staff make you feel welcome? Next, you'll want to come up with some questions for the health care provider to help you make your decision. Here are some to get you started:

- When is the health care provider available by phone?
- What hospital(s) does the health care provider use?
- Where should you go if you become seriously ill or injured? If the hospital is a teaching hospital with interns and residents, find out who would actually care for you if you were to be admitted.
- Who covers the practice when the health care provider is unavailable?
- What are the fees? What insurance plans does the practice accept?

During your first visit, tell your health care provider that you'd like to be health care partners when it comes to treatment decisions. Pay attention to how you feel during the visit. Does the health care provider listen? Do you think you could build a good working partnership with this person? If the answers are "no," keep on looking. If "yes," you've found your health care provider.

How available will your new health care provider be?

Odds are, chest pains won't happen in the middle of a workday afternoon. Because it seems that health problems rarely develop when it's convenient, it's important to find out how easily you'll be able to reach your health care provider in an emergency. During your introductory visit, tell the clinic receptionist that you're looking for a new health care provider and ask these questions:

- What are the office hours?
- Is this health care provider available when needed?
- If I called right now for a routine visit, how soon could I be seen?
- How much time is allowed for a routine visit?
- Will the health care provider discuss health problems over the phone?

After you've finished your interview, ask yourself if you felt comfortable with the health care provider and the staff. Are you satisfied that the health care provider will try to be accessible to you when you need to see him or her, and not only when it's convenient for the health care provider?

"I don't want to be a partner!"

Not everyone wants to be a health care partner. Maybe you don't like to ask your health care provider questions and you don't want to share in any decisions. Would you rather just let your health care provider tell you what is best for you? If that's

Bright Idea
Find out if your health care provider uses nurse practitioners, physician assistants, or nurse midwives. These allied health providers have special training to manage routine medical problems and can often see you sooner and spend more time with you.

what you prefer, say so. Most health care providers have patients who don't want to be a partner. Let the health care provider know what you expect.

Be a patient your health care provider loves

Good health care isn't a one-way street. You should have high expectations for your health care provider—but you also need to be a good patient. Here's a list of tips on how to be the kind of patient your health care provider will love:

- Educate yourself: Read up-to-date information on the Internet, in medical journals, and from patient support groups and national medical organizations. A good health care provider won't mind if you bring along an article to discuss. However, watch out how you present information. There's a difference between patients who say "I read this on the Internet—what do you think?" and patients who say "I read this on the Internet—you don't know what you're talking about." Most reasonable physicians will accept the former and be put off by the latter. Wouldn't you?

- Keep appointments or notify your health care provider when you have to cancel.

- Schedule several visits if you can't get all of your complaints taken care of at once. Let the health care provider know all of your concerns and then the two of you can decide which ones to tackle first.

- Start with your major concern first. Waiting until the end of an appointment to discuss an important problem may mean it won't get proper attention.

- Be specific about your symptoms and pay attention to details. Things that don't seem important to you may be important to your health care provider.

- Take notes: If your treatment details are complex, let the health care provider write them down for you. If you don't understand the treatment, you won't be able to carry out the health care provider's orders.

- If you're extremely ill, bring along someone else to listen to the health care provider. You don't want to miss important information because you were too sick to take it all in.

- Be honest about your medical history. Health care providers have seen it all—odds are, nothing you tell them will be too shocking. Don't feel you need to please the health care provider or hide things.

- Before you leave the office, know what you should do when you get home. It's difficult to remember everything a health care provider tells you, especially if you're nervous or worried. Know who and when to call if you run into any problems.

- Accept the responsibility for refusing treatment or not following instructions.

- Pay your bills promptly.

Before your office visit

Most medical appointments are scheduled for only 10 to 15 minutes, so the better organized you are, the more you'll get from the visit. Before you go for your appointment

- Update your list of symptoms. Write down your primary complaint (your health care provider will want to hear that first).
- Practice describing your complaints.
- Write down your hunches about what's wrong.
- Write down three questions you most want to have answered. (There may not be time to ask a long list of questions.)
- Prepare a list of the prescription and nonprescription medications you are taking and the pharmacy telephone number, together with all the herbs and vitamins you use.
- Be very familiar with your health care plan—do you need a referral? Which labs and X-ray facilities are available to you? Do you have a co-pay? Is your prescription plan mail away, and what are your limitations? It is impossible for your health care provider's staff to know this information! It is your responsibility.

Unofficially...
The American Society of Internal Medicine has concluded that 70 percent of correct diagnosis depends solely on what the patient tells his or her health care provider.

During your office visit

Once you get to the office, be honest and straightforward. Don't hold anything back because of embarrassment. Tell the health care provider

- The list of medications and herbs you're taking (many health care providers like you to bring all your medications to the office).
- Your primary complaint, including when it started, the symptoms, and where the pain is; be sure to describe the pain clearly (Is it stabbing? dull? aching?). Is the pain constant or intermittent? Rate the pain on a scale of 1 to 10. Is it relieved by anything? Is it aggravated by

anything? Have you every had a similar pain at any other time in your life? Have you tried any remedies thus far? What were your results?

- Your temperature (if you have a fever).
- Whether you've had this problem before and what you did for it, if anything.
- About changes in your life (stress, medications, food, exercise).
- Other lifestyle info: Do you take recreational drugs, what's your energy level, sleep patterns, and so on?
- Does anyone else at home or work have these symptoms?
- If you're having alternative care (such as acupuncture or chiropractic treatments, nutritional counseling, or biofeedback).

Do you have a good partnership?

To help figure out whether you and your health care provider are a good fit, ask yourself the following questions:

- Are you comfortable with your health care provider?
- Can you openly discuss your feelings and talk about your most personal concerns? Are your concerns handled compassionately?
- Do you believe your health care provider will stand by you, no matter how difficult the problems become?
- Does your health care provider listen to you and answer all your questions rather than being impatient and vague?

Bright Idea
Take notes. Write down the diagnosis, the treatment and follow-up plan, and what you can do at home. Then read it back to the health care provider to be sure you've got it right.

- Does your health care provider thoroughly evaluate the problem rather than attributing it to "just old age," for example?
- Does your health care provider deal with the real cause of your medical problems or just automatically prescribe drugs?
- Does your health care provider speak so that you can understand him or her?
- Does your health care provider return your calls promptly or tell you when is the best time to call if you have questions?
- Are you usually kept waiting long when you have an appointment?
- Is your health care provider willing to work with you to find an alternative treatment?

Working together as a team

Ideally, you and your health care provider should work together on your health problems as a team, making decisions together with your best interests in mind. These days, health care choices aren't always simple—there is often more than one option. Good partnerships are based on a common goal, shared effort, and good communication.

If you and your health care provider can make these things happen, you'll get better care and your health care provider will be able to practice good medicine. For example, you have mild asthma that is only triggered by certain allergens during specific times of the year. Your health care provider recommends that you use steroid inhalers every day to prevent attacks. However, you believe the inhalers weaken your immune system, making you vulnerable to other infections. Since you only have an asthma attack once or twice a year, you'd prefer to treat the attack once it occurs with oral steroids. Your health care provider agrees.

Your nine year old has a sore throat with no fever, nausea, or white patches on the throat. The health care provider says it's probably nothing to worry about, but you know your child is prone to strep throat. You'd like to bring her in for a strep test. The health care provider agrees.

You've been suffering from carpal tunnel syndrome for several months. Your health care provider recommends a wrist splint and a steroid injection. You'd rather try just the splint with aspirin first. If that doesn't work, you'll consider other medications. Your health care provider agrees.

In each case, the treatment will have an effect on your life. How do you choose what's best for you? With a combination of your health care provider's medical expertise and your personal values and experience, the two of you can usually come up with a good solution. If you have a good relationship with your health care provider and both of you are willing to listen to the other, you should make a good health care team. Here's how:

Unofficially... Accept responsibility for your choices. When you make shared decisions with your health care provider, both of you must accept the responsibility for the outcomes.

- Let your health care provider know that you want to help make decisions about what to do for your health problems.

- Do your own research. Sometimes you have to do some reading on your own before you can really understand what your health care provider is saying.

- Always ask why before agreeing to any medical test, medication, or treatment. This may help you find another option that better meets your needs.

- Find out if there are alternative choices. Learn enough to understand the options your health care provider thinks are sensible.
- Can it wait? Ask your health care provider if it would be risky or costly to wait (a day, a week, or a month) before treatment.
- Let your health care provider know what you think if you prefer one option over another based on your personal values.
- Discuss side effects, pain, recovery, and so on.

If you're unhappy with your health care provider...

If you're unhappy with the way your health care provider treats you, it may be time for a change. Before you start looking for a new health care provider, tell your current health care provider how you would like to be treated. Most health care providers aren't mind readers, and would welcome a chance to find out if they've done something that has displeased you. If you keep your mouth shut and just abandon the health care provider, he or she will never know what the problem was and won't have a chance to fix it.

If you need a specialist

If you have a simple ear infection, it makes more sense to get help from your family health care provider rather than running off to a otolaryngologist (an ear, nose, and throat doctor).

You should use specialists only for special problems. *Specialists* are health care providers with in-depth training and experience in a particular area of medicine. A visit to a specialist may cost more than a visit to your family health care provider, and the tests and treatment you receive may be more expensive.

If you have a major health problem, specialists are the best choice. When your primary health care provider refers you to a specialist, a little preparation and good communication can help you get your money's worth.

Before you go see a specialist:

- Know the potential diagnosis.
- Understand the basic treatment options.
- Know what your family health care provider would like the specialist to do (take over the case, confirm the diagnosis, conduct tests).
- Make sure that all your records are sent to the specialist.
- Ask your regular health care provider to remain involved in your case.
- Ask the specialist to give all new test results or recommendations to both you and your family health care provider.

"What's this test designed to do?"

We're fortunate in the United States to have some of the best state-of-the-art medical tests available; however, medical tests are important tools, but they do have limits. Some women think that if one test is good, five are better. In fact, tests carry costs and risks as well as benefits. If your health care provider is considering tests for you, there are some things you'll need to do. First and foremost, educate yourself:

- What's the name of the test and why do you need it?
- If the test is positive, what will the health care provider do differently?

- What could happen if you don't have the test?
- How accurate is the test?
- What is the rate of false positives (a test that indicates a problem where none exists) and false negatives (a test that indicates there is no problem, when, in fact, there is one)?
- Is the test painful?
- What can go wrong?
- How will you feel afterward?
- Are there less risky alternatives?
- How much does the test cost?
- Is there a less expensive test that might give the same information?
- What does the health care provider expect the test will do for you? Is that realistic?
- What if you're pregnant or have other medical conditions?

You can say no!

Some women have problems with confrontation. Socialized to please others and to "go along," especially in the presence of someone they perceive as an authority figure, some women don't feel comfortable saying "no."

You have the right to refuse any procedure, drug, or test, for whatever reason. If you feel uncomfortable about a certain treatment or diagnostic tool, discuss your concerns with your health care provider. Ask your health care provider if you can avoid a test if it seems too expensive or risky and it doesn't seem as if it would really change the recommended treatment. Remember, no test can be done without your permission.

If you agree to a test

Once you and your health care provider decide that a particular test is a good idea, your responsibility doesn't end there. Ask what you can do to lower the chance of errors. Should you avoid any particular food (especially sugar), beverages (especially caffeine or alcohol), exercise, or medications?

After the test:

- Ask to see the results.
- Make notes about it for your home records.
- If the results are unexpected and the error rate of the test is high, consider redoing the test before basing further treatment on its results.

Home medical tests

Many common medical tests are now available in home kits. Combined with regular visits to your health professional, home tests can help you monitor your health and, in some cases, detect problems early.

Home medical tests must be very accurate (over 95 percent) to be approved by the U.S. Food and Drug Administration. However, they must be used correctly to give accurate results. If you're going to use a home test, follow the package directions exactly.

Home medical tests are especially helpful if you have a chronic condition that requires frequent monitoring, such as diabetes, asthma, or high blood pressure. Ask your health care provider which home medical tests would be appropriate for you.

Urinalysis

Some of the more common medical lab tests on urine can be done at home. These tests can help you monitor diabetes.

Blood glucose

If you have diabetes, you probably know all about monitoring your blood sugar levels (glucose) with a finger prick and a test strip or an electronic monitor. This test should always be used under a health care provider's supervision. Never adjust your insulin dose based on a single abnormal test, unless your health care provider has specifically instructed you to do so. Check with your health care provider if you have symptoms of abnormal blood sugar levels, even if the test is normal.

Blood pressure

Blood pressure never stays the same—even among the healthiest women, your blood pressure constantly rises and falls in response to stress, exercise, even speaking. But if you have consistent hypertension, it's important to monitor your blood pressure frequently.

With a little practice, you can easily monitor your blood pressure at home. This way, you can check your pressure when you're relaxed and you'll be able to track how your blood pressure responds to medications. (Of course, you should never change your medications based on your home blood pressure readings without consulting your health care provider.)

Check your blood pressure at different times during the day to see how rest and activities affect it. For regular readings, check it at the same time of day each day. Blood pressure is usually lowest in the morning, rising during the day.

For the most accurate reading, sit quietly for five minutes before taking a reading. Adjust the blood pressure device yearly.

Bright Idea
If you have questions or concerns about a home medical test, ask your pharmacist or check the label for the company's toll-free phone number.

Blood in stool

It's possible to do a fecal occult blood test at home to detect hidden blood in the stool, which may indicate colon cancer or other problems. It is usually quite accurate at detecting the presence or absence of blood, but the presence or absence of blood does not necessarily mean the presence or absence of cancer. The occult blood test is recommended for all adults. Your health care provider may recommend a more accurate screening test for colon cancer called a flexible sigmoidoscopy. This test is recommended for women over 50 or for those with a positive occult blood test. (See Chapter 3 for more information.)

Home pregnancy tests

Probably the best-known home medical test is the home pregnancy test, which offers a reliable (99 percent) and simple way to find out if you're pregnant. This test measures the presence of a hormone called human chorionic gonadotropin (hCG). hCG is most commonly present as the result of pregnancy, but there can, on occasion, be other reasons for its presence. Follow the package instructions and report all positive results to your health care provider. When positive, home tests are usually very accurate. If negative, it could mean that you are just taking the test too early. A home pregnancy test costs about $10. A urine test in the doctor's office is probably at least $20 and a blood test is at least $30.

In-home ovulation predictor kit

In-home ovulation prediction kits are 98 percent accurate and more and more couples are using them to help get pregnant. These should be used after you know the length of your cycle and the time frame when you can expect to ovulate. In-home ovulation prediction kits help determine the woman's fertile period by detecting the increase in the concentration of hormones in her urine prior to and during ovulation. A significant increase in the intensity of the color over baseline means a hormone surge. Different ovulation prediction kits contain supplies for between five and nine tests. Theoretically, the earlier testing begins in a cycle and the more consecutive days tested, the greater the chance of predicting the day of ovulation.

Take two pills and call me in the morning

When it comes to medications, you should always know exactly why you need each drug before you ever put it in your mouth. Ask your health care provider the following questions:

- What is the name of the drug and why do you need it?
- How long does it take to work?
- How long should you take it?
- Are there any rules about how to take it (with or without food, any foods to avoid)?
- Are there nondrug alternatives?
- How much will this drug help?
- What are the side effects or other risks?
- Could this drug react with other drugs, vitamins, or herbs that you're currently taking?
- How much does it cost? Is an equivalent generic drug available?

There are some things you should tell your health care provider before getting a new prescription:

- Your concerns about the drug
- What you expect it will do
- All other substances you're taking (including illegal drugs, vitamins, herbs, and over-the-counter drugs)

Bogus cures

If you learn as much as you can about your medical problem, you may turn up new options—but you may also uncover some questionable treatments and downright quack cures. Think you're too savvy for that? Millions of people are taken in each year by medical fraud and worthless health products.

Bogus "cures" are advertised for many chronic problems—especially arthritis, cancer, baldness, and impotence. Unfortunately, these cures rarely help and can cause harmful side effects. How do you know if a treatment is bogus? You should be suspicious of products that

- Advertise by testimonials.
- Claim to have a secret ingredient.
- Aren't evaluated in well-known, peer-reviewed medical journals.
- Make statements that seem too good to be true (they probably are).
- Are available only by mail.

If you need surgery...

Every surgery has risks. You're the only one who can balance the benefits with those risks. Are you willing to live with your problem or do you want to have the operation? Once you understand the costs, risks, and benefits of surgery, the decision is up to you.

Moneysaver
Start with a smaller prescription for just a few pills if there's any suspicion that you might not be able to tolerate the drug. That way, if you have a reaction to the drug, you won't have wasted a lot of money.

CHAPTER 1 ▪ MAKING SAVVY HEALTH CARE CHOICES

If you're facing surgery, your health care provider should be willing to answer these questions:

- What is the surgery called and what happens during the operation?
- Why do you think I need it?
- Is this surgery the typical treatment for this problem? What are my other options? Is there an alternative?
- How many similar surgeries have you done?
- What's the success rate (and define "success")?
- What can go wrong? How often does this happen?
- How will I feel afterward?
- How long will it be until I'm fully recovered?
- How can I prepare for the surgery?
- What type of anesthesia do you plan to use? Are there alternatives?
- Can it be done on an outpatient basis?
- Ask your primary health care provider or surgeon to recommend another specialist.
- Have your test results showing you need surgery sent to the new health care provider.
- Consider getting an opinion from a different type of health care provider who treats similar problems. If you do get a second opinion from another kind of doctor, remember that the two different specialists may not be trained in the same techniques or have the same amount of experience. For example, ob/gyns and urologists both treat female urinary incontinence, but it's considered to be a significant part of the gynecologist's practice where it is only a small

Unofficially... Many HMOs and other managed health care plans will pay for a second opinion. Find out what your insurance plan will cover before getting a second opinion, but be prepared to pay for it yourself if you have to.

part of the urologist's training. Most urologists have little experience in treating this problem while there is a whole subspecialty of gynecology devoted to this area.

If you want a second opinion, get one. Your health care provider won't be hurt (and if yours is, then he or she isn't for you). Second opinions are a good idea if you have any doubts about whether the proposed operation is the best solution for your problem. However, even if you feel that the second doctor is better than the first, don't expect him or her to take over your care. Many doctors feel to do so would be unethical.

Managed care: Working the system

Managed care has changed the face of medical care in the twentieth century. In the United States today, more than half the population receives health care through managed care systems such as health maintenance organizations (HMOs). But the change has caught many women unaware. If you participate in a managed care plan, you're both a health care provider's patient and an HMO member. You need to learn how managed care works, how you can be more responsible for your own medical care, and how you can get the most out of being an HMO member.

An HMO provides health care coverage through a network of health care providers, clinics, and hospitals that work together to coordinate patient care and contain costs. Members of an HMO must choose from a list of physicians and facilities with fixed fees for all services. Employers often provide health insurance through HMOs because they offer comprehensive health care at cheaper rates. Because managed care is cheaper, many employers offer only HMO plans.

Within an HMO, the health care provider you choose to be responsible for your health care is called your primary care physician. He or she will be your health care advocate—your most important link to satisfaction in the HMO. Your primary care health care provider coordinates all your medical care (routine checkups, preventive services, referrals, and hospital visits).

The downside of HMOs

HMOs sound great on paper, but in reality, many people are unhappy with their managed care plans because they feel their health care providers are slow to recommend effective treatment and even slower to refer them to specialists if they need extra care.

Typically, many HMOs use less expensive (and sometimes less effective) methods of treatment, but the patient never knows because the health care provider may not tell the patient about all the options. In an effort to cut expenses, HMOs often contract with low-cost providers for medical services (like lab tests), which can lead to inaccurate diagnoses. Often, the managed care company even tells a health care provider how much time he or she can spend with a patient, and controls which specialists the health care providers may refer patients to.

The fact that a health care provider depends on income from an HMO sets up a conflict of interest between the health care provider and the patient. Most HMOs can dismiss health care providers without cause, so that if a health care provider gives too many referrals or orders too many tests (which cost the HMO money), he or she can be booted out without explanation. In addition, many HMOs give health care providers year-end bonuses if they keep

> HMO patients must learn to take care of themselves.
> —Physicians Who Care, a patient advocacy organization with about 3,500 physician members nationwide

their costs in line (for example, by limiting referrals or tests). As a result, patients are sometimes not offered the care they need. This risk is greatest with health care providers who are paid under capitation (a system where the health care provider gets a set fee per patient each month, whether or not he sees the patient).

Fortunately, this risk has lessened as managed care has placed more emphasis on accountability. Even health plans that are capitated now use underutilization reviews to find health care providers who are working the system against the patient's benefit. An underutilization review means that the HMO will actually keep track of the number of tests performed per diagnosis; if Dr. Jones orders three tests for every diagnosis of chest pain and Dr. Smith orders six tests for every diagnosis of chest pain, the managed care department of the HMO will review outcomes to see which health care provider's patients do better (Jones versus Smith).

Before you join an HMO...

Some women don't have much choice about their insurance—perhaps your employer contracts with one group, and that's all you can use. Other women have a choice—either their employer presents them with several options, or you and your spouse can choose whether to sign with his plan or yours. Or, some women are self-employed and must find their own coverage.

If you do have a choice, and you're thinking of joining an HMO or any other type of managed care (and especially if you're now in a traditional medical plan), you should try to make an educated choice between plans by asking questions. If you don't get an answer, or if you don't like the answers you do get, don't join. Interview other HMOs until you find one that fits your needs.

Before you make any decision, get answers from the HMO to these questions:

- Tell me exactly how you reward your health care providers for cost containment. I want to be sure that your system won't keep me from having needed tests or seeing a specialist.
- Describe how you make sure I'll always be treated by a competent, well-trained physician.
- Who decides what is "medically necessary" in my case?
- How can I appeal a medical decision that I don't think is correct? How soon I will get your answer?
- Will I have free choice of physicians within the plan?
- Who pays if I want to see a health care provider outside your plan?
- How much of your income goes to treat patients and how much is spent on marketing, administration, and profit?
- How do you decide what drugs to provide for your patients? Some generic drugs are not bioequivalent to brand names. What's your policy on this? Do you use a drug formulary?
- Do you cover contraceptives?
- How do you decide when I can see a specialist?
- How can I let you know what I think about the quality of care your staff provides?
- What care will I get in a medical emergency?
- Will you charge me if I have to go outside your system?

- What is the length of time that it will take you to reimburse for my medical care? If I have an emergency out of state, what are your guidelines for my obtaining care?
- Do you recognize alternative medicine?
- Will you pay for second opinions?

If your current health care provider is not affiliated with the HMO you're thinking of joining, call your plan's member services department to learn more about the health care providers who are available.

Are you satisfied?
HMOs often survey their members to measure patient satisfaction. It is so important to HMOs that many of them have several programs to promote patient satisfaction and to explain health care coverage or decisions about treatment.

It's a good idea to ask about any appeals process available to members and to understand these procedures before joining an HMO. Many HMOs publish information about their member satisfaction surveys. Find out what the HMO members say about how satisfied they are with their coverage and care.

Understanding your HMO coverage
Read your disclosure form. This document, sometimes called the *evidence of coverage,* will outline all the plan's policies and rules. Just because your best friend's HMO covers mental health care and hospice visits doesn't mean that yours will. Coverage can vary widely among HMOs and can also vary widely within the same HMO (or other insurance) depending on what exact policy or coverage the employer elects to provide. HMO X, for example, may provide contraceptive coverage for the widget

factory, but not for the local Catholic church's employees.

Keep your membership card handy. You'll need it when you visit your health care provider, have medical tests, fill a prescription, or go to the ER. The card tells how to reach your health care provider and the HMO responsible for your health care, and proves that you're insured.

Know where to find the phone number for member services. (It's usually printed on your membership card.) Member services reps are available to explain and answer questions about your coverage. If your health care provider can't resolve a problem, contact member services.

With doctors participating in many plans, it's essential for you to know the details and requirements of your plan. Your doctor's office will expect you to know whether you need a referral for certain things, at what interval yearly gynecological exams are covered, what lab to use, and so on. It's unfair to expect your doctor to keep track of this for you.

How to get the best HMO care

The managed health care industry is still young and experiencing growing pains. Some people view it as unresponsive and slow-moving. It takes a lot of persistence and energy to get satisfaction in working with any large organization. Unless you stand up for your rights, you may end up getting lost in the system and receiving less than the best possible care.

Be persistent in getting the best health care from your HMO and your physician. Don't accept the first response if it doesn't meet your needs.

If you're in an HMO, here are some tips to getting the best care you can:

Bright Idea
For great tips on dealing with HMOs, get a free brochure from Physicians Who Care (PWC) called "Are You Thinking of Joining an HMO?" To get a copy, write PWC at 10615 Perrin Beitel, Suite 201, San Antonio, TX 78217.

- When choosing your HMO health care provider, discuss your preferences about office locations, training, and education with the member services representative; this will help you narrow the field of health care providers.
- Find a health care provider who knows how to work with the system. Your health care provider has the right to seek exceptions to HMO rules when he or she finds it medically necessary.
- Be your own advocate. Demand appropriate, necessary care. Ask your health care provider: "What are my options in terms of treatment?"
- Ask your plan to consider the care you think is necessary, even if it's not covered. It doesn't hurt to ask, and you may get better care this way.
- Be suspicious if your health care provider is hesitant to discuss treatment options with you.
- Ask your health care provider outright: "Are you getting paid more money for not treating me?"
- Ask for the name of the lab and the pathologist who will be doing your medical tests, and then call the lab to find out the level of the technician's training.
- Get a second opinion from a health care provider who is outside the HMO—even if you must pay for it yourself.
- If you're denied care, use your HMO's formal complaint process and call your state's department of insurance and your state legislator to report any problems.
- Don't put off getting care if you have a serious medical emergency because you're afraid your HMO won't cover the cost. Know your HMOs

rules for emergencies, but realize it may be impossible to reach an affiliated hospital in time.

Getting checkups and following your health care provider's advice will show you to be someone who is willing to take extra steps for your own health. When you need ongoing medical treatment or surgery, your relationship with your health care provider will help you gain access to the most appropriate care possible.

Women who know what they need are more likely to get what they want. Do research to back up arguments about your care. Clip articles from journals about new treatments. Search the Internet for information about your condition. Show that you're a savvy woman who's interested in getting the best health care possible, but present this information in the right way—don't be hostile or assume that you automatically know more than the doctor because you read it on the Internet. And also understand that just because you read about it online, doesn't mean it's accurate. Get your health information from reputable sites maintained by well-known research organizations, hospitals, and health groups, not from personal Web sites, companies selling products, or private bulletin boards.

For further insight into the HMO-health care provider/patient relationship, check out *The Insider's Guide to HMOs,* by Dr. Alan J. Steinberg (see Appendix B).

If you've got a problem getting care...
Speak up immediately when you have concerns about the quality of your care. You may be able to get valuable information about treatment options

from nonprofit health advocacy groups, such as the American Cancer Society, the American Lung Association, or Internet Web sites. (See Appendix B.) They often have data on the effectiveness of new treatments, and this information may help you decide whether to file an appeal or a grievance.

If you think you have been denied necessary care, the first step is always to work with the plan. Here are steps you can take to get the care you need:

1. Keep written records of all contacts and correspondence, and make use of your health care provider as well, who may be an advocate for you.

2. Talk to your primary care health care provider first.

3. If your health care provider doesn't have an answer, call your HMO's member services department. Your plan's representatives may be able to get you the benefit you need. Your employer's health benefits administrator also may be able to help—this person should be a strong advocate. After all, the administrator is the HMO's real customer.

4. If your complaint can't be resolved, file an appeal with your HMO to ask that your request be reconsidered. The member services department will explain how to file an appeal.

5. If you aren't satisfied with the outcome of your appeal, send a letter to the plan's medical director and the head of its member services department. Ask them to respond to you within a certain number of days, and tell them that you will seek regulatory or legal help if necessary.

6. If you can't resolve a problem with your HMO, you can file a grievance with your state's HMO

regulatory agency. Your HMO's member services department will give you the agency's name and phone number.

7. Ask the regulatory agency how to file a grievance about an unsatisfactory treatment decision by your HMO. The National Association of Insurance Commissioners' Web site has a list of all health insurance complaint contacts at state departments of insurance (www.naic.org/consumer/state/healthcn.htm).

8. If you still don't get results, think about contacting a news organization. Many have consumer advocacy reporters and journalists who may be interested in consumer concerns related to health care.

9. As a last resort, consider talking to a lawyer. Sometimes just a letter from an attorney will prod your HMO into action. If you can't afford a lawyer, call a legal aid organization in your area.

HMO membership contracts almost always require binding arbitration to settle most disputes. This means your case will be decided by a panel of qualified individuals instead of being heard in court. If your claim is subject to binding arbitration, you waive your right to a court or jury trial. Experts say you should not begin the arbitration process without the advice of an attorney.

Most HMOs require you to file a demand for arbitration and pay a fee to begin the arbitration process. You may also be liable for arbitration costs, which can run into thousands of dollars. But none of the requirements or the potential cost should dissuade you from pursuing a valid claim. (Some HMOs have provisions for waiving some of the costs of arbitration in cases of extreme hardship.)

Bright Idea
The National Association of Insurance Commissioners has a consumer guide to resolving health care insurance disputes available online at www.naic.org/geninfo/0909nbl.htm.

Patients who need help with HMO-related problems may call the hot line at Physicians Who Care (800/800-5154) and leave a voice message. PWC will respond by mail.

External review boards
Independent, external review boards designed to settle disputes between patients and managed care organizations have been established by legislation in 18 states. But only two out of every 1,000 health plan enrollees turn to state-run independent review boards to mediate disputes with health insurance companies, researchers report.

Experts suspect that most people don't use state-run independent review boards because they don't know their rights. In addition, independent review is a complicated process for someone who doesn't have a lot of education or is sick or incapacitated. In many states, there really aren't too many resources at the consumer's disposal.

You should realize that external review boards don't always decide in the patient's favor. About half the time, the plan's denial is upheld. The other half, the denial is overturned and they find in favor of the consumer. For more information, contact your state insurance commissioner.

Emergency! The ins and outs of the ER visit

In life-threatening situations, modern emergency services are essential. However, far too many people use an emergency room in place of their family health care provider. At 2 a.m. in many ERs, you'll see people sitting around with colds, the sniffles, slight temperatures—all things that should have been taken care of by a regular health care provider.

Emergency rooms charge two to three times more for routine services than a health care provider's office. In addition, the ER health care provider won't have access to your records, so these health care providers have no information about your medical history.

Hospital ERs are designed to handle trauma and life-threatening cases—they aren't set up to care for routine illnesses, and they don't work on a first-come, first-served basis. During busy times, people with minor illnesses may wait for hours. Always ask yourself if you can take care of a problem safely at home and wait to see your regular health care provider. If you don't have a regular health care provider, get one. However, if you feel that what you're facing is an emergency situation, go to the emergency department. If you decide to visit the ER:

- Call ahead, if possible, to let them know you're coming.

- Call your family health care provider (if possible). He or she may meet you at the ER or call in important information. Many patients don't want to bother their health care provider with "minor" things at night and go to the ER instead. The doctor who knows you is almost always in a better position to advise you, except in dire emergency situations. If you call your health care provider first, he or she may well be able to handle the problem on the phone, meet you at the office, or refer you to an urgent visit center, which is less expensive and usually more responsive than an ER.

- Take your home medical records with you and use them to discuss your medications, past test results, or treatments. Information about your allergies, medications, and conditions may be critical.

- As soon as you arrive, tell the emergency room staff what your emergency is.
- If you're a member of an HMO, as soon as possible (within 48 hours), make sure that you (or a family member) contact your primary care health care provider and health plan. This will help you receive the best coverage your plan provides in emergency situations and ensure that your health care provider is kept up-to-date on your case and involved in decisions about your care.

Choosing the best place for your treatment and recovery

Gone are the days when a patient could lounge around in a hospital for two or three weeks undergoing a few tests. Today, modern insurance directives dictate exactly how long you should be in the hospital for any particular problem. It's often better for you, as well; studies show that people recover better from surgery at home.

Remember that a stay in a modern hospital costs far more than a vacation at most luxury resorts (and it's a lot less fun). Try to avoid additional days in the hospital by bringing in extra help at home. Ask about home nursing services to help while you recover. If you've got help at home, you may be able to shorten your hospital stay.

Community hospital or specialty center?

Today, you have choices about which hospital to go to. For example, if you've been diagnosed with cancer, you might have the choice of going to a local community hospital, a regional teaching hospital, or a regional cancer center. Which should you choose?

Typically, a local community hospital is a good place to go for the basics—simple, uncomplicated deliveries and basic operations. Research has also shown that a smaller community hospital may score more points for their human dimensions of care.

If you are critically ill or need a complicated surgery, you might prefer to go to a larger teaching hospital that specializes in the type of care or complicated surgery you require. Indeed, studies have shown that elderly patients are more likely to survive a heart attack and certain other illnesses if they're admitted to a teaching hospital, according to two reports published in a January 1999 issue of the New England Journal of Medicine. This is because teaching hospitals (where health care providers train) are more likely to do research and to have high-technology facilities than other hospitals. Other research has shown that it's best to have your surgery in a hospital that performs the highest number of that type of surgery. The better results are most likely due to the fact that there are physicians present 24 hours a day in teaching hospitals.

When it comes to treatment for cancer, many women prefer the special care they can find in a comprehensive cancer center, which typically can offer not only up-to-the-minute treatment, but also a range of experimental treatments and clinical studies. Comprehensive cancer centers also often offer unique services for women, such as risk assessment programs, free breast cancer gene testing, and the opportunity to participate in a range of clinical studies. Comprehensive cancer centers also offer a unique "team approach" to cancer treatment aimed at providing the support of a health partnership.

When being at home is the right choice

Hospitals aren't the only choice for people with terminal illnesses. Many people choose to spend their remaining time at home with people they know and love. Special arrangements for the needed care can be made through hospice care programs in most communities. Look for "Hospice" in the Yellow Pages or ask your health care provider for more information.

Moneysaver
You may be able to save money or a day in the hospital by having routine tests (blood count, urinalysis, etc.) performed in your health care provider's office.

Getting the care you need while in the hospital

You've probably heard your share of horror stories about grumpy and short-staffed nurses, unfeeling technicians, and inedible food in modern-day hospitals. However, even if you're in the hospital, you're not helpless. There are things you can to do help improve the quality of care you receive. (If you're going to be very sick, ask your spouse or a friend to help watch out for your best interests.) Here's what you can do to take control:

- Ask why. Don't agree to anything unless you have a good reason. Agree only to those procedures that make sense for (and to) you.

- Make sure your hospital armband has the correct information on it.

- With staffs in short supply, people make mistakes. Provide an extra level of quality control by checking drugs, tests, injections, and other treatments to see if they are correct.

- Be friendly with the nurses and aides and they may pay more attention to your needs and speed your recovery. Sharing fruit baskets or candy with the staff is an easy way to get them on your side. If you're going to be in for a while, have a relative buy a box of candy, some donuts, popcorn, and so on for the staff on your floor. It will work wonders!

- Be sure the hospital staff understands that you want to know immediately about any changes in your condition or your treatment.

- Be aware of the medicines you are given, what they are for, and what side effects they may cause. You may also want a family member to know this information.

- Find out when your health care provider plans to visit so you're not napping or you can have a family member to be present at that time. Have your questions written down.

- Know your rights. Most hospitals have adopted the Patient's Bill of Rights developed by the American Hospital Association. Ask your hospital for their copy (see below).

- Keep a pad and pen handy to write down questions for your health care provider and/or nurse and take notes on information given to you.

- If you get an itemized bill, check it and ask about any charges you don't understand. If you don't get an itemized bill, demand one.

Patient's Bill of Rights

Most hospitals have adopted the Patient's Bill of Rights, developed by the American Hospital Association. A patient has the right

Bright Idea
If you prefer privacy during your hospital stay, the difference between your insurer's reimbursement for a private and semi-private room may be less than you imagine and worth making up for out of your own pocket.

- To be treated with courtesy and respect, with appreciation of his or her dignity, and with protection of a need for privacy.
- To a prompt and reasonable response to questions and requests.
- To know who is providing medical services and is responsible for his or her care.
- To know what patient support services are available.
- To know what conduct rules and regulations apply.
- To be given information such as diagnosis, planned course of treatment, alternatives, risks, and prognosis.
- To refuse any treatment, except as otherwise provided by law.
- To be given full information and necessary counseling on the availability of known financial resources for care.
- To receive—prior to treatment—a reasonable estimate of charges for medical care.
- To receive a copy of an understandable itemized bill and to have the charges explained.
- To impartial access to medical treatment or accommodations.
- To treatment for any emergency medical condition that will deteriorate as a result of not providing treatment.
- To know if medical treatment is for purposes of experimental research and to give consent or refusal to participate in such research.
- To express grievances regarding any violation of his or her rights.

A living will

A living will (lawyers like to call them "advance directives") is a document that states your wishes should you become seriously ill or irreversibly incompetent and need life support systems or heroic measures to keep you alive. It spells out to your health care provider, the hospital, your family, and to everybody else what measures you want and don't want, so that you can die with dignity and without unwanted intervention.

What follows is a sample living will. If you wish, you may also consult with your own attorney about laws in your state.

Unofficially...
There are also medical or health directives that give general directions to your family and the hospital. Many hospitals and medical facilities want you to sign their medical directive form when you are admitted.

Living Will Declaration

I, (Declarant's Name), being of sound mind, willfully and voluntarily make this declaration to be followed if I become incompetent. This declaration reflects my firm and settled commitment to refuse life-sustaining treatment under the circumstances listed below.

I direct my attending physician to withhold or withdraw life-sustaining treatment that serves only to prolong the process of my dying, if I should be in a terminal condition or in a state of permanent unconsciousness.

In addition, if I am in the condition described above, I feel especially strong about the following forms of treatment:

I ( ) do ( ) do not want cardiac resuscitation.

I ( ) do ( ) do not want mechanical respiration.

I ( ) do ( ) do not want tube feeding or any other artificial or invasive form of nutrition (food) or hydration (water).

I ( ) do ( ) do not want blood or blood products.

I ( ) do ( ) do not want any form of surgery or invasive diagnostic tests.

I ( ) do ( ) do not want kidney dialysis.

I ( ) do ( ) do not want antibiotics.

I realize that if I don't specifically indicate my preference regarding any of the forms of treatment listed above, I may receive that form of treatment.

Other instructions:

I ( ) do ( ) do not want to designate another person as my surrogate to make medical treatment decisions for me if I should be incompetent and in a terminal condition or in a state of permanent unconsciousness. Name and address of the surrogate:

Name and address of alternate surrogate (if surrogate designated above is unable to serve):

I make this declaration on the _____ day of _____, in _____ (year).

Declarant's signature:

> Declarant's address:
>
> _____
>
> _____
>
> The declarant knowingly and voluntarily signed this writing by signature or mark in my presence.
>
> Witness' signature:
>
> _____
>
> Witness' address:
>
> _____
>
> _____

Just the facts

- You and your health care provider should work together in a health care partnership.
- Be honest, well-informed, and straightforward with your health care provider, and don't be afraid to ask questions about things you don't understand or have concerns about.
- Before you join an HMO, find out how they reward health care providers for cost containment.
- You do have options if your HMO has denied you treatment you feel you deserve.
- The Patient's Bill of Rights provides you with certain rights regarding the type of care you receive and the information which must be disclosed to you about your care.

GET THE SCOOP ON...
Anorexia, bulimia, and binge eating ▪ Women's special diet needs ▪ Making your own exercise plan ▪ Lipo-ing the fat away ▪ Tummy tucks ▪ Breast size

Body Image

Any woman who has ever stood naked in front of a department store mirror under those merciless fluorescent lights knows the reality of "body image." American culture is particularly hard on women—the self-image that most girls and women have has nothing to do with reality and everything to do with Madison Avenue's glorification of reed-thin models and impossible ideals of beauty.

When your mirror lies: Negative body image

Studies are quite clear that American women are almost always dissatisfied with the way they look—we're convinced we're too fat, too thin, too hairy, too ugly, too pimply, too tall, too busty, too short, too flat-chested . . . well, you get the picture. Most men seem to be blissfully unaware of their own physical flaws, no matter how pronounced—or if they're aware of them, they don't seem to care much. Not so with women.

"I hate my body"

Sadly, the conviction that we are never "just right" begins very early in life, during the prepuberty years of 9, 10, and 11. Very few of us outgrow that feeling. Prior to puberty, boys and girls have about the same percentage of body fat—about 9 to 12 percent. By the end of puberty, body fat has usually doubled in girls (about 25 percent of body weight), while boys grow leaner and more muscular. These dramatic changes in the female body seem to predispose girls to be preoccupied and dissatisfied with their weight.

For many of these girls, poor body image is not just a passing disappointment but a lifelong passion, overriding all other aspects of their lives. It becomes something that affects their self-esteem and well-being—for some girls, poor body image is not just about what they look like, but who they are.

While almost all teenage girls feel awkward about their bodies and self-conscious about their development (or lack of it), there is a great deal their families can do to help offset some of the worst of the self-criticism. If a girl's family makes her feel attractive and accepts her as she is (especially her father, according to research), she'll be much more likely to establish a positive image of herself as a developing woman. Mothers can do their part, too, by showing their daughters they are comfortable with their own bodies.

However, if nothing is done about a young girl's poor body image, she's at risk of developing eating disorders in an effort to control her appearance. As she gets older, she may struggle with chronic self-esteem issues, develop sexual problems, and traipse from doctor to doctor in search of surgical solutions to perceived physical problems.

It's often a problem that doesn't go away. Aging is fraught with psychological risk for the woman who has never been able to accept her own body, or whose self-image and self-esteem is tied up in how she looks. Americans tend to associate sexual attractiveness with youth so that for many women, growing old gracefully is impossible.

Body dysmorphic disorder

In severe cases, a negative body image may be diagnosed as body dysmorphic disorder (BDD)—an unhealthy, delusional obsession with imagined or slight physical imperfections. The condition can push some teens into depression, isolation—even suicide.

Sadly, this often debilitating disorder is still underrecognized and even unknown to many doctors, according to researchers at Brown University, who published a study on the disorder in the April 1999 issue of the *Journal of the American Academy of Child and Adolescent Psychiatry*.

BDD involves a morbid preoccupation with perceived (but often minor or nonexistent) imperfections in skin, hair, facial features, or other body parts. It can occur any time, but seems to peak in midadolescence. Women with BDD are delusional, since experts who speak with BDD-affected patients note that the flaws so apparent to the affected teens seem to be normal to others. Moreover, changes made to the problem body parts (such as a nose job or ear pinning) don't seem to alter the woman's distorted ideas about her looks.

Treatment with drugs like Prozac and Paxil seems to help, which suggests that the cause of BDD may be an abnormal level of brain chemicals.

Unofficially...
In a typical case of BDD, a 17-year-old girl who has been obsessed with her body since about the age of 13 says she thinks about her appearance every second. Her BDD led to a severe depression, and she attempted suicide via a drug overdose.

Exploding the diet myths

Everywhere you turn—books, magazines, TV talk shows—you'll hear about the latest food fads, what diets work, and which ones promise the quickest results. The thing to remember here is that if it sounds too good to be true, it probably is. Here are a few dietary myths that are just that:

- You can lose weight with special wraps, lotions, and pills.
- Special vitamins can erase cellulite.
- Special foods can make you young.
- Starchy foods are particularly fattening.
- Cottage cheese and grapefruit have magical weight loss properties.

Why weight loss diets don't work

Grapefruit and cottage cheese . . . bacon and strawberries . . . rice . . . high protein, low carbo . . . high carbo, low protein . . . many women bounce from one diet to the next like a tennis ball at Wimbledon. When they're not successful, they blame themselves.

They should really blame the diets. Most weight loss diets don't work because they're poorly designed and they don't help you keep the weight off, period. In fact, any diet that emphasizes limiting calories for a set period of time, or that focuses on crash dieting, will fail. You may lose weight temporarily—after all, you are starving yourself—but as soon as you stop the diet, the pounds return. This sort of yo-yo dieting will make it even harder to lose weight the next time you break out the diet books—and it may be dangerous to your health.

There is a way to lose weight and keep it off, and it doesn't involve joining a club, visiting a fat farm, or filling your refrigerator with celery sticks. It's just this: You must change your eating habits permanently and get more exercise.

If you're not obese and have no risk factors for obesity-related illness, focus on preventing further weight gain by increasing your exercise and eating healthy foods, rather than trying to lose weight. If you do need to lose weight, you should be ready to commit to lifelong changes in your eating behaviors, diet, and physical activity.

Eat out and lose weight

It's certainly possible to find a low-fat, healthy meal even if you're dining out, as long as you avoid the high-fat delectables. Even if you're going to Chinese, Mexican, Italian, or fast food places, you can still choose wisely and eat sensibly:

- Chinese: Choose more rice and vegetables, skip extra sauce and lots of meat. Avoid the fried appetizers (try steamed dumplings or soup instead).
- Mexican: If the rice and beans aren't refried in fat, they can be a healthy choice. Skip the fried taco shells and taco salads, cheese, sour cream, and guacamole, and choose chicken soft tacos and fajitas.
- Italian: It's not the pasta that loads on the pounds, it's all those creamy and cheesy sauces. Pick pasta with a tomato-based sauce and replace that oily garlic bread with a salad (dressing on the side).
- Fast food: You don't have to choose a hamburger with the works; opt for a plain burger (no cheese) or a grilled chicken sandwich (if it's not breaded first). Visit the salad bar instead

Bright Idea
If you're obese, don't let fear of yo-yo dieting stop you from achieving a modest weight loss. Health problems associated with weight cycling haven't been proven, but the health-related problems of obesity are well-known.

of choosing a large order of fries, and when you're there, take raw vegetables instead of sauce-filled prepared pasta or bean salads.

For women only: Special nutritional needs

Starting at puberty and continuing all the way into menopause, women have special health and nutrition needs that men don't—but most of us don't pay much attention to our changing needs. These unique requirements are related to hormonal changes and experiences that occur throughout the course of a woman's adult life:

Bright Idea
To get the best and healthiest produce, either grow your own or buy local-grown at roadside stands.

- Menstruation: If you're losing blood every month, you need to replenish lost iron. (After you go through menopause, your iron needs fall.) You may want to choose a daily multivitamin supplement with iron. Dietary sources include meat, eggs, vegetables, and fortified cereals.

- Premenstrual syndrome (PMS): Cut back on caffeine and alcohol to reduce irritability, fatigue, depression, and headaches; curtail salt intake to ease fluid retention; eat calcium-rich foods to reduce bloating and moodiness and consume complex carbohydrates to increase serotonin; take a multivitamin (avoid supplements in unusually high doses); increase soy to reduce hormonal difficulties.

- Before pregnancy: If you're trying to get pregnant, it's imperative that you eat a healthy diet. Usually, you may not realize you're pregnant during the first few weeks, and that's a critical time in the development of a fetal spine and brain. Folic acid is especially critical—it is necessary for the development of normal brain tissue and to prevent neural tube defects such as spina bifida. Folic acid is especially important just before conception. Since birth control pills have been shown to actually reduce the levels of folic acid in your body, if you're on the pill but planning to get pregnant soon, you should actually start taking folic acid supplements (one mg. per day) before you even go off oral contraceptives. If you're not using contraception, be sure to get enough folic acid (or take a daily supplement of one mg. per day). Folic acid is also found in liver, leafy vegetables, oranges, peanuts, peas, beans, and lentils.

- Pregnancy: Everybody knows you need to eat healthy while you're pregnant—but you don't need to "eat for two." Instead, ingest about 300 calories more each day. Plan to gain between 25 and 35 pounds (overweight women should gain only about 15 pounds during pregnancy). Your doctor may prescribe a multivitamin supplement; if you're vegetarian, work with your doctor to plan a good diet.

- After pregnancy: You're not doomed to carry around that extra weight if you start a sensible weight loss plan right after your baby's birth. (Don't plan to lose too much weight while you're breastfeeding.) Remember that whatever you eat and drink usually goes into your breast milk.

- Menopause: If you lose too much calcium and protein, your bones will become brittle; many doctors recommend 1,500 mg a day of calcium. (Five Tums a day is a good calcium source.) Dietary sources include green leafy vegetables, tofu, fish with bones, and dairy. Supplements may be a good idea as well. Cut down on carbonated soft drinks high in phosphorus (it flushes calcium from the system).

- Older women: As you age, you need fewer daily calories because your metabolism slows down. You may want to use more spices to tempt a palate that is losing its ability to taste and smell.

Whatever your age, it's never too late or too early to form healthy eating habits that are suited to your special dietary needs. Women generally have less muscle and more body fat than men—and, therefore, lower metabolisms. That means women need significantly fewer calories than men to maintain a satisfactory body weight. For most women, between 1,200 and 2,200 calories a day is appropriate. A woman's body requires about 11 calories per pound each day to maintain body weight. Excess physical activity will increase the needs, but not by much (a 150-pound person will only use up 100 calories by walking or running a mile).

Many women struggle with their weight, sometimes resorting to new diet fads and pills along the way. These are short-term fixes that don't hold up over time, and some of them may be downright dangerous to a woman's health. To enjoy a healthy diet that provides high-quality nutrition and a reasonable number of calories, the best thing to do is follow the USDA Food Pyramid Guidelines on the following page.

Watch Out! Multivitamins with iron are an important daily habit if you're menstruating—but keep those pills out of the hands of youngsters! Accidental overdose of iron is the leading cause of poisoning death in kids under six.

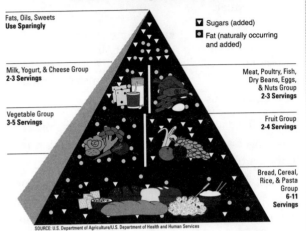

Figure 2.1: Food Guide Pyramid

Obesity

One of the most common complaints women have when they look in the mirror is that they weigh too much—and in fact, more than 55 percent of American women weigh more than 20 percent over their optimum weight (the definition for obesity). While women may not like what they see when they've put on too many pounds, obesity isn't just a cosmetic problem—it's a health hazard. Someone who is 40 percent overweight is twice as likely to die prematurely as an average-weight person after 10 to 30 years of being obese. Obesity has been linked to

- Diabetes.
- Heart disease.
- High blood pressure.
- Stroke.
- Higher rates of certain types of cancer.
- Gallbladder disease and gallstones.

- Osteoarthritis, a disease in which the joints deteriorate (possibly as a result of excess weight on the joints).
- Gout, another disease affecting the joints.
- Breathing problems (including sleep apnea, a condition which causes a person to stop breathing for a short time during sleep).

But for many obese women, the health concerns take a back seat to the emotional suffering they face at the hands of their thinner compatriots. American society places great emphasis on physical appearance and equates attractiveness with slimness, especially in women. Many Americans assume that obese people are gluttonous, lazy, stupid, and self-indulgent.

The idea that women with weight problems just aren't "trying hard enough" to diet, or that they lack the backbone to stick to an eating plan, is contradicted by recent research. Nevertheless, obese women face daily prejudice and discrimination at work and school, while job hunting, and in social situations. Feelings of rejection, shame, and depression are common.

For most of these women, obesity is a long-term condition that requires a lifetime of attention, even after formal weight loss treatment ends. Obese women need to aim for permanent lifestyle changes of healthier eating, regular physical activity, and an improved outlook about food, because without a long-term commitment, body weight will drift back up. Activity of any sort helps

- Relieve stress.
- Build and maintain healthy bones, muscles, and joints.

- Control weight, build lean muscle, and reduce fat.
- Reduce the risk of developing high blood pressure, and lower existing high blood pressure.
- Reduce the risk of dying prematurely, dying from heart disease, and developing diabetes and colon cancer.
- Ease depression and anxiety.
- Older adults become stronger and better able to move about without falling.

Get physical

Dieting is a great way to lose weight—but no matter how vigilant you are about throwing out those bags of potato chips, you need to exercise at the same time. Losing weight by dieting alone will weaken your muscles, making you more tired and less energetic than you were before. And if you drop the pounds too quickly by dieting alone, you can lose muscle mass—and that can be harmful.

The best plan: Try to lose about a pound a week so that the loss won't harm your body. Team that with an exercise program to burn fat, build muscle, and increase cardiovascular fitness.

Designing your own plan

If you want to make exercise a part of your life, you'd better choose something you enjoy or it just won't happen. If, for example, the only place you have to jog takes you down a busy highway past several construction sites and you can't stand the catcalls, odds are you won't enjoy your run. Too many women assume that "exercise program" means you need to work out as if you were training for the New York City marathon. It's just not true. Like the

Bright Idea
You'll need a good sports bra to make your workouts more comfortable. Choose a tight, well-fitting bra without wires or seams. Wear special pads to prevent nipple chafing and use lanolin to keep nipples soft.

outdoors? Then join a walking group, take a hike on the weekends, or learn to cross-country ski.

If you live in the city and you can't make yourself pop that exercise video in the VCR, invite a friend over or join an exercise group.

Even low to moderately intensive activity can help lower your risk of heart disease. Examples of such activities are pleasure walking, stair climbing, gardening, yard work, moderate-to-heavy housework, dancing, and home exercise. To get heart benefits from these activities, do one or more of them every day.

More vigorous exercises improve the fitness of the heart, which can lower heart disease risk still more—these aerobic activities include jogging, swimming, and jumping rope. Walking, bicycling, and dancing can also strengthen your heart, if you do them briskly for at least 30 minutes, three or four times a week. Whatever you choose, keep the intensity moderate and you'll be more likely to continue the program. Set realistic goals and monitor your progress.

Once you've chosen your activity, go slowly. Build up your activity level gradually. If your idea of exercise is to stand up and walk to the TV instead of grabbing the remote, you'll want to set a gradual pace—begin exercising regularly but slowly, with a 10- to 15-minute walk three times a week. As you become more fit, you can increase the sessions to every day or make each session longer.

If you choose a fairly vigorous activity, begin slowly with a five-minute period of stretching and slow movement to give your body a chance to warm up. At the end of your workout, take another five minutes to cool down with a slower exercise pace.

Listen to your body. A certain amount of stiffness is normal at first. But if you hurt a joint or pull a muscle or tendon, stop for several days to avoid more serious injury. Most minor muscle and joint problems can be relieved by rest and over-the-counter painkillers.

Check the weather report: On hot, humid days, exercise during the cooler parts of the day. Wear light, loose-fitting clothing and drink lots of water before, during, and after the activity. On cold days, wear one layer less of clothing than you would wear if you were outside but not exercising. Also wear gloves and a hat.

Don't give up. Unless you get sick or injured, stay with it. Set small, short-term goals for yourself. If you get bored, try doing the activity with a friend or family member, or switch to another activity.

See your doctor if...

Most women don't need to see a doctor before they start a gradual, sensible program of physical exercise. But do consult your doctor before you start or increase physical activity if you

- Have heart problems or you've have had a heart attack.
- Take medicine for high blood pressure or a heart condition.
- Are more than 50 years old and aren't used to energetic activity.
- Have a family history of developing heart disease at a young age.

Got kids?

Women with school-age children (especially during the summer!) may find it extremely hard to find any time at all to fit in an exercise regimen—and because they can't find two hours three times a week to exercise, they don't exercise at all. If this is your situation, try one of these suggestions:

Watch Out!
While regular exercise strengthens your heart, some activities may worsen existing heart problems. Warning signals include sudden dizziness, cold sweat, paleness, fainting, or pain or pressure in your upper body just after exercising.

Unofficially... Nearly half of American kids 12 to 21 aren't vigorously active on a regular basis—and young girls have the worst exercise rates of all. Participation in all types of physical activity declines strikingly as age or grade in school increases.

- Are you a morning person? Get up 30 minutes early, pop in an exercise video, and work out without the sound. Or start a yoga routine as the sun rises.
- Night owls can pop in the same video in the evening, ride a stationary bike at night while watching TV, and so on.
- Make a date with a friend to go for a walk every morning if your spouse can watch the kids.
- Park your car half a mile from the office and walk to and from.
- Sign up with a gym that offers free childcare.
- Swap childcare with your spouse or a friend; you exercise Mondays, Wednesdays, and Fridays while they watch the kids; you watch the kids while they work out Tuesdays, Thursdays, and Saturdays.
- If your kids are older, join in together—ride bikes, take hikes, or play tennis or badminton.
- If you've got a new baby, take a walk in the park with a stroller—it may be fun, but it's also exercise.

Exercise for seniors

There are many benefits to appropriate exercise for older women, but be sure to talk with your health care provider before starting any new exercise plan. Physical activity and exercise programs should meet your needs and skills. The amount and type of exercise depends on what you want to do. Different exercises do different things—some may slow bone loss, others may reduce the risk of falls, still others may improve the fitness of your heart and lungs. Some may do all three.

You can exercise at home alone, with a buddy, or as part of a group. Talk to your doctor before you begin, especially if you are over 60 or have a medical problem. Move at your own speed, and don't try to take on too much at first. A class can be a good idea if you haven't exercised for a long time or are just beginning. A qualified teacher will make sure you are doing the exercise the right way.

Older women benefit from lots of stretching, strength training, and aerobic (also called endurance) exercises. People who are weak or frail and may risk falling should start slowly. Begin with stretching and strength training; add aerobics later.

Aerobics are safer and easier once you feel balanced and your muscles are stronger. Aerobic exercises strengthen the heart and improve overall fitness by increasing the body's ability to use oxygen. Swimming, walking, and dancing are low-impact aerobic activities. They avoid the muscle and joint pounding of more high-impact exercises like jogging and jumping rope.

Eating disorders: Are you at risk?

Body image, weight loss, dieting . . . it's true that we want to look our best and maintain our health by watching what we eat. Unfortunately, millions of women in the United States spend far too much time watching what they eat. These are the millions of women who are affected by serious and sometimes life-threatening eating disorders, the vast majority of whom (more than 90 percent) are adolescent and young adult women.

One reason that women in this age group are particularly vulnerable to eating disorders is their tendency to go on strict diets to achieve an "ideal" figure. Researchers have found that stringent dieting can play a key role in triggering eating disorders.

About 1 percent of teenage girls develop *anorexia nervosa,* a dangerous condition in which girls can literally starve themselves to death. Another 2 to 3 percent of young women develop *bulimia nervosa,* a destructive pattern of excessive overeating followed by vomiting or other purging behaviors to control weight. (These eating disorders also occur, although much less often, in older women.) Still another 3 percent develop binge eating, an eating disorder similar to bulimia in which girls gorge themselves on food, but don't vomit to lose weight.

The consequences of eating disorders can be severe. For example, 1 in 10 girls with anorexia dies from starvation, heart attack, medical complications, or suicide. Fortunately, increasing awareness of the dangers of eating disorders, backed by medical studies and extensive media coverage, has led many women to seek help. Nevertheless, some women with eating disorders refuse to admit there's a problem and reject treatment. Family members and friends can help recognize the problem and encourage these young women to seek treatment.

In trying to understand the causes of eating disorders, scientists have studied the personalities, genetics, environments, and biochemistry of people with these illnesses. As often happens, the more we know, the more complex the roots of eating disorders appear.

So why do some women diet off and on without any problems, while others develop eating disorders? Genetic studies have found that anorexia nervosa is five times as likely to co-occur in identical twins than

Watch Out! Women with eating disorders who use drugs to stimulate vomiting, bowel movements, or urination may be in considerable danger of heart failure.

in fraternal twins or non-twin siblings, suggesting there's a genetic component. In fact, there's an increased risk for both anorexia and bulimia in close relatives of women with eating disorders.

Certain personality characteristics seem to be associated with these two disorders:

- Fear of losing control
- Inflexible thinking
- Perfectionism
- Self-esteem heavily linked to body shape and weight
- Dissatisfaction with body shape
- An overwhelming desire to be thin

Anorexia nervosa has also been linked to obsessive-compulsive tendencies, such as a preoccupation with food, while bulimia seems to be associated with mood disturbances (such as depression or social anxiety).

We're beginning to understand why eating disorders develop, but a "cure" has been elusive and even treatment is a problem, since many women with eating disorders resist getting help. In fact, women with eating disorders often have trouble admitting they have a serious problem, and in many cases, particularly with anorexia, family or friends must persuade the individual to seek treatment.

Family support is extremely important in treating both anorexia and bulimia nervosa. In many cases, anorexic and bulimic women and their families attend family counseling sessions. Even after the eating disorder has been controlled, follow-up counseling for the patient, as well as her family, may be recommended.

While many people with an eating disorder will fully recover, relapse is common and may occur months or even years after treatment. About 5 to 10 percent of anorexics will die from the disorder, usually from starvation, suicide, or electrolyte problems. Women with anorexia do better if they are younger when they become sick, or are more mature, have better self-esteem, and don't deny their condition as much.

The outcome for bulimia isn't as well documented and mortality rates aren't yet known. Experts do know that it is a chronic disorder which comes and goes. Of those women who are treated for the disorder, three years later less than one-third will be fully recovered, more than one-third will show some improvement in their symptoms, and about one-third will have resumed chronic symptoms.

A variety of specialists may be well trained in the treatment of eating disorders, including

- Internal medicine physicians
- Psychiatrists
- Psychologists
- Clinical social workers
- Nurses
- Dietitians

Anorexia nervosa

Anyone who believes that you can never be "too thin or too rich" has never watched a young anorexic lying in a hospital bed, hooked up to an IV drip. In fact, you can be too thin, and far too many young American women every year are just that.

For reasons not yet understood, girls suffering from anorexia nervosa become terrified of gaining any weight. Anorexia, which usually begins around puberty, is diagnosed when a girl is at least 15 percent below her normal body weight. Food and weight become obsessions. For some, the compulsiveness shows up in strange eating rituals or the refusal to eat in front of others. Some anorexic girls and young women obsess about food, collecting recipes and preparing lavish gourmet feasts for family and friends while refusing any food themselves. They may adhere to strict exercise routines to keep off weight.

As the girl's weight plummets, vital organs, such as the brain and heart, can be damaged. As the body begins to starve, it shifts into "slow gear" to protect itself—monthly menstrual periods stop; breathing, pulse, and blood pressure rates drop; and thyroid function slows. Nails and hair become brittle; the skin dries, yellows, and becomes covered with soft hair called lanugo. Girls notice excessive thirst and frequent urination. Dehydration contributes to constipation, and reduced body fat leads to lowered body temperature and the inability to withstand cold. In addition, mild anemia, swollen joints, reduced muscle mass, and lightheadedness also commonly occur with anorexia.

If the disorder becomes severe, women may lose calcium from their bones, making them brittle and prone to breakage. They may also experience irregular heart rhythms and heart failure. Some women's brains shrink, causing personality changes.

Fortunately, these symptoms can be reversed once normal weight is reestablished. The first step in treating anorexia is to get the woman to put on weight. The greater the weight loss has been, the more likely the woman will need hospitalization. Outpatient programs have become common in

Unofficially...
Scientists have found that many women with anorexia also suffer from other problems; most are clinically depressed, but some suffer from anxiety, personality, or substance abuse disorders, or obsessive-compulsive disorder, an illness characterized by repetitive thoughts and behaviors.

recent years; some centers have day programs requiring patients to stay eight hours a day, five days a week.

Anorexic patients are given a carefully prescribed diet, starting with small meals and gradually increasing the caloric intake. A woman is given a goal weight range, and as she approaches her ideal weight, more independence in her eating habits is allowed. If, however, she falls below the set range, greater supervision may be reinstated.

As she begins to gain weight, she will usually begin individual and group psychotherapy. Counseling typically involves education about body weight regulation and the effects of starvation, clarification of dietary misconceptions, and work on the issues of self-control and self-esteem. Follow-up counseling for anorexia may continue for six months to several years after healthy weight is restored.

Bulimia nervosa

Unlike their food-resistant sisters, women with bulimia nervosa eat large amounts of food—and then get rid of the excess calories by vomiting, abusing laxatives or diuretics, taking enemas, or exercising obsessively. Some use a combination of all of these. Because many women with bulimia binge and purge in secret and maintain normal or above-normal body weight, they can often successfully hide their problem from others for years.

Bulimia becomes a serious problem when a girl is bingeing and purging at least twice a week for three months while becoming excessively worried about her body shape and weight. Dieting heavily between episodes of bingeing and purging is common; eventually, half of girls with anorexia will develop bulimia.

As with anorexia, bulimia typically begins during adolescence and occurs most often in women. Many women with bulimia, ashamed of their strange habits, don't seek help until they reach their 30s or 40s—but by this time, their eating behavior is deeply ingrained and more difficult to change.

Girls and women with bulimia aren't as successful at dieting as anorexics. They may be able to deny their hunger and restrict their food intake for several days or weeks at a time, but sooner or later (say, when something upsets them), women with bulimia crack. They begin to eat and can't stop eating until they have stuffed themselves. Experts think this overeating compensates for the prior calorie restriction. Binge eating may also be related to problems with feeling satisfied after meals, since many bulimics report that they have trouble feeling full unless they eat large amounts of food.

Bulimia patients (even those with normal weight) can severely damage their bodies by frequent binge eating and purging. In rare instances, binge eating causes the stomach to rupture; purging may result in heart failure because of loss of vital minerals, such as potassium. Vomiting causes other less deadly, but serious, problems—the acid in vomit wears down the outer layer of the teeth, the esophagus becomes inflamed, and glands near the cheeks become swollen. As with anorexia, bulimia may lead to irregular menstrual periods. Interest in sex may also diminish.

Some women with bulimia struggle with addictions, including abuse of drugs and alcohol or compulsive stealing. Like individuals with anorexia, many bulimics suffer from clinical depression, anxiety, OCD, and other mental health issues. These

Unofficially...
Bulimia means "ox hunger," referring to the large amount of food consumed during binge episodes.

Unofficially...
A drop in serotonin levels in the brain may trigger the symptoms of bulimia in susceptible women, according to research published in the February 1999 issue of the *Archives of General Psychiatry*.

problems, combined with impulsive tendencies, place them at increased risk for suicidal behavior.

In treating bulimia, doctors must first deal with any serious physical complications. In some cases, when the binge-purge cycle is so severe that the woman can't stop on her own, hospitalization may be necessary, followed by individual counseling (sometimes combined with medication). Counseling involves exploring issues similar to those discussed in the treatment of anorexia, and usually lasts for about four to six months. In addition, group therapy is especially effective for bulimics. Antidepressants may be an effective way of treating bulimia, as well.

In outpatient treatment, bulimic patients are often asked to keep a food-intake diary, making sure they eat three meals a day of moderate caloric intake, even if they are still binge eating. Exercise is limited, and if the patient becomes compulsive about it, it is not permitted at all.

Binge eating

Binge eating disorder is an illness that resembles bulimia but without the purging. Women with binge eating disorder feel that they lose control of themselves when eating, gorging themselves with huge amounts of food until they are uncomfortably full. Usually they have more problems losing weight and keeping it off than do women with anorexia or bulimia. In fact, most women with the disorder are obese and have a history of weight fluctuations.

Women with binge eating disorder are usually overweight, so they are prone to the serious medical problems associated with obesity, such as high cholesterol, high blood pressure, and diabetes. Obese individuals also have higher risk for gallbladder disease, heart disease, and some types of cancer.

Women with binge eating disorder also have high rates of co-occurring psychiatric illnesses, especially depression.

Like mother, like daughter

Daughters born to mothers with past or present eating disorders may be at high risk of developing an eating disorder themselves, according to Stanford University researchers. Mothers with eating disorders "interact differently" with their daughters than other mothers when it comes to feeding and weight issues, according to researchers in the April 1999 issue of the *International Journal of Eating Disorders*. This suggests that the risk factors for the later development of an eating disorder may begin very early in life.

The new study found that the baby daughters of women with eating disorders sucked significantly faster, whether breast- or bottle-fed, and were weaned from the bottle an average of more than nine months later than offspring of noneating disordered women. When their children were age two or older, moms with a history of eating disorders fed their children on a less regular schedule, used food as a reward or to calm the child, and showed greater concern about their daughters' weight than did other mothers.

These differences "may pose a serious risk for the later development of an eating disorder," according to the team, led by Dr. Stewart Agras of the Department of Psychiatry at Stanford University in Palo Alto, CA.

For more information...

To find an eating disorders clinic, check with your local hospitals or university medical center. In addition, Appendix A contains a listing of organizations

Unofficially...
Binge eating disorder is found more often in women than men. Recent research shows that binge eating disorder occurs in about 30 percent of people participating in medically supervised weight control programs.

that can provide more information on eating disorders and referrals.

Plastic surgery

Dieting and exercise work well in toning and strengthening the body, but sometimes there are areas that just don't respond. In these cases, some women turn to plastic surgeons to reshape the parts of their body that they feel need some extra help.

Here's an average of what some common operations may cost; in some parts of the country, procedures may be less or more expensive:

- Breast size reduction: $4,500
- Breast size augmentation: $4,500
- Collagen injections: $250 per injection
- Eyelid surgery with bag removal: $2,500
- Liposuction: $2,000 per site
- Rhinoplasty (nose job): $3,000
- Tummy tuck: $3,500
- Face-lift: $4,000

For more information about specific procedures and to get referrals to a plastic surgeon by geographical location, consult one of the organizations listed in Appendix A.

Cosmetic breast surgery

Let's face it—most women just don't seem to be happy with the size of their breasts. Tiny-breasted women long to look like Dolly Parton, and Dolly Parton look-alikes ache to look like Twiggy. Enter breast augmentation and breast reduction.

Are they too small?

Breast augmentation (making a smaller breast bigger) is the more popular of the two. Women want to

Moneysaver
Plastic surgery is expensive, so try to see if your insurance plan will cover the cost of treatment. Don't count on it though—you should be prepared to foot the bill yourself, especially if there isn't a medically necessary reason for the surgery.

enlarge their breasts for many reasons besides just wanting to be bustier: some women lose breast volume after pregnancy, after weight loss, or as they got older, while others have a difference in size between the right and left breasts, and still others need reconstruction after breast surgery.

In the past, fluids were directly injected into the breast to plump it up—with some dreadful results. Today, a prosthesis (a saltwater-solution implant, known as a saline implant) is implanted into a pocket either directly under the breast tissue or underneath the major chest muscle.

Not so long ago, the most common implants were silicone gel, but after numerous medical reports questioning their safety and linking them to connective tissue disorders, saline inflatable implants have now become more popular. A third type features an implant made of a gel-filled inner portion surrounded by a saline inflatable outer jacket.

Breast augmentation is usually performed in an office facility, surgery center, or hospital outpatient facility. Either local or general anesthesia can be used for this procedure. The incision through which the implant is inserted will be made in such a way as to make it as inconspicuous as possible—either above the crease under the breast (the most popular choice), near the nipple, or high in the armpit. The armpit incision leaves no scar on the breast itself, but it's more risky since the incision is far from the area in which the surgeon is working. After the procedure, the breast should look and feel natural. Scars are usually not noticeable.

The surgery typically takes one to two hours to complete. Most women can return to work within a few days, depending on the nature of their jobs.

Unofficially...
Soybean oil-filled implants are now used in Europe for breast augmentation but are not approved yet in the United States.

Breast augmentation is relatively safe, but like any surgery, there are certain risks and specific complications associated with this procedure that you need to discuss with your doctor. So far, there has been no evidence that breast implants will affect your fertility, pregnancy, or ability to nurse. However, there are problems with breast hardness caused by scar tissue that forms around the implant in up to 30 percent of women. This hardness may appear soon after surgery or years after the procedure. Other risks are rare, but include loss of nipple sensitivity (5 to 10 percent), infection, or poor healing of scars. There is no evidence that breast implants cause breast cancer.

Breast implants do make it technically difficult to get or read mammograms. Special mammogram views or extra exams by ultrasound may be needed if you've had breast implants. While soybean oil-filled implants don't interfere with mammograms, they aren't yet available in the United States.

Are they too big?

Women with the opposite problem—breasts they feel are too large—choose breast reduction to have a smaller bustline. The problem of overlarge breasts is more than a cosmetic one; heavy, pendulous breasts can actually cause physical discomfort. Breast reduction may be recommended when any of the following conditions are present:

- Cystic breast infections
- Pain from weight of large breasts that is not relieved by a supporting bra
- Back pain, neck pain, or shoulder pain
- Headache resulting from weight of large breasts
- Breast pain

- Numbness in the breasts
- Sleeping problems resulting from large breasts
- Poor posture caused by large breasts
- Arm or finger numbness caused by large breasts
- Pigmented bra-strap groove
- Scarlike lines on the breasts

It's not recommended if you have breast cancer, uncontrolled diabetes, cellulitis, hardened breast skin, or dry or broken skin.

A breast reduction usually requires a hospital stay and general anesthesia. The surgeon will remove excess breast tissue, raise the nipple position, and trim the skin to fit the new shape. There are many ways to perform a breast reduction, and the method must be tailored to the patient. However, a common method of surgery is to mark the new nipple position and, with the blood supply of the nipple preserved on a tissue flap, remove the excess breast tissue. The nipple is then moved into its new position and the new breast shape is constructed. The incision is often around the nipple and on the under surface of the breast, much like an upside-down "T."

After reduction, a bulky gauze dressing is wrapped around the breasts and chestor a surgical bra may be used. Pain is controlled by medication and will subside in a day or two. Some doctors perform the operation on an outpatient basis; others require hospitalization for a day or two. Within two weeks of surgery, sutures will be removed. You should limit exercise in order to prevent stretching of the scars, but some activity may be allowed in a day or two following surgery. Your plastic surgeon will recommend a schedule for resuming your usual routine (usually after about eight weeks). To permit

Moneysaver
Because breast reduction is not always simply cosmetic, your insurance company may cover at least part of the cost of the operation.

proper healing, avoid overhead lifting for three to four weeks.

The dressing will be replaced by a soft bra within seven days, and in turn must be worn for several weeks. Generally, within a few days the swelling and discoloration around the incisions will subside. Expect some scarring (usually around the nipple, under the breasts, and between the nipple and the second scar). The scars are permanent and often remain highly visible for a year following surgery, after which time they fade to some degree. Every effort is made to place the incisions so that scars are as inconspicuous as possible, and the scars should not be noticeable, even in low-cut clothing.

There may be temporary loss of sensation in the breast skin and nipples after surgery, but this condition will improve with time. In addition to the general risks of surgery and anesthesia, there is a chance that you'll have large scars requiring prolonged healing time, uneven position of the nipples, and the inability to nurse a baby after surgery. The emotional risks may include feeling that the breasts look imperfect, or that the reactions of others are not what you'd hoped for. As with breast augmentation, there is no evidence of a higher risk of breast cancer in women who have had breast reduction. Odds are, you'll be very happy with your appearance after surgery as your looks and lifestyle are improved and the pain or skin symptoms disappear.

Nose job (rhinoplasty)

Surgery to reshape your nose is one of the most common of all plastic surgery procedures. It can reduce or increase the size of your nose, change the shape of the tip or the bridge, narrow the span of the nostrils, or change the angle between your nose and your upper lip. It may also correct a birth defect or injury or help relieve some breathing problems. The best candidates for rhinoplasty are people who are looking for improvement, not perfection. If you're physically healthy, psychologically stable, and realistic in your expectations, you may be a good candidate. Many surgeons prefer not to operate on teenagers until after they've completed their growth spurt—at around age 14 or 15 for girls. It's important to consider a teen's social and emotional adjustment, too, and to make sure it's what they—not you, the parent—really want.

When rhinoplasty is performed by a qualified plastic surgeon, complications are infrequent and usually minor. However, there is always the possibility of complications, including infection, nosebleed, or a reaction to the anesthesia. You can reduce your risks by closely following your surgeon's instructions before and after surgery.

In about 1 case out of 10, a second procedure may be needed to correct a minor deformity. Such cases are unpredictable and happen even to patients of the most skilled surgeons. The corrective surgery is usually minor.

Rhinoplasty is usually done on an outpatient basis, although complex procedures may require a short inpatient stay. It can be performed under local or general anesthesia, depending on the extent of the procedure and on what you and your surgeon prefer. With local anesthesia, you'll usually be lightly sedated, and your nose and the surrounding area will be numbed; you'll be awake during the surgery, but relaxed and insensitive to pain. With general anesthesia, you'll sleep through the operation.

Rhinoplasty usually takes an hour or two, although complicated procedures may take longer. During surgery, the skin of the nose is separated from the bone and cartilage and then sculpted to the desired shape. The nature of the sculpting will depend on your problem and your surgeon's preferred technique. Finally, the skin is redraped over the new framework. Many plastic surgeons perform rhinoplasty from within the nose, with an incision inside the nostrils. Others prefer an "open" procedure (especially in more complicated cases) using a small incision across the vertical strip of tissue separating the nostrils. When the surgery is over, the surgeon will apply a splint to help your nose maintain its new shape. Nasal packs or soft plastic splints also may be placed in your nostrils to stabilize the dividing wall between the air passages.

The first day after surgery, your face will feel puffy, your nose may ache, and you may have a dull headache. The swelling and bruising around your eyes will increase at first, peaking after two or three days. Most of the swelling and bruising should disappear within two weeks or so. (Some subtle swelling may remain for several months, but almost no one but you will notice.) A little bleeding is common during the first few days following surgery, and you may continue to feel some stuffiness for several weeks. If you have nasal packing, it will be removed after a few days and you'll feel much more comfortable. By the end of one or, occasionally, two weeks, all dressings, splints, and stitches should be removed.

You'll probably be up and about within two days and able to return to school or sedentary work a week or so following surgery. Your surgeon will give you more specific guidelines for gradually resuming your normal activities but, usually, you're asked to avoid strenuous activity (jogging, swimming, bending, sex) for two to three weeks. You can wear contact lenses as soon as you feel like it, but you can't wear glasses normally for about six to seven weeks. (Once the splint is off, they'll have to be taped to your forehead or propped on your cheeks for another six to seven weeks, until your nose is completely healed.)

Suck the fat away

There you are in your new bathing suit, which looks just terrific on you . . . except for those pouchy little pockets of fat on either hip. If you've tried dieting, exercise, stretching, pounding—all to no avail—then liposuction might be next on the list.

Liposuction has become the most popular cosmetic procedure in the United States—even more popular than face-lifts. More than 292,000 liposuction procedures were done in the United States in 1996, an increase of more than 300 percent in six years. But is it safe? That depends . . . .

Diet and exercise are usually the best ways to reduce body fat and improve muscle tone, but if you have a few isolated large fat deposits, they may not respond to exercise and diet. Enter liposuction, the process that doesn't just shrink fat cells, leaving them lying there ready to plump up when you eat that next cheeseburger—it gets rid of them permanently.

The procedure does work, because fat cells don't regenerate after they are destroyed or removed. (For example, if you gain weight after liposuction, you don't regain significant amounts of weight in areas where your fat had been removed.)

However, liposuction has limitations, some fairly serious. Complications of liposuction can be deadly, and the procedure should not be viewed as trivial, according to a report in the May 13, 1999, issue of *The New England Journal of Medicine*. It has the potential to kill otherwise healthy people from drug interactions, fluid overload, clotting problems, and the volume of fat removed. The report was prompted by five deaths of liposuction patients referred to the Office of the Chief Medical Examiner of New York City, between 1993 and 1998.

There are other risks. Since the surgical incision is so small, it will be hard for your surgeon to see under the skin to figure out how much blood and fluid has been lost. If the surgeon sucks out too much fat, the associated blood loss can lead to life-threatening shock; fortunately, this risk is much less now that surgeons have become more experienced with the procedure, but it does still occur. There is also a small risk of having a *fat embolism*—a bit of fat that may migrate to an organ, where it could be fatal.

The best candidates for liposuction are those women in their 30s and 40s who are healthy, at near-normal weight, with good skin elasticity—this will help your skin drape properly after the fat is removed. (Of course, you may be thinking that these are precisely the women who may not need liposuction, and you may be right.) Provided you keep your weight on an even keel after surgery, your results will be permanent.

Liposuction works best if you've got fat in certain localized areas, covered by nice, taut skin. Once the fat is removed, your skin will reshape itself; if the skin is too loose, you'll have extra skin hanging

Watch Out! Certainly, liposuction is not for everybody. If you're over age 50, have chronic health problems, and you're seriously overweight, you're a poor candidate for liposuction.

down which may be less attractive than the original fat. In this case, you may be in the market for an additional skin tuck (see below).

While some surgeons perform liposuction under general anesthesia, it's most often done with use of a local. A doctor infuses a solution of fluid under the skin that contains the pain-killing drug lidocaine, which allows deposits of fat to be removed through special instruments without pain.

Next, the surgeon inserts a tube through a small skin incision; the tube is attached to a suction pump and is moved through fat, removing the cells. As the tube moves, it creates tunnels that scar, resulting in a permanent flattening of the area. With newer anesthesia techniques, the risk of blood loss is low and the procedure is easy to perform. The surgery lasts between 30 minutes and three hours and you can be back to work within a day to a week (depending on how extensive the surgery was).

This is usually outpatient surgery, and you'll be encouraged to get up and walk soon afterwards. If you've had a liposuction of the thighs and buttocks, you may not want to sit much for a week or so, because you'll feel bruised and uncomfortable.

You should avoid exercise for several weeks after surgery. You can expect bruises to last between one and six months; the final appearance isn't apparent until the healing process is complete. Liposuction costs vary from city to city and from doctor to doctor, but on average, it can cost $2,000 for a single site.

Now for the side effects. The most frequent side effect is a ridging of the skin's surface (an external reflection of the tunneling created underneath). Ridging may be unattractive, but it's not apparent

Watch Out!
The local anesthetic lidocaine can cause low blood pressure and a slowing of the heartbeat, and doses of lidocaine used during liposuction may be high compared to doses of the drug used for other procedures.

when you're fully dressed. Other side effects include soreness, temporary bruising and swelling, and numbness. There is the risk of infection, local irregularity of contour, or blood loss.

Tummy tucks

Known medically as *abdominal recontouring*, this procedure is often favored by women after pregnancy who didn't bounce back to their original shape, despite proper diet and exercise. It's also a favorite of women who've had liposuction but were left with some envelopes of hanging skin that didn't retract appropriately. Cosmetic repair of the abdomen can help improve your appearance, especially after massive weight gain and loss. A tummy tuck can help flatten the lower abdomen, tighten stretched skin, and strengthen abdominal muscles.

Under general anesthesia, the surgeon makes a long, curved incision at above the pubic line, freeing the loose skin and fat of the abdomen to be tightened. The surgeon may also tighten the underlying muscles with stitches, or by sewing them closer together. Your navel is detached and then reattached after the abdominal skin and fat have been tightened up. The incision is stitched (sutured) closed. Small flat tubes (drains) may be inserted and used for a few days after surgery to allow fluid to drain out of the incisions. A firm elastic dressing is applied to the abdomen. If you had stretch marks with your pregnancy, this procedure won't erase them unless they are on a part of the skin that was cut away.

You can expect to feel some pain and discomfort for several days after surgery, which can be eased with pain medications. Resting with the legs and hips bent will reduce pressure on the abdomen during the recommended two- to three-day hospital stay. An elastic support (like a girdle) worn over the abdomen for two to three weeks provides extra abdominal support while healing. You should avoid strenuous activity and straining for three to four weeks. The scars will become lighter in color and flatter during the next three to six months.

If you're considering body contouring, you need to realize that this is a major procedure that entails some risk, just as liposuction does. It isn't a substitute for weight loss. There are risks of bleeding and infection, as in all surgery, with additional risks of blood clots and poor healing.

Just the facts

- Treatment approaches may vary, but it's important to find an expert well trained in handling eating disorders.
- The roots of eating disorders involve psychological, biochemical, genetic, and social factors.
- Dieting is a good way to lose weight, but if you don't exercise at the same time, you may weaken your muscles and suffer from fatigue.
- It's better to succeed with short, doable exercises than fail at a mammoth marathon activity program.
- There is no good easy way to lose weight.
- Liposuction works best for younger, healthy women of average weight.
- Insurance may cover part or all of the costs of breast reduction surgery since the reasons for having it may not be entirely cosmetic.

GET THE SCOOP ON...
Which screening tests you need to have at each stage of your life ▪ How to find the right specialist ▪ What do the experts say about vaccine safety? ▪ What to expect for a girl's first pelvic exam ▪ What's happening to your body at each stage of your life ▪ Special concerns at each stage of your life

Checking Up Through All Stages of Life

Susan was a 42-year-old mother of two with high blood pressure and a very stressful job. With a family history of high cholesterol and heart disease, Susan suggested to her doctor that perhaps she needed a cholesterol level check. "We don't give those tests," she was told, "unless you have symptoms of high cholesterol." Susan was frustrated, and yet unsure. Did she have the right to demand a cholesterol test, given her family history and high blood pressure?

Yes, she did. In fact, a baseline cholesterol check wouldn't be a bad idea for Susan, no matter what her family history and current lifestyle. But far too many women just like Susan don't really know what tests they should have, and when and why.

Sure, we all know that checkups are important. But how many of us visit the doctor as often as we should? Experts tell us that most women are lucky if they get Pap smears and breast exams as often as they should. In fact, too many of us really don't understand what tests and vaccinations we should have. This can be of particular importance as some health maintenance organizations become more resistant to scheduling these preventive tests.

Knowing what to expect with each decade of life, which vaccines are important, and which tests should be scheduled should be a part of every woman's health care habit. Ideally, this emphasis toward prevention—with adequate vaccinations and checkups—should begin at birth.

How to choose a specialist

The selection of a pediatrician or family practitioner who is "right" for your family can be daunting, especially if you're expecting your first child. Whichever doctor you choose, it's a good idea to make your selection before your baby is born.

Pediatricians are graduates of four-year medical schools with three additional years of specialty training in pediatrics. Many pediatricians are board certified, meaning they've passed a rigorous exam given by the American Board of Pediatrics. Family practitioners are also good choices for newborn and child care—they have an additional advantage of knowing other family members. In some communities, there are few pediatricians and the family practitioners take care of most babies and children.

Before selecting specialists to interview, take into consideration the type of practice you prefer: Are you looking for a single doctor, partner, or group practice? Where is the office and how long does it take you to get there?

Bright Idea
To find a good pediatrician or family practitioner, ask your obstetrician for referrals or ask other parents, neighbors, or friends with children. Or contact the chief resident in pediatrics at the nearest teaching hospital.

Once you've answered these questions and you have the names you want to consider, arrange a get-acquainted visit during your final months of pregnancy. When you get to the doctor's office, take a look around. Is the office oriented toward children, with lots of toys and books? Does the staff make you feel welcome? Is there a "sick child" waiting room so those visiting the office for well-baby/child checkups or immunizations aren't exposed to contagious illnesses?

Next, you'll want to come up with some sample questions to help you make your decision. Here are some suggestions:

- Ask about the doctor's philosophy on child rearing, (including issues such as breastfeeding versus bottle feeding, circumcision, and preventive medicine). Are the answers close to your own views?

- Ask whether the doctor has hospital privileges at the hospital you're using in case of complications at the time of your delivery. Another philosophical issue to consider: is the doctor willing to give advice over the phone (as opposed to your coming in for an appointment)? There isn't any "right" or "wrong" here—it's a matter of matching styles. If you're the type who would like to take your child to the doctor whenever there is any question, pick a doctor who's willing to go along with that. If you're comfortable being reassured over the phone and reserving office visits for more significant problems, make sure the doctor agrees with that, too.

- How soon after birth will the pediatrician see your baby? Unless you had complications during your pregnancy or delivery, your baby should be examined during the first 24 hours of life. Ask the pediatrician if you can be present during the initial exam.

- When is the doctor available by phone? Many pediatricians have a specific call-in period each day when you can phone with questions. Ask the doctor for guidelines to help you determine which questions can be answered with a phone call and which require an office visit.
- With which hospital is the doctor affiliated?
- Where should you go if your child becomes seriously ill or is injured? If the hospital is a teaching hospital with interns and residents, find out who would actually care for your child if he or she were to be admitted.
- Does the pediatrician take his or her own emergency calls at night? If not, how are they handled? Does the pediatrician see patients in the office after regular hours or must you take your child to an emergency room?
- Who covers the practice when the doctor is unavailable?
- What are the fees? What insurance plans does the practice accept?
- How often will the pediatrician see your baby for checkups and immunizations?

After these interviews, assess the experience: Do you feel comfortable with the doctor and the staff? Do you feel that your questions will be answered clearly and your concerns handled compassionately? Did the pediatrician show an interest in you and your child?

Unofficially...
The American Academy of Pediatrics recommends well-baby checkups at 1, 2, 4, 6, 9, 12, 15, 18, and 24 months; annual checkups are recommended after two years of age.

Birth to 11 years

Now that you've got a pediatrician and your son or daughter is born, it's important to understand that his or her first years are crucial to getting a good start. You'll need to concentrate on frequent well-baby checkups and a series of vaccinations that today can prevent most of the common childhood illnesses.

Vaccinate!

In just the last few years, scientists have made dramatic strides to protect today's infants from diseases that only recently were commonplace in nurseries and day care centers around the country. Just as pertussis and polio were almost wiped out for children in the 1950s, chicken pox, rotavirus, and perhaps even ear infections will soon be unheard of.

Chicken pox: Is it safe?

The arrival of the chicken pox vaccine marked the end of one of the last childhood diseases. Less serious than measles, mumps, and rubella, chicken pox is still more than simply a "rite of passage" for kids. Each year, secondary complications from chicken pox put 14,000 kids and adults in the hospital and kill about 100 otherwise healthy people. Most complications are caused by bacterial infections (such as staph and strep), but sometimes kids can also develop encephalitis, pneumonia, or other brain disorders after contracting chicken pox.

When the chicken pox vaccine was approved by the FDA in 1995, some experts worried that the shot would trigger shingles, a painful skin-blister condition caused by the same virus that causes chicken pox. But according to experts at the National

TABLE 3.1: VACCINATIONS DURING YOUR CHILD'S FIRST YEARS

Vaccine	Birth	1m[1]	2m	4m	6m	12m	15m	18m	4–6yr	11–12yr
Chickenpox[2] Var. (varicella)						xxxxxxxxxxxxxxx				xxxx
Hep B	xxxx Hep B1 xxxx	xxx Hep B2 xxx			xxxxxxx Hep B3 xxxxxxx					Hep B3
Diptheria, Tetanus, Pertussis[3]			DTaP or DTP	DTaP or DTP	DTaP or DTP		DTaP or DTP	xxxxxx	DTaP or DTP	Td
H. influenzae type B (Hib)			Hib	Hib	Hib	xxx Hib xxx				
Polio			Polio	Polio	xxxx Polio	xxxxxxxxxxxx			Polio	
Measles, Mumps, Rubella (MMR)						MMR xxxxxx			MMR	

Approved by the American Academy of Pediatrics and the American Academy of Family Physicians

[1] m = month.

[2] Susceptible children may receive varicella vaccine at any visit after the first birthday, and those who have never had it should be immunized during the 11 to 12 year visit. Susceptible children 13 years of age and older should receive two doses at least one month apart.

[3] DtaP (diphtheria and tetanus toxoids and acellular pertussis vaccine) is the preferred vaccine for all doses including completion of the series in shildren who have received 1 or more doses of the whole-cell DTP. The fourth dose may be given as early as 12 months of age provided 6 months have passed since the third dose. Tetanus and diphtheria toxoids (Td) is recommended at 11–12 years and every 10 years thereafter.

Institute of Allergy and Infectious Diseases, the vaccination actually lowers, rather than increases, the risk of shingles.

Experts were also concerned that the effects of the vaccine would wear off, leaving a child vulnerable to disease at an older (and more dangerous) age. However, research has found that this does not occur. As a result, a chicken pox vaccine is now recommended for children.

There are no recommendations for chicken pox booster shots.

Polio vaccines: Give it a shot

It's one of the enduring memories of the 1950s: Long lines of kids snaking around school cafeterias waiting to take a tiny sugar cube coated with the polio vaccine. The mass vaccinations marked the end of one of the most frightening medical nightmares in America, when mysterious epidemics of polio would sweep across the country in the summer, sickening and paralyzing children without warning.

After the initial relief from finding a vaccine faded, however, these oral polio vaccinations—which featured a live, weakened, vaccine—became caught up in controversy. It became apparent that the oral polio vaccine was still capable of causing polio in about six to eight children a year (or 1 out of every 2.5 million doses). On the other hand, the "killed" polio shot caused none. While some experts argued that those cases of vaccine-induced polio were very few and far between, many Americans believed that even one child with polio was one too many.

Eventually, after extensive lobbying by parents whose children had been infected with polio, experts recommended the use of a safe, injected polio vaccine to be given to infants at two and four months of age. Researchers anticipate that soon the oral polio vaccine will probably be phased out altogether.

DTP versus DTaP

This isn't the first time that a newer, safer vaccine has been developed to replace one that has caused

Unofficially...
A Kaiser Permanente study in Oakland, CA, found that a pneumococcal vaccine given to 35,000 children was 90 percent effective against illnesses caused by the bacteria. The only side effects were a mild fever and pain at injection.

a few unpleasant side effects. In the past, some parents and experts have charged that the diphtheria, tetanus, and pertussis vaccine (DTP) is unsafe. The pertussis part of the vaccine, which contained whole bacteria, was linked to a range of side effects and serious neurological complications.

Today, experts recommend a DTaP vaccine that contains only pieces of the disease's bacterial cell. This "acellular" vaccine causes fewer side effects and is now given to all children in place of the older DTP shot.

Goodbye, ear infections!

Not content with preventing measles, mumps, rubella, chicken pox, diphtheria, polio, tetanus, and pertussis, scientists next went to work on the scourge of childhood—ear infections. Within a year or two, the government is expected to approve a vaccine that could protect your child from the most common cause of ear infections—a bacteria called pneumococcus. In addition to ear infections, the bacteria also causes a host of other serious illnesses ranging from meningitis, pneumonia, and blood infections, which kill 1.5 million children around the world every year.

Sniff away the flu

In other new developments, a pain-free alternative to the flu shot for kids is expected to be approved in time for the fall 2000 flu season—a nasal spray that is 93 percent effective against the flu, and 98 percent effective against ear infections.

At the moment, flu shots are only recommended for kids with chronic health conditions (such as asthma or heart disease) or those with weak immune systems. But because kids help spread the flu—and because they can also develop complications such as pneumonia—experts decided a painless way to prevent the disease in kids would be helpful. Flu shots are only effective for a short period of time, are only developed against the one or two strains of flu expected to be most prevalent that season, and must be readministered every year.

The teenage years (12 to 19)

By the age of 12, teenagers will probably be spending much less time in the doctor's office now that yearly "well-child" visits are no longer required. Still, there are some basics—vaccinations and physicals—that still need to get taken care of, in addition to the first gynecology visits.

Vaccinations

By age 12, most girls should have had all their recommended vaccinations. If you haven't already gotten them, there are still a few you need to be sure to have no later than age 12:

- Final hepatitis B shot
- Final measles/mumps/rubella (MMR)
- Tetanus/diphtheria (Td) booster at some point between ages 11 and 15
- Chicken pox vaccine (for girls who have never had chicken pox or who have not yet been vaccinated)

What to expect in a physical

We've all heard the advice—be sure to get a physical every two or three years. But if all your doctor does is listen to your heart and take your blood pressure, is that good enough?

To be really helpful, a physical should include at least some of the following:

- Blood glucose check: This blood test screens for diabetes or hypoglycemia.

- Blood pressure check: Almost every doctor will do this basic test every time you visit.

- Breast exam: This annual manual exam is an essential screen for breast cancer.

- Complete blood count (CBC): This test screens for anemia and measures blood components.

- Immunizations: Depending on your age, at least some of these vaccinations should be discussed.

- Pap smear: This is usually done as part of an annual pelvic exam (see below).

- Skin cancer check: This visual inspection of your entire body for skin cancer should be done at least every three years (or more often if you have a family history of skin cancer or many moles); ideally, it can be performed by a dermatologist, but family practitioners, gynecologists, nurse practitioners, and other health care providers are also trained to check for abnormal skin growths.

- TB test: This test checks for exposure to tuberculosis and should be done every year for people at high risk, or as suggested by your doctor.

- Urinalysis: Screens for urinary tract infections and kidney disorders, in addition to other diseases (such as diabetes) But in the later teenage years, it may be time to begin thinking about finding a gynecologist. The current recommendation for a first gynecological exam is at the first appearance of a gynecological problem, after having sex for the first time, or by age 18 (whichever of these comes first).

Choosing a gynecologist

In addition to the general physical listed above, as a young woman enters the teenage years it's time to think about finding a gynecologist. Some young women simply begin seeing their mother's gynecologist. Alternatively, you may want to get a referral from a friend or your former pediatrician, or attend a clinic (such as Planned Parenthood). If you do choose your mother's gynecologist, it's important to discuss confidentiality issues up front.

Your family doctor provides comprehensive medical care for everyone in the family, treating all problems and making referrals to specialists as necessary. However, a gynecologist is a physician who specializes in diagnosing and treating problems of the female reproductive tract, including problems related to menstruation and menopause. A gynecologist also offers advice on contraception. Once you start having sex or you turn 18, you should see a gynecologist every year for a pelvic exam.

Once you've gathered all this information, you can narrow your choice to the doctors who have the most convenient locations, whose office hours are most convenient, who accept your type of insurance, who are affiliated with a good hospital, and whose office staff seem pleasant and well informed.

Your first Pap smear

You should have your first Pap smear once you become sexually active or when you turn 18—whichever comes first. No cancer screening test in history is as effective for the early detection of cancer. In fact, since the Pap exam began after World War II, deaths from cervical cancer have dropped 70 percent in the United States. What's more,

Timesaver
To find a gynecologist, you also can check your local library for the *Compendium of Certified Medical Specialists* or the *Directory of Medical Specialists*. These sources list physicians' credentials and whether or not they are board certified.

80 percent of women who die from cervical cancer had not had a Pap smear in the previous five years.

Remember that the Pap is just a screening test, so it can have a high false positive rate (meaning an "abnormal" Pap smear does not necessarily mean you have cancer or anything precancerous). Unfortunately, the Pap also has a high false negative rate. Any one Pap test can miss up to 40 percent of abnormalities but the more Pap smears you have that are normal, the better the chance that everything is okay. In addition, since precancerous and cancerous changes of the cervix are slow growing, having a Pap smear every year gives the best chance of preventing cervical cancer.

A Pap smear is a simple, painless test in which your doctor obtains some cells from your cervix during a pelvic exam. The cells are sent to a lab, which examines them for any abnormalities.

For the best sample:

- Schedule a Pap smear during the two weeks right after the end of your period.
- Don't have sex 48 hours before the Pap smear is done.
- Don't use a vaginal douche 48 hours before.

You should also be ready to answer the following questions your doctor will ask:

- Have you ever had an abnormal Pap smear?
- Are you sexually active? Have you ever been exposed to a sexually transmitted disease?
- Have you had vaginal infections or abnormal discharge?
- When was your last period?
- Have you had any abnormal bleeding?

- Are you taking medications (like antibiotics, birth control pills, hormone pills, or heart disease medications)?
- Have you had surgery, chemotherapy, or radiation treatment?
- Are you pregnant?

Bright Idea
To find out if your insurance company's lab is accredited, call 800/LAB-5678.

Pap smears are highly effective tests, provided they are done by a lab accredited by the College of American Pathologists (or another accrediting group). If the lab is not accredited, you can request that your Pap smear be sent to an accredited one. To be sure, ask your doctor. (Of course, if the Pap is sent to a lab that isn't on the insurance provider list, you may have to pay for the test yourself.) You can also ask him or her the following questions:

- What's the name of the lab and where is it located?
- Do you (the doctor) have good communication with the pathologist at the lab where the Pap smear will be checked?
- Can I see a copy of the report?
- Will the lab inform you (the doctor) if the cell sample isn't adequate, so another sample can be taken?

Your first pelvic exam

Many doctors recommend that a girl get her first pelvic exam by age 18 (or when she becomes sexually active, whichever is sooner). There are a number of different specialists who have special training in the health and diseases of a woman's reproductive organs, including gynecologists, nurse midwives, and gynecological nurse practitioners. (For information about how to find a good health professional, see Chapter 1.)

Teenage girls who decide to go to a doctor's office may need to involve an adult for insurance purposes. However, girls who can't (or prefer not to) involve their parents may visit a health clinic such as Planned Parenthood, which has a fully trained staff to care for teenagers (usually at a lower cost).

Many private doctors will also treat teens without parental consent, depending on state law. Some states allow competent teens to consent for care for pregnancy, STDs, safe sex counseling, and birth control. Most doctors will see an adolescent and provide STD screening, contraceptive and safer sex counseling, and the contraception without notifying parents (although most encourage girls to discuss sexual activity with parents). Often, the doctor will charge a reduced rate comparable to what a clinic may charge.

When making that first appointment for a pelvic exam, be sure you won't have your period the day of the exam. (You can have an exam during your period, but it's hard to get a Pap smear while you're menstruating.) If your period is very light, or is just starting, some doctors say it's okay to have a Pap smear. If you're in doubt, call ahead and ask.

When you go into the exam room, a nurse or assistant will record your weight and take your pulse and blood pressure. You'll need to know the date of your last period. After the nurse leaves the room, you'll then change out of all your clothes (including your bra and underwear) and put on a paper or cloth gown.

After a few minutes the doctor will come in—if this is your first exam, be sure to tell that to the doctor. Feel free to ask as many questions as you

Moneysaver
To find lower-cost care at a clinic, your county health department's family planning or STD screening clinic, or Planned Parenthood near you, visit Planned Parenthood's Web site (www.plannedparenthood.org) for a listing of local clinics by zip code.

like. This is also the time to ask when you can talk about birth control. The doctor will then ask you to lie back on the table; a paper sheet will cover the lower half of your body. The doctor (or nurse practitioner) will do a breast exam by pressing his or her fingers on your breast. The doctor will probably show you how to do this exam yourself so that you can check your breasts every month.

Most physicians will talk to a new patient in the office first to take a history, while she is fully dressed, before doing the exam. Most will also discuss the findings of the exam in the consultation room. Most patients are more comfortable talking things over when they are clothed and on the same level as the physician.

Now comes the pelvic exam. The doctor will ask you to scrunch down to the edge of the table, bend your knees, and place your feet in the two metal stirrups on either side of the table. It's normal to feel a bit odd in this vulnerable position, but it's the best way for the doctor to examine your internal organs. First comes the external exam of your vagina, to make sure there are no sores or swelling. Next, the doctor will slide a speculum (a thin piece of metal) into the vagina (it may feel a bit cold, but many doctors try to warm them up first).

Once the speculum is in place, it can be opened so that the doctor can see inside. Inserting the speculum doesn't hurt, but some women say they feel some pressure. You'll feel less pressure if you can avoid tensing the vaginal muscles. (Sometimes this takes a conscious effort to relax on your part.) Some women say that breathing exercises help them to relax.

Unofficially...
Teenage girls who are sexually active should be screened for chlamydia every six months, according to Johns Hopkins University researchers in a study published in the Journal of the American Medical Association.

The doctor will look for inflammation, discharge, or sores, and will do a Pap smear. To do the Pap smear, the doctor uses a long thin stick and brush to gently scrape some cells from the outside of the cervix as well as from the cervical canal (it doesn't hurt). The cells are sent to a lab to make sure there are no abnormalities which might indicate an infection or cancer.

Next, the doctor will feel your uterus and ovaries by inserting two fingers into the vagina; with the other hand, he or she will press on the outside of the lower abdomen. This will help show that your organs are the right size and position. The health care provider will then do a rectal exam and note hemorrhoids, polyps, and other rectal problems. A test for occult blood can also be done at this time.

You're done! The whole exam should only take about five minutes. The doctor will leave you alone to get dressed. Some women like to put a panty liner in their underwear after an exam, since you may bleed a bit after the Pap smear. If you do bleed, it will only be a tiny amount and it won't last.

About a month after your exam you'll be notified of the results of the Pap smear and STD tests. If you're worried about other people finding out, most clinics will agree to send the results in a plain envelope that doesn't indicate the name of the clinic or the doctor.

If everything checks out fine, you won't need to go back for another year. Most doctors are very sensitive to dealing with teenagers, but if you feel uncomfortable with the doctor or nurse practitioner for any reason, it's perfectly okay to find a new doctor for your next annual visit.

Eat healthy, stay healthy

Teenage girls need more calories and nutrients than at any other time in their lives. Because your body mass will almost double, you're especially vulnerable to even slight drops in nutrition. Yet this dramatic increase in food requirements comes at a time when many girls develop irregular eating habits. Many girls, concerned as their bodies begin to change and become more mature, start to diet. A few girls take dieting too far and develop eating disorders. (See Chapter 2.)

Despite what your mother tells you, many fast foods (if not eaten to excess) are perfectly adequate sources of energy: Pizza, hamburgers, ice cream, fishburgers, and chocolate all can help meet your dietary needs. It's when you eat only one kind of food—for example, fast food burgers six days a week—that you can get into trouble. Fast foods are okay if they are an occasional part of a well-balanced diet that includes lots of fruits and veggies. You can get into nutritional trouble (and into a larger jeans size!) by eating different fast foods every day (McDonald's on Monday, Taco Bell on Tuesday, Arby's on Wednesday . . .), as well as way too much sodium and fat. At the same time, skipping meals and crash dieting may mean you're not getting the nutrients you need to stay healthy. It's especially important that teenage girls get enough iron-rich foods (lean red meat, dark green vegetables, and dried beans) to replace iron lost during menstrual periods.

Bone development and calcium requirements really peak during these years. In fact, how much calcium you get now will establish the lifelong pattern for how healthy your bones become.

As young girls start to make their own food choices, many stop drinking milk and switch to soda (which further depletes calcium). If you don't drink milk, then you should at least eat three daily servings of calcium-rich food (low-fat yogurt, cheese, cottage cheese, ice cream, and salmon with bones, for example).

Most physicians feel that all women should take a calcium supplement regardless of their age or milk intake. Some recommend taking two or three Tums twice a day. This is probably the cheapest form of calcium supplementation available.

Young adulthood (20 to 39)

Young women in their 20s and 30s have a range of new health concerns to consider with each new decade. While cancer is still relatively unlikely, infectious diseases, sexually transmitted diseases, and issues of birth control, pregnancy, and infertility move into prominence.

What to expect in your 20s

Your body is now producing estrogen, progesterone, and androgen at peak levels in preparation for pregnancy. You're adding both fat and muscle to your body, and your metabolism rate is high. (This means that you probably can get away with the occasional cheeseburger or hot fudge sundae.) Most likely you have strong bones and good flexibility and if you don't regularly exercise now, you should start to get in the habit.

Your skin is young and healthy, with plenty of collagen and elastin to keep it looking strong and flexible. Try to avoid skin-damaging habits like smoking, drinking, and sun exposure. Start now with a routine of good cleansing, moisturizing, and

Watch Out! New research suggests that women in their mid- to late 30s with symptoms of PMS may actually be experiencing the onset of early menopause (perimenopause). You should bring any troubling symptoms to the attention of your gynecologist.

using sunscreen—if you do, you'll have to worry less about wrinkles and skin cancer when you are older.

What to expect in your 30s

As you move into your 30s, your eggs begin to age and you will gradually be less and less fertile. This doesn't mean you can't get pregnant, however. Indeed, the number of first-time moms in their 30s has more than tripled since 1975.

Your metabolism begins to slow down in your 30s, as the percentage of lean muscle tissue in your body decreases and fat increases. You'll need to be sure to start exercising now as it will become easier to put on weight—even a gain of 5 to 10 pounds can mean a significant increase in health problems.

You're still young, but don't be surprised if you start seeing some wrinkles around your eyes and mouth, as the rate of facial skin-cell renewal starts to slow down. Exfoliating may help here.

What you can do to stay healthy

Be sure to eat a healthy, balanced diet and avoid those fad diets that allow you nothing to eat but grapefruit and hard-boiled eggs.

Once you pass age 30, your bones begin to lose calcium. One in four American women will develop osteoporosis in their lifetime. To make sure you're not that one, be sure to take:

- Calcium—at least 1,000 mg a day will prevent hip and spine fractures.

- Vitamin D—it helps bones absorb calcium and maintain bone density.

- Vitamin C—it helps absorb calcium and iron to maintain tissues, bones, and teeth (and to prevent cataracts).

Bright Idea
Hate milk? You can boost your calcium levels by eating salmon and leafy greens instead of guzzling glass after glass of milk. (If you don't like or can't afford salmon, flavored Tums are excellent.)

Don't forget your folic acid. (You'll find it in liver, yeast, whole-grain cereals, and leafy greens.) Folic acid may help prevent heart disease and it will definitely help prevent birth defects. Finally, remember to eat enough iron (you can get iron from poultry, meat, fish, dried beans, nuts, dried fruits, and whole grains). All women of reproductive age should take 0.4 to 0.8 mg of folic acid daily. The FDA has recently mandated that folic acid be added to breads and cereals, so if you eat two slices of bread a day, you'll get enough folic acid.

Do you need a special doctor?

Many women tend to rely on their gynecologist for all their health care needs. But as you get older and your health care needs broaden, you may want to find an internist or family care physician as well.

As they enter their late 30s, some women experience perimenopause, the stage of life when hormones begin to change and menopausal symtpoms start. If this is happening to you, you may prefer to locate a doctor who is an expert in the field of menopause. A reproductive endocrinologist may be a good choice if you have severe symptoms during perimenopause. If you prefer to find a specialist yourself without a referral from your other doctor, you can obtain a list of qualified specialists from the American Fertility Society.

Unless you live in a metropolitan area or near a large medical center, you may need to travel to find a good specialist, who also tends to be more expensive. However, it's possible to have most of your needs taken care of by your regular doctor, and simply rely on the specialist for diagnosis and consultations. Most reproductive endocrinologists don't provide regular, ongoing gynecological care anyway, but will refer you back to your original doctor once your situation has stabilized.

Types of specialists

Your family doctor provides comprehensive medical care for everyone in the family, treating all problems and, when necessary, making referrals to specialists who are qualified to treat particular health concerns:

- Internist: A specialist in the diagnosis and treatment of adult diseases, especially those related to the internal organs. Internists often provide primary care.
- Reproductive endocrinologist: A gynecologist or obstetrician-gynecologist who has extra training in the specialty of reproductive endocrinology, menopause and infertility, who specializes in problems involving reproductive hormones, such as the problems you face during early menopause and menopause.

Locating a doctor

Once you've decided what sort of doctor you're looking for, you can start by asking friends and family for recommendations. You also could call your local hospital for a list of affiliated physicians.

You can check your local library for books such as the *Compendium of Certified Medical Specialists* or the *Directory of Medical Specialists*. These sources list physicians' credentials and whether or not they are board certified. A reproductive endocrinologist should be board certified in reproductive gynecology (many are not, so check).

If you're looking for a doctor to treat menopause or early menopause symptoms, you can contact the North American Menopause Society (NAMS); it will send you a list of NAMS members categorized by geographic location and specialty. NAMS members include physicians, nurses, psychotherapists, social workers, and others who describe themselves as "menopause clinicians." For a list of members of the North American Menopause Society, write to NAMS, P.O. Box 94527, Cleveland, OH 44101. NAMS can also be reached by fax at 216/844-8708, e-mail at nams@apk.net, or phone at 900/370-6267 (there is a charge for this call).

Once you've gathered all this information, you can narrow your choice to the doctors who have the most convenient locations and office hours, who accept your type of insurance, who are affiliated with a good hospital, and whose office staff seems pleasant and well informed.

Tests you should have

As a young woman in your 20s or 30s, you should be sure to have certain tests and exams performed at recommended intervals. The following table indicates which tests and exams you should have and how often you should have each done.

Vaccines for your 20s and 30s

There are several vaccines recommended for women in their 20s and 30s. A discussion of each follows.

- Lyme disease: The first vaccine against Lyme disease (LYMErix) has recently been licensed by the FDA; a second vaccine (ImuLyme) is still awaiting FDA approval. You must be over age 15 in order to have the vaccine, which requires three injections over a 12-month period to build immunity to its peak level. It has not yet been determined whether additional booster shots will be needed in subsequent years. If you're

Unofficially...
By the age of 24, one in three sexually active people contracts an STD. STDs such as gonorrhea and chlamydia often cause no noticeable symptoms in young women.

TABLE 3.2: TEST AND EXAMINATION FREQUENCY

Exam or test	Frequency
Breast exam	Yearly (usually at the same time as your Pap smear and pelvic exam).
Breast self-exam	Every month.
Pelvic exam	Every year.
Pap smear	You should have a Pap smear every year beginning with the time you are sexually active. (See above for details on finding out if the lab your doctor uses is accredited.)
STDs check	Every year if at risk for STD.
Mammogram	Baseline mammogram at age 35 to 40 followed by mammograms every 1 to 2 years starting at age 40 until age 50, and then annually. If there is a family history of breast cancer in a first degree relative, begin screening mammograms 5 years earlier than the age at which the family member was diagnosed and get a mammogram yearly after that. This is only part of a screening program for breast cancer — the screening program must include monthly self-breast exams and an annual exam by the health care provider. A palpable mass despite a negative mammogram requires evaluation.
Blood work	Every five years.
Cholesterol	Every five years after age 35 (or more often if your level is above 200).
Physical	Every one to three years.
Blood pressure	Every year from age 30 on.
Electrocardiogram	It's a good idea to have a baseline ECG done in your 30s followed by another at age 45 to check the health of your heart.
Stool screening	Check for fecal occult blood every other year beginning at age 40.

Bright Idea
Every woman over age 20 should examine her breasts every month to check for lumps, thickening, dimpling of the skin, or an unusual discharge from the nipple.

reasonably at risk for Lyme disease or you live in an area where the disease is common, you should talk to your doctor about having this vaccination. These vaccines are preventative, and can't be used to treat actual symptoms of Lyme disease. They won't be effective against other tick-borne diseases (such as ehrlichiosis, babesiosis, and Rocky Mountain spotted fever).

- Flu shot: Each year scientists at the World Health Organization and the Centers for Disease Control predict which strains of the flu should be in that year's flu shot; if they're correct, the shot is up to 90 percent effective in preventing infection (if you're among the unlucky 10 percent who get sick anyway, the shot is 80 percent effective in preventing death).

- Tetanus booster: You should continue to get a tetanus shot every 10 years to protect against tetanus, a life-threatening central nervous system disease contracted when bacteria invades an open wound. If you haven't had a tetanus booster within the past 10 years, schedule a visit to the doctor.

Contraception: What's your choice?

Proper types of birth control are crucial if you're going to avoid unwanted pregnancies and also for protecting yourself against STDs. (For a detailed discussion of birth control, see Chapter 5.)

Contraception ranges in effectiveness from implants (Norplant) at 99 percent to spermicides alone (79 percent):

- Norplant—99 percent
- The Pill—99.7 percent when used correctly (not skipping pills, etc.)
- IUD—99 percent
- Condom—88 percent
- Diaphragm—82 percent

Unofficially... Historically, the flu shot was recommended for older people or those with chronic conditions. But new research shows that younger folks are also at risk for complications from influenza and should get a yearly flu shot.

- Cervical cap—82 percent if you've never had a child (only 64 percent if you've had a child before)
- Spermicide—79 percent

Ask your doctor about...

In addition to the guidelines on annual tests and vaccinations, if you have special illnesses (diabetes, liver, kidney disease, high blood pressure or cholesterol, etc.), the frequency of these tests will change and your doctor will order certain special tests. In addition, you may want to ask your doctor about his or her recommendations on the following:

- Skin exam for cancer
- Risk of osteoporosis
- Aspirin treatment to prevent heart disease
- Special testing for toxic exposures at work or home

Your mature years (40 to 64)

What were once considered the "middle ages" are now rapidly becoming the best years of a woman's life, as she settles into her career and her life. Nevertheless, these years also can be stressful as women in their 40s and 50s become sandwiched between raising a family and caring for aging parents.

What to expect

The pressures involved in juggling the obligations of daughter, wife, mother, and career woman can be overwhelming—and can lead to stress-related disorders such as depression, high blood pressure, and heart disease. Now is the time to be sure to get enough rest and exercise, and to eat a good diet—and be sure to keep up with your social support network.

What you can do to stay healthy

In a word—exercise! The National Institutes of Health says that exercise is the most effective anti-aging drug ever discovered. Women facing menopause may find that exercise is the single best thing they can do to boost their physical and emotional health. Among other things, exercise can

- Regulate cholesterol
- Control weight
- Strengthen bones
- Lower your cancer risk
- Ease depression
- Ease unpleasant symptoms of menopause

Menopause: How to choose a specialist

As you enter menopause, you may want to find a doctor who is an expert in the management of this special time of life. If you're looking for a doctor to treat menopause or early menopause symptoms, you can contact the North American Menopause Society; they will send you a list of NAMS members categorized by geographic location and specialty.

(See the section above entitled "Locating a Doctor" in the discussion about young adulthood for information on contacting NAMS.)

Tests

You should have certain tests and exams performed at set intervals in your mature years, as well. The following table details this information for you.

Bone density tests

Unfortunately, 80 percent of the 20 million American women with osteoporosis have no idea they have the disease. There are several kinds of tests you can take to measure your bone density.

TABLE 3.3: TEST AND EXAMINATION FREQUENCY

Exam or test	Frequency
Breast exam	Yearly.
Breast self-exam	Every month.
Pap smear	Yearly (even after you've reached menopause or if you've had a hysterectomy).
Rectal exam	Yearly.
Sigmoidoscopy	This procedure to inspect the last 12 inches of the large intestine should be done about every four years after age 50.
Mammogram	Every year for all women over age 40.
Stool screening	Check for fecal occult blood every three years until age 50; after 50, get an annual exam (have the test every year after age 40 if you have predisposing factors or a family history for rectal/colon cancer).
Electrocardiogram	You should have an ECG at age 45 to check the health of your heart.
Blood work	Every five years (including a cholesterol check).
Physical	Every one to three years.
Blood pressure	Every year.
Bone density baseline	If you're in menopause, you take corticosteroids, or you have a fractured vertebrae, or you're thin, petite, smoke, have a family history or don't exercise, you should have a bone density test (see below for more details).
Eye exam	Every five years until age 50; after that, schedule an exam every four years (exams should include a glaucoma screen).

They don't take much time and they usually can be finished within 30 minutes (in many centers, you don't even need to change clothes). The best is the dual-energy X-ray (DEXA) absorptiometry, although dual-photon absorptiometry is also used.

The machines measure current bone mineral content at the hip, spine, or wrist (the most common sites of fractures by osteoporosis). You lie fully clothed on the table as the scanner passes above you, emitting radiation at an intensity of only half of what is contained in a typical chest X-ray.

The DEXA can help show whether you're losing or building bone mass (or staying the same). Your bone density is compared with someone else's of your age and size, and also with the estimated peak bone density of a healthy young adult woman. (Generally, the lower your bone density, the higher your risk for a fracture.)

You can also check your bone density with an ultrasound of your heel; it's much faster and less expensive than densitometry, and is radiation free. Alternatively, you could get a CAT scan or a single-photon densitometry, both of which evaluate bones in the wrist. You could also get a lab test to check the amount of calcium in your urine.

Not all insurance companies pay for these tests, which range from inexpensive to very expensive. (For example, the dual-photon test can cost from $50 to $250, depending on where in the country the test is done.) Recently, a federal law was passed covering DEXA for all women over 65.

Vaccinations

You should keep up with your vaccinations in order to continue protection against some illnesses:

Timesaver
To find the nearest bone density testing site near you, call the National Osteoporosis Foundation Action Line at 800/464-6700.

- Pneumococcal (pneumonia) vaccine: One dose of vaccine to prevent infection with *Streptococcus pneumoniae* is recommended if you have a chronic illness or a weakened immune system, and if you're a member of certain Alaska Native and American Indian populations. One shot provides permanent immunity.

- Flu shot: You should get a yearly shot if you're in a high risk group (some experts say any woman in this age bracket should get a yearly shot).

- Lyme disease: If you're at high risk, consider this new vaccine which is given in a three-shot dose over one year. (High-risk individuals include those who work daily in woods and high grass, especially in the northeast and who are likely to come into daily contact with ticks.

- Tetanus booster: You should continue to get a tetanus shot every 10 years to protect against tetanus, a life-threatening central nervous system disease contracted when bacteria invades an open wound. If you haven't had a tetanus booster within the past 10 years, schedule a visit to the doctor today and get one.

Ask your doctor about...

In addition to the guidelines on annual tests and vaccinations, if you have special illnesses (diabetes, liver, kidney disease, high blood pressure or cholesterol, etc.) the frequency of these tests will change and your doctor will order certain special tests. In addition, you may want to ask your doctor about his or her recommendations on the following:

- Skin exam for cancer
- Hormone therapy after menopause
- Risk of osteoporosis
- Aspirin treatment to prevent heart disease
- Special testing for toxic exposures at work or home

Your older years (over 65)

Just because you've hit the big "5-0" doesn't mean you have to get out the shawl and walker and retreat into old age. As life expectancy increases, your odds of being healthy and energetic into old age likewise increase.

Unofficially...
Two out of three people over age 50 lack adequate immunity to tetanus, according to researchers at the University of Florida.

What you can expect

During your 60s, the balance between your female hormones (estrogens) and male hormones (androgens) shifts. As a result:

- Hair on your head may thin.
- Body hair may get darker or thicker.
- Hairs may appear on your face or chin.
- Sexual interest may wane.

The weight gain you noticed during your 40s and 50s may slow, but if you're already carrying too much weight in the abdomen, you're running the risk of high blood pressure, heart disease, and diabetes. Exercise (think about weight training) can help prevent all three of these conditions, while also building strength and muscle tone.

As you approach your 70s, you may lose your appetite as your metabolism slows down. Be sure to keep taking a multivitamin and a calcium supplement to combat loss of muscle strength and bone density. Keep moderately active to stay flexible and strong.

Your skin also begins to change as cells in the top layer become irregular. You may notice precancerous lesions now. (For information on how to check your skin, see Chapter 11.) You'll also notice pigment changes (liver spots), with skin getting thinner and more wrinkly.

Tests you need

Older women need to continue being tested and examined at regular intervals. The following table tells you what you need and how often you need it.

Get your shots!

You should keep up with your vaccinations in order to continue protection against some illnesses:

TABLE 3.4: TEST AND EXAMINATION FREQUENCY

Exam or test	Frequency
Thyroid tests	Measure the level of thyroid stimulating hormone (TSH), and check for tumors or thyroid malfunction every two to three years.
Hearing tests	Yearly.
Eye tests	Schedule eye exams every four years (don't forget to check for glaucoma and cataracts).
Pap smear	You should continue to have a Pap smear every year, even after you have reached menopause or if you've had a hysterectomy (some experts say that women over age 65 who have had no abnormal Pap smears three consecutive times may schedule an exam every three years).
Breast exam	Yearly.
Breast self-exam	Every month.
Mammogram	Yearly.
Sigmoidoscopy	This procedure to inspect the last 12 inches of the large intestine should be done about every four years.
Rectal	Yearly.
Stool screening	Check for fecal occult blood every year.
Urinalysis	Yearly.
Blood pressure	Every year.
Blood work	Every five years (including a cholesterol check).
Physical	Every one to three years.

- Pneumococcal (pneumonia) vaccine: A one-time dose of vaccine to prevent infection with *Streptococcus pneumoniae* is recommended for all women over age 65.
- Flu shot: Yearly.
- Tetanus booster: You should continue to get a tetanus shot every 10 years to protect against tetanus.

Watch Out!
If you're getting an X-ray, forewarn your doctor about any supplements you've been taking. Certain undissolved pills (such as calcium, multivitamins, iron, and estrogen) appear as white dots on X-rays and can lead to an incorrect diagnosis.

- Lyme disease: If you're at high risk (those working in the outdoors, for example in areas of high brush), consider this new vaccine which is given in a three-shot dose over one year.

What you can do to stay healthy

As you get older, it's crucial that you maintain your social support network and stay busy and involved with life. Studies are clear that memory stays sharp when you're surrounded by an enriched environment and when you keep on challenging yourself mentally and physically.

Spending time with family and friends—even pets—will keep you healthier and help stave off depression. If you do get sick (even chronically ill) or suffer life crises, having social support will help you survive.

Ask your doctor about...

In addition to the guidelines on annual tests and vaccinations, if you have special illnesses (diabetes, liver or kidney disease, high blood pressure or cholesterol, etc.) the frequency of these tests will change and your doctor will order certain special tests. In addition, you may want to ask your doctor about his or her recommendations on the following:

- Skin exam for cancer
- Hormone therapy after menopause
- Risk of osteoporosis
- Aspirin treatment to prevent heart disease
- Special testing for toxic exposures at work or home

Special vaccinations

Keep in mind that each year, as many as 70,000 adults die—and many others needlessly suffer—from vaccine-preventable illnesses. There are a number of illnesses that baby-boomer women may not have contracted in childhood, when vaccinations against them were not available. If you've escaped childhood without these diseases and have not been vaccinated, you may need to be vaccinated now as an adult:

- Measles, mumps, rubella (MMR): Any woman who has not had measles, mumps, or rubella should be vaccinated. All three of these diseases can cause miscarriage or birth defects if caught during pregnancy. Get vaccinated at least three months before becoming pregnant.

- Chicken pox: Since adults who get chicken pox are at much greater risk of complications or death than children, if you're over age 21 and never had chicken pox, you should talk to your doctor about getting vaccinated.

- Hepatitis A: The two-shot series against hepatitis A is recommended for anyone who may be exposed to someone with the disease, or travelers to countries where the water and food may not be clean and the virus is common, such as Africa, Asia, the Caribbean, Central and South America, Eastern Europe, the Mediterranean Basin, and the Middle East.

- Hepatitis B: The three-shot series is now recommended for adults who may be exposed to the virus through sexual activity, injected drug use, contact with infected blood, contact with infected persons, or exposure to areas where the disease is very common such as Alaska, the Pacific Islands, Asia, Eastern Europe, the Middle East, and the Amazon Basin.

You can find out more about immunizations by contacting the following organizations:

- The Centers for Disease Control and Prevention (information line for international travelers): 404/332-4559; www.cdc.gov/travel
- Centers for Disease Control and Prevention National Immunization Program: 800/232-0233 (Spanish Immunization Hotline); 800/232-2522 (English Immunization Hotline); 800/CDC-SHOT (vaccines and referrals); www.cdc.gov/nip

Just the facts

- Checking your own breasts and skin each month for signs of cancer is every woman's responsibility.
- Getting enough exercise, a healthy diet, and regular checkups can help prevent heart disease, cancer, and osteoporosis later in life.
- Stay current with your vaccinations throughout all the stages in your life, not just in childhood; talk to your doctor about the newest vaccines for chicken pox, rotavirus, hepatitis A and B, and Lyme disease.

PART II

Reproductive Health

GET THE SCOOP ON...
Menstrual problems ▪ Managing PMS symptoms ▪ Uterine fibroid and cysts ▪ Identifying endometriosis ▪ Ovarian infections ▪ New treatments for polycystic ovarian syndrome

Keeping Your Reproductive System Healthy

You thought you learned all the stuff you'd ever need to know about your reproductive organs back in seventh grade health, right? Your teacher probably covered the basics, but, most likely, you didn't learn what to do about your reproductive health when things go wrong—and there is a lot you can do!

Menstrual problems

Let's start with something we probably all understand—menstruation, the normal part of your reproductive cycle that begins when an ovary releases an egg. At the same time this happens, estrogen is released, stimulating the lining of the uterus to thicken with blood. If the egg isn't fertilized, progesterone levels drop and blood vessels constrict, the uterine lining sheds and the menstrual flow begins. This cycle repeats itself every 28 days or so until interrupted by pregnancy or ended by menopause.

All women are different and the degree of discomfort or pain your period causes depends on many things. Your period may occasionally be heavier or more painful than usual. Such problems (while unpleasant), generally don't mean you've got a disease. But you should be aware that these same complaints—heavy flow or pain—can sometimes indicate more serious conditions, such as endometriosis or an ovarian cyst.

The three main categories of menstrual irregularities include absence of a period (amenorrhea), painful periods (dysmenorrhea), and heavy periods (menorrhagia).

Absent periods

If you're not menopausal and your period suddenly skids to a halt, odds are you're either pregnant, under stress, exercising too much, or you've lost too much weight. You may have developed hyperprolactinemia (a common condition of the pituitary) or a thyroid disorder, either of which can cause your period to stop. Most of the time, an occasional missed period isn't any cause for concern—but sometimes it's the sign of an underlying problem. Amenorrhea might be telling you that your estrogen levels are low, which could mean you're at a greater risk of developing osteoporosis. Or it may signal low levels of progesterone, so that you're at a greater risk for endometrial problems such as endometrial cancer (see Chapter 12).

Primary amenorrhea means you're older than 16 and you've never had a period. While a girl may not reach puberty until age 17 and still be completely within the normal range, delayed puberty in a girl who is very thin or who exercises too much could be one symptom of anorexia nervosa. In rare cases, a girl who has never menstruated might actually lack ovaries or a uterus. Or perhaps a tumor, injury, or structural defect might be interfering with some aspect of the menstrual cycle.

If you've been menstruating right along and temporarily stop, you have secondary amenorrhea. This could be caused by:

- Pituitary disorders
- Primary ovarian failure (early menopause)
- Pregnancy
- Thyroid problems
- Structural abnormalities
- Ovarian cysts
- Stress
- Weight problems

If you've never had your period and you're under 16 or 17, your doctor may wait for you to mature. But if you're older than that, investigation is usually begun. If you exercise strenuously or you're very thin, your doctor might want you to train less or gain weight. Treatment for anorexia nervosa might also be necessary. If your doctor suspects a hormonal irregularity, he or she might prescribe drugs to replace missing hormones. Rarely, you might need surgery to remove a growth or to correct a structural problem.

The treatment for amenorrhea depends on the cause of the problem. If you're under a lot of stress, identifying and eliminating the stressors may restore your cycle. If you're underweight, you may need to gain weight. If you've been diagnosed with a condition that may be causing amenorrhea (such as an ovarian cyst), your periods may return once you are treated for that condition. If your absent period is related to the onset of menopause, your doctor may prescribe natural estrogens or hormones. Being overweight can also produce secondary amenhorrhea, and so weight loss may get your cycles back on track.

Painful periods

Dysmenorrhea, better known as menstrual cramps, is very common; one in every two women suffers from it each month, and about one in four are in so much pain they must take time off work or school. Cramps are usually entirely normal, but occasionally they may be a symptom of

- Endometriosis.
- Polyps.
- Fibroids or other uterine lesions.
- An intrauterine device (IUD).
- Adenomyosis, a cousin of endometriosis where the uterine lining cells penetrate the wall of the uterus an abnormal amount, causing increased bleeding and pain.
- Cervical stenosis (a narrowing of the cervical outflow pathway).

Unofficially... Reducing fat, exercising, and eating a vegetarian diet can significantly decrease menstrual pain, according to researchers at the Physicians Committee for Responsible Medicine and Georgetown University Medical Center in Washington, D.C.

Each month, as the lining of the uterus breaks down during menstruation, hormones called prostaglandins are released, which trigger the muscles of the uterus to contract and expel the lining. The muscles are the same ones that push a baby out during childbirth, so they're mighty strong—which is why cramps can hurt so much. Women with severe cramps have significantly higher prostaglandin levels in their menstrual fluid than do other women.

For quick relief of your cramps, your doctor will probably recommend prostaglandin-inhibiting drugs such as ibuprofen (Motrin or Nuprin). They may work best when taken three to four days before the onset of your period since this prevents the buildup of prostaglandins. The birth control pill is another option, as it stops ovulation and decreases prostaglandin levels. "Natural" remedies may include

- Calcium: Sesame seeds or supplemental calcium in combination with magnesium (begin with 500 mg calcium and 250 mg magnesium).
- Herbal teas: Chamomile, ginger, red raspberry leaf, lemon balm, and catnip.
- Exercise: Strengthening the pelvic floor muscles may help reduce menstrual pain—try yoga, bicycling, dancing, martial arts, and various sports.
- Heat: Try a hot bath, hot water bottle or a steam room (a sauna might be too extreme).
- Touch: Massage or acupressure can ease pain; try firm fist or finger pressure along the lower (lumbar) spine; a foot massage; or rubbing and pressing the tissue on the hand between your thumb and first finger.

Bright Idea
If menstrual pain occurs in your back, try a daily regimen of sit-ups to strengthen back muscles. To ease cramps, steady rhythmic exercise (such as swimming) loosens muscles, decreases discomfort, and releases tension, which can alleviate pain.

Heavy flow

Menstrual flow is considered to be abnormally heavy or prolonged if it soaks through at least a pad or tampon an hour for several consecutive hours. It can be caused by a number of problems, but the most common is fibroids.

Hormone imbalances cause frequent or irregular bleeding. In a normal menstrual cycle, there is a balance between estrogen and progesterone to regulate the buildup of blood and tissue in the uterine lining. Irregular or unusually heavy menstrual flow can occur if the levels of estrogen and progesterone become unbalanced, so that the endometrium keeps building up. Thus when it finally sheds, bleeding is heavier than usual. Heavy or irregular bleeding is common during adolescence and also as women approach menopause, because hormone imbalances are common at these times. Other, less common causes of irregular bleeding include

- Endometrial cancer.
- Inflammation or infection of the vagina, cervix, or pelvic organs.
- Thyroid conditions.
- Liver, kidney, or blood diseases.
- Blood-thinning drugs.
- Stress.
- An IUD.

It's certainly true that not all women's menstrual periods are the same in length or severity, but there are certain ways to tell if you're bleeding too much. You should call your doctor if you

- Have heavy menstrual flow that fills a tampon or sanitary napkin within an hour or that lasts more than a seven days.
- Suddenly have periods less than 18 to 20 days apart (many women menstruate normally every 21 days).
- Experience anemia from a heavy flow.
- Have a late flow that is unusually heavy (this could indicate a miscarriage).
- Experience sharp abdominal pain before periods or during intercourse (you could have endometriosis).
- Have any vaginal bleeding after menopause.

Watch Out!
Although cancer is not a common cause of heavy bleeding, it should be ruled out in women over age 35 or in younger women who have been exposed to unapposed estrogen. Anyone over age 35 with abnormal uterine bleeding should have a tissue sample to rule out endometrial cancer.

When you visit your doctor, expect to answer questions about your past health and bleeding patterns. Your doctor will do a pelvic exam and a Pap smear to try to find the reason for the heavy bleeding. There also may be blood, urine, and stool tests to check on your gastrointestinal and urinary tract. A pregnancy test is likely if you're sexually active. Your doctor may remove a small amount of tissue from the endometrium for testing. You may also be tested to determine if you are ovulating or have any sexually transmitted diseases (STDs). A standard pelvic ultrasound may also be needed to rule out fibroids, polyps, ovarian cysts, and even malignancy.

Your doctor will treat any underlying medical condition that is causing your heavy flow. If a hormone imbalance is responsible for abnormal uterine bleeding, your doctor may recommend hormonal or nonhormonal treatment options to ease the problem.

Abnormal bleeding

In general, any girl or woman experiencing unexpected, irregular vaginal bleeding should go to her doctor. Irregular vaginal bleeding may include

- Spotting of small amounts of blood between periods (often seen on toilet tissue after wiping).
- Heavy periods where you soak a pad or tampon every hour for several hours.
- Vaginal bleeding of any amount for weeks at a time.
- Bleeding after intercourse.

Irregular bleeding may also depend on your age or whether you're taking hormones. Check out the following scenarios:

- Premenopausal women: Light spotting a couple of days before your period is common and not worrisome.

- Starting the Pill: You may experience occasional spotting the first few months.

- Menopausal or postmenopausal women on cyclic hormone replacement: If you take oral estrogen daily plus oral progestin for 10 to 12 days a month, you may experience some expected "withdrawal" bleeding starting two to three days after finishing the progestin, resembling a period for a few days out of the month. If you have any vaginal bleeding other than the expected withdrawal bleeding, you should see your doctor.

- Menopausal or postmenopausal women on continuous homone replacement therapy (HRT): If you're taking a low-dose combination of estrogen and progestin daily, you shouldn't be spotting. If you are, you should see your doctor. While it may take several months on continuous HRT for irregular spotting to go away, 80 percent of women will have no bleeding after 12 months.

- Menopausal or postmenopausal women who aren't on HRT: Any vaginal bleeding means you should go see your doctor.

- Prepubertal girls: Any vaginal bleeding is cause for concern.

- Newborn girls: Vaginal bleeding a few days after birth is normal, but any vaginal bleeding beyond that should be checked out.

Irregular vaginal bleeding is a possible symptom of the following:

- Menstrual dysfunction
- Fluctuating hormone levels
- Vaginitis, a common and treatable vaginal infection
- Tumors, polyps, or fibroids of the vagina, cervix, uterus, or fallopian tubes
- Cervical disorders
- Cancer of the uterus, cervix, vagina, or vulva
- Some STDs, such as chlamydia, gonorrhea, or genital warts
- Vaginal injury from trauma or sexual abuse
- Early pregnancy-associated bleeding or an ectopic pregnancy (the fertilized egg becomes implanted outside the uterus)
- Complications from pregnancy (such as miscarriage)

If you have irregular vaginal bleeding, you should schedule an appointment with your doctor and then write down when the bleeding occurs during the month. Try to determine if the bleeding is vaginal or anal. If you're taking birth control pills or you're on HRT, follow your doctor's instructions. However, if you're pregnant and you start to bleed vaginally, contact your doctor immediately.

Premenstrual syndrome

Everybody gets a little cranky now and then. But for many women, the week or so prior to their period is fraught with a range of upsetting and uncomfortable symptoms, appearing like clockwork each month.

Premenstrual syndrome (PMS) is a term given to the physical and behavioral changes that may affect some women a week or so before menstruation, including everything from fatigue to tension to moodiness. Although PMS was first reported in the medical literature way back in the 1930s, its validity as a medical condition has been hotly debated ever since. Feminists themselves have been afraid that to acknowledge PMS would allow critics of sexual equality to say women were too emotionally and physically unpredictable for certain jobs or responsibilities.

Today most experts accept that PMS is a physical condition characterized by a variety of symptoms that typically recur during a particular phase of the menstrual cycle, usually a week to 10 days before a woman's period begins. Practically every woman experiences at least one PMS symptom sometime in her life, and between 10 and 50 percent of women in the United States regularly suffer from PMS.

Fortunately for teenagers (who are already struggling with quite enough life stress and hormonal upheaval), PMS usually doesn't appear until a woman's mid- to late 20s. Women most often affected by PMS are those who've experienced a major hormonal change, such as childbirth, miscarriage or abortion. Women who stop taking birth control pills may also notice an increase in PMS symptoms until their hormone balance returns.

PMS or bad temper?

Specific symptoms vary from woman to woman. Some 5 to 10 percent of women experience symptoms severe enough for them to seek medical help. The symptoms of PMS usually appear from 7 to 10 days before your period begins and may include any of the following:

- Bloating and fluid retention
- Breast swelling and pain
- Acne, cold sores, or susceptibility to herpes outbreaks
- Weight gain of five pounds or more (from fluid retention)
- Headaches, backaches and joint or muscle aches
- Moodiness, anxiety, depression, or irritability
- Food cravings, especially for sugary or salty foods
- Insomnia
- Drowsiness and fatigue, or conversely, extra energy
- Hot flashes or nausea
- Constipation, diarrhea, or urinary disorders

A small number of women with PMS may experience more intense symptoms:

- Crying
- Panic attacks
- Suicidal thoughts
- Aggressive or violent behavior

What is it?

Experts have come up with many unproven theories to explain some or all PMS symptoms. Many researchers once believed PMS was the result of a hormonal imbalance, such as an overproduction of the hormone estrogen—except that most women don't get symptoms at the middle of their menstrual cycle, when estrogen levels are at their peak. More recently, controlled studies have ruled out a single hormone (such as estrogen, progesterone, testosterone, or prolactin) as the cause. Instead, scientists are now investigating other possibilities (but these are still not proven in any way):

- Neurotransmitters: Monthly fluctuations in these brain chemicals (including the mood-altering endorphins) could be a possible cause, but studies have been inconclusive.

- Diet deficiencies: PMS symptoms of mood swings, fluid retention, bloating, breast tenderness, food cravings, and fatigue have been linked to a deficiency of vitamin B6 or magnesium. Some researchers think that one type of PMS characterized by headache, dizziness, heart pounding, increased appetite, and a craving for chocolate is caused by a magnesium deficiency brought on by stress. According to this theory, the craving for chocolate, which is rich in magnesium, helps balance the deficiency; unfortunately, the sugar in chocolate also raises blood insulin levels, which can worsen other symptoms.

- Genetics: The fact that identical twins are more likely to share PMS symptoms than are fraternal twins suggests that PMS may have a genetic component.

Diagnosing the problem

If you're wondering whether your symptoms could be PMS, the first step should be a thorough physical examination by a gynecologist to eliminate any other medical or psychological causes. If it turns out that you're healthy, the next step depends on you.

There's no simple blood test that can detect PMS; instead, you'll need to help accurately diagnose PMS by keeping a daily diary of your symptoms for at least two months. Keep a calendar record of when your menstrual period begins and ends. Each evening mark on the calendar any PMS symptoms you've had that day. Your doctor can then use this written record to confirm a diagnosis and to come up with a possible treatment plan.

What you can do

If you do have PMS, there are many lifestyle changes you can make that may help ease your symptoms:

- Exercise: Studies have shown that regular exercise lessens PMS symptoms, perhaps by stimulating the release of endorphins and other brain chemicals that help relieve stress and lighten your mood.

- Sleep well: Getting enough sleep is also important for the successful treatment of PMS. Lack of sleep can exacerbate fatigue, irritability, and other emotional symptoms.

- Diet: Try to eat a low-fat, high-fiber diet. Avoid salt, sugar, caffeine, white flour, and dairy products 7 to 14 days before your menstrual period.

- Small meals: Eating six or more small meals throughout the day rather than three large ones eases symptoms, perhaps by keeping insulin levels more constant.

- Vitamins: Nutritionists recommend supplements of vitamin B6 (50 to 100 mg) and magnesium (250 mg) daily.

- Fatty acids: Many women report that taking evening primrose oil (a substance that contains essential fatty acids) is effective. Consult your health care provider for the correct dosage for you.

Bright Idea
If you have trouble getting enough rest, stick to a regular sleep schedule. By going to bed and waking at the same time each day, even on weekends, you may find it easier to get the sleep you need.

- Manage food cravings: Giving in to chocolate cravings may make your symptoms worse; eat fruit instead of sugary treats.
- Hot baths: As your period approaches, take long, hot baths to ease tension and stress.
- Heat for pain: Use a hot water bottle, a heating pad, or castor-oil packs to ease backaches and muscle aches associated with PMS.
- Avoid alcohol: Don't drink before your period; alcohol can worsen PMS depression, headaches, and fatigue and can trigger food cravings.
- Get support: Join a PMS support group to get constructive feedback and exchange information. Check your phone book or call a local hospital for the name of a group in your area.
- Calcium: Recent studies show that calcium supplements reduce the physical discomfort and minimize the emotional rollercoaster suffered by millions of women who have PMS; a dosage of 1,200 mg daily, plus about 500 mg of magnesium was proven effective in well-controlled studies. Calcium is one of the most important treatments for PMS.

Unofficially... Taking daily calcium supplements of 1,200 mg for two to three months lowers PMS symptoms by more than 50 percent, according to researchers from St. Luke's-Roosevelt Hospital in New York City.

Do drugs work?

Medication can help manage PMS symptoms. The two broad groups of prescription medications doctors use are hormonal drugs (including oral contraceptives) and antidepressant/anti-anxiety medications. Recent research has cast doubt on the effectiveness of hormones, such as progesterone, which were found to be no better than a placebo for treating PMS, according to researchers at the University of Pennsylvania. The anti-anxiety drug Xanax was more effective at reducing symptoms.

While Xanax offers relief to some women with severe PMS, it can be addictive. For this reason, when treating PMS, Xanax is usually only given during the five or six days a month before menstruation. Under those conditions, the risk of addiction is very low.

The newest class of antidepressants (selective serotonin reuptake inhibitors), including Prozac, Zoloft, and Paxil, have been fairly extensively studied and found to be very effective in the treatment of PMS symptoms. These drugs are a mainstay of therapy and act by increasing levels of the neurotransmitter serotonin (associated with depression) levels in the brain. In addition, some doctors recommend the herb St. John's wort (hypericum) to be effective in PMS. Several European studies have found St. John's wort to be more effective than placebo in the treatment of depression and equally effective as some antidepressants.

In patients whose symptoms are mostly bloating and other signs of water retention, a mild diuretic starting five to seven days prior to the period is frequently quite helpful.

Uterine fibroids

If you gather 10 women into a room, odds are four of them will have uterine fibroids—single nodules or clusters of harmless tumors made of smooth muscle and connective tissue that develop within the wall of the uterus, protruding into the interior or toward the outer surface. In rare cases, they may sprout up on stalks projecting from the surface of the uterus.

There's no need to panic if your doctor finds a fibroid during your next exam—these are benign tumors and they won't develop into cancer, nor do they increase your risk for uterine cancer.

Unofficially...
As many as one woman in every four will someday develop uterine fibroids, often without realizing it.

Watch Out!
In rare cases, a fibroid can compress and block the fallopian tube, preventing fertilization and migration of the egg; after surgical removal of the fibroid, fertility is generally restored.

Is it a fibroid?

Most of the time, you'll never know you're carrying around fibroids deep inside, since they usually don't cause any symptoms. However, some women who have uterine fibroids may experience symptoms such as:

- Excessive or painful bleeding during menstruation
- Bleeding between periods
- A feeling of fullness in the lower abdomen
- Frequent urination resulting from a fibroid that compresses the bladder
- Pain during sexual intercourse
- Lower back pain

Tests your doctor may do

Odds are you won't have any idea that you have a fibroid. Most of the time, they are discovered during a routine gynecologic exam or during prenatal care. If your doctor suspects fibroids based on your symptoms or an exam, he or she may suggest:

- An ultrasound to rule out other reasons for uterine changes such as pregnancy, ovarian cysts or cancer
- Endometrial biopsy to help rule out cancer or determine the cause of heavy or irregular menstrual periods
- Dilatation and curettage (D&C) to help rule out cancer or determine the cause of heavy or irregular menstrual periods

To treat or not to treat?

Most of the time, you won't have any symptoms or problems associated with fibroids, so they don't require any intervention or—at most—may require limited treatment. If your fibroids aren't causing problems and they aren't growing rapidly, the best therapy is watchful waiting. Your doctor will probably want to see you once or twice a year to monitor the fibroids' growth. These regular checkups (with occasional ultrasounds) can determine if there are uncommon or hidden problems, such as an enlarging fibroid blocking the ureter.

However, if they start to grow bigger or they move into sensitive areas of the uterus, fibroids may begin to cause problems such as severe pelvic pain, heavy bleeding, or even infertility and miscarriage.

Some doctors may suggest a nonsurgical option aimed at shrinking fibroids—drugs called gonadotropin releasing hormone agonists, or GnRH agonists, which interfere with estrogen production and produce a temporary artificial menopause. GnRH agonists are most useful for shutting down the ovaries for three months, which stops the bleeding and in turn allows the patient to build up her blood count by taking iron. Then the doctor can go ahead with the surgery and the patient is much less likely to need a blood transfusion. These drugs (Lupron or Synarel) are usually used for only about six months They can produce side effects similar to menopause, including insomnia, thinning of vaginal tissue, hot flashes and decreased bone mass. Only about 15 percent of women using lupron will be cured of their fibroids, pain or endometriousus, and even then symptoms may recur in a year or two. However, some women who have taken these drugs report significant and long-lasting effects while critics argue that studies investigating these drugs were very small and inconclusive.

Unofficially...
The small amount of estrogen in estrogen replacement therapy does not appear to have any significant effect on fibroid growth in most women.

If your fibroids are causing problems, you may need some form of surgery to remove them. If at least half of the small fibroid is protruding into the uterine cavity, it may be removed from the uterus through the vagina in an outpatient procedure called hysteroscopy. In this procedure, the fibroid is removed using a thin, telescope-like instrument inserted through the vagina and into the uterus. If the fibroid doesn't protrude into the uterine cavity, it can't be reached by hysteroscopy.

Alternatively, you may opt for myomectomy to remove the fibroids. A myomectomy is a more involved surgical procedure than a hysteroscopy, with higher rate of risks—the main difference is that with myomectomy, you keep your uterus. The fibroids are removed through an abdominal incision called a laparotomy. There is still a recurrance rate as well as a complication of uterine scarring with hysterescopy; the most common type of fibroids—large growths of the intramural or serosal variety—are best handled through laparotomy (myomectomy).

In the past, hysterectomy was the only option if you wanted to get rid of fibroids—and even today, if your fibroids are too large, this may be your only option. If you're over 35 and you don't want children, this may be an option for you. In fact, nearly half of all hysterectomies performed on women over 35 are because of fibroids. However, while hysterectomy can completely remove fibroids, there are some drawbacks:

- It may take up to two months for you to recover (although other women can recover much quicker than that).

- As major surgery, it carries all the risks of any surgical procedure (such as infection and bleeding).

Watch Out! Fibroids return in about 10 to 25 percent of women who undergo a myomectomy or hysteroscopy; the procedure is least effective for women with multiple fibroids or individual growths that are deeply embedded in the uterus.

- Some women report a decrease in sexual function.

On the horizon...

The newest (and most controversial) way to treat fibroids is a procedure called fibroid embolization, a process that shrinks the fibroids by blocking their blood supply. Instead of enduring major surgery and weeks of recuperation, you are given a local anesthetic in a hospital and can go home the next day. It appears to work best on fibroids of a certain size and location that myomectomy or hysteroscopy can't remove. This procedure is done by a radiologist.

There are many questions still remaining about this procedure, however. For example, most women who undergo embolization are over 40 and the procedure's effect on fertility is unclear. About 1 to 2 percent of women who've had the procedure experience premature menopause afterward, perhaps as a result of ovarian damage. The reason for the premature menopause is thought to be related to the fact that the embolization works by cutting off the blood supply to the fibroid and, in doing so, also cuts off blood supply to the ovaries and may stimulate permanent damage. Because of the risk of infertility, the procedure isn't normally recommended for women who still want to get pregnant, unless they also face infertility with any other fibroid surgery.

The procedure is considered to be experimental and, because it's so new, most insurance companies won't cover the costs, although some doctors say they can often persuade insurers to cover it on an individual basis by showing them research. Those who must pay for the procedure on their own may need to come up with about $15,000.

Bright Idea
The amount of estrogen in birth control pills may cause fibroids to grow. If you're taking birth control pills, ask your doctor to check your fibroids to make sure your condition doesn't worsen. The onset of menopause will usually cause the tumors to shrink.

Can you prevent fibroids?

No risk factors have been found for uterine fibroids other than being a female of reproductive age; although they're diagnosed in African-American women two to three times more frequently than in others. They're seldom seen in young women who have not begun menstruating and they usually stabilize or regress in women who have passed menopause.

About the only thing you could do to prevent fibroids might be to have at least two children, since some studies suggest that having two liveborn children cuts the risk of uterine fibroids in half. (However, researchers aren't sure if having children actually protects a woman from developing fibroids or whether fibroids contributes to the infertility of childless women.)

Endometriosis

Endometriosis is a serious medical condition in which tissue that looks and acts like endometrial tissue is found outside the uterus, usually inside the abdominal cavity. The problem is that this misplaced tissue acts as it would if it were inside the uterus. Endometriosis does not necessarily respond to hormones the same way that normal endometrium does. Frequently, normal endometrium will be in the premenstrual state and the endometriosis will be in a pre-ovulatory state. It may not bleed at the time of the period and it may bleed when the patient is not having a menstrual flow.

No one knows why this happens, but scientists have many theories, ranging from tissue backup to genetics:

- Tissue backup: During menstruation, some experts think menstrual tissue backs up through the fallopian tubes into the abdomen, where it implants and grows. (Some experts on endometriosis believe all women experience some form of this "tissue backup," but that an immune-system problem or hormonal glitch allows this tissue to grow in women who develop endometriosis.)

- **Genetics:** Other experts suggest that endometriosis may be a genetically based, or that certain families may be predisposed to endometriosis.

- **Systemic:** Still others suspect that the endometrial tissue doesn't back up through the fallopian tubes, but travels from the uterus to other parts of the body via the lymph or blood system. There are a few cases that may be brought on in this manner.

- **Embryonic:** Some scientists theorize that remnants of tissue from a woman's own embryonic development may later develop into endometriosis, or that some tissues retain the ability they had in the embryonic stage to transform into reproductive tissue under certain circumstances.

How to tell if it's endometriosis

Some women with endometriosis have no symptoms, but most commonly, the symptoms of endometriosis start years after you've begun menstruating, gradually worsening as the misplaced tissue grows, until menopause, when the tissue shrinks again and symptoms subside. Most women with endometriosis have pain, especially really bad menstrual cramps in the abdomen or lower back before and during menstruation. Pain also may occur during or after sex.

Bright Idea
If you are wondering if you might have endometriosis, you can order the "How Can I Tell If I Have Endometriosis?" kit from the International Endometriosis Association at 8585 N. 76th Place, Milwaukee, WI 53223 ($3.75), or call 800/992-3636.

Other symptoms may include

- Fatigue.
- Painful bowel movements during your periods.
- Diarrhea and/or constipation and other intestinal upsets during your periods.

Rarely, the irritation caused by endometriosis may lead to an infection or abscess, causing pain at times other than your period. There may be intestinal pain because of patches of tissue on the walls of the colon or intestine. But the degree of pain is not necessarily related to the seriousness of the condition; some women with severe endometriosis have no pain, while others, with just a few small growths, experience incapacitating pain.

Complications

Severe endometriosis with extensive scarring is one of the three major causes of female infertility, occurring in about 30 to 40 percent of women with the condition. However, while many infertile women have unsuspected or mild endometriosis, how this type of endometriosis affects fertility is still not clear. While the pregnancy rates for women with endometriosis are lower than those of the general population, most women with endometriosis don't have fertility problems.

There are all degrees of endometriosis. Most women with endometriosis can conceive, and the pregnancy can actually improve the disease.

Endometrial cancer (cancer of the uterine lining) is very rarely associated with endometriosis, and occurs in less than one percent of women with the disease. When it does occur, it's usually found within more advanced patches of endometriosis in older women and the long-term outlook in these unusual cases is reasonably good. However, endometriosis does not turn into endometrial cancer; endometriosis is a benign condition.

Other complications depend on the location of the tissue growths and can include

- Rupture of growths (which can spread endometriosis to new areas).
- Adhesions, intestinal bleeding, or obstruction (if the growths are in or near the intestines).
- Interference with bladder function (if the growths are on or in the bladder); the worst cases interfere not just with the bladder, but with the ureters and kidneys as well.

Tests your doctor should perform

While there are symptoms that are highly suggestive of endometriosus, the only definitive way to diagnose it is with laparoscopy. First, your doctor will evaluate your medical history and perform a complete physical exam (including a pelvic exam). Then the doctor will perform a laparoscopy, a surgical procedure in which a lighted tube is inserted into a small incision in the abdomen under general anesthesia.

The laparoscope is moved around the abdomen, which has been distended with carbon dioxide gas to make the organs easier to see. The surgeon can then check the condition of the abdominal organs and see the endometrial lesions. This procedure will reveal the locations, extent and size of the growths, and will help you and your doctor make better-informed decisions about treatment.

Confirmation of the problem is important since ovarian cancer sometimes has the same symptoms as endometriosis.

Surgery: Yes or no?

While the preferred treatment for endometriosis has varied over the years, doctors now agree that if the symptoms are mild, nothing further than medication for pain may be needed. If you have mild, or minimal, endometriosis and you want to become pregnant, depending on your age and the amount of pain you have, the best thing to do may be to have a trial period of unprotected intercourse for six months to a year. If you don't get pregnant within that time, further treatment may be needed.

If you experience only occasional pelvic pain or discomfort, a mild, over-the-counter anti-inflammatory or painkilling drug often helps. More troubling cases may require stronger drugs, which are available by prescription. The following treatments are also available:

- Hormone suppression: If you don't want to get pregnant, your doctor may suggest hormone suppression treatment, which can stop ovulation for as long as possible, and can force endometriosis into remission during treatment—sometimes for months or years. Hormone suppression treatments include estrogen and progesterone, progesterone alone, a testosterone derivative (Danazol) or GnRH (gonadotropin releasing hormone). However, as with all hormonal treatments, side effects are a problem for some women and you won't be able to get pregnant during therapy. Hormonal suppression is usually a short-term treatment that will often cause the endometriosis to regress (or at least stop growing). It can only be used for a short time (three to six months); afterwards, the endometriosis usually starts to grow again.

- Laparoscopy: Depending on the severity of the endometriosis, you may seek surgical treatment to remove the diseased tissue without risking damage to healthy surrounding tissue. This technique is performed in a hospital under general anesthesia as an alternative to full abdominal surgery. Laparoscopy is quickly replacing major abdominal surgery in the U.S.

- Hysterectomy: Hysterectomy and removal of all growths plus removal of the ovaries (oophorectomy) to prevent further hormonal stimulation is necessary in cases of long-standing, troublesome endometriosis.

- Pregnancy: Because pregnancy often temporarily eases symptoms, and because infertility is more likely the longer you have endometriosis, your doctor may advise you not to postpone pregnancy.

Once you hit menopause, mild to moderate endometriosis usually subsides. Even after radical surgery or menopause, however, a severe case of endometriosis can be reactivated by estrogen replacement therapy. For this reason, some experts warn that no replacement hormones should be given for between three to six months after hysterectomy and removal of the ovaries for endometriosis. Others believe that it's okay to start endometriosis patients on ERT before they leave the operating room.

Ovarian problems

The ovaries are a pair of almond-shaped organs located deep within the pelvis on each side of the uterus, and are responsible for producing one egg a month during ovulation. The egg then floats down

Watch Out!
Women with endometriosis have higher rates of ectopic pregnancy and miscarriage, and one study has found they have more difficult pregnancies and labors.

to the uterus through one of the the fallopian tubes in a journey that takes about three days. The ovaries also produce the hormones estrogen and progesterone. While the egg is maturing, the follicle releases estrogen to help thicken the lining of the uterus in case the egg is fertilized and grows into an embryo. After the follicle ruptures, it produces progesterone to help the uterus prepare for a fertilized egg. If no pregnancy occurs, the level of progesterone and estrogen decreases, menstruation occurs, and the cycle repeats itself.

Several problems can develop in the ovaries:

- Infection: The ovaries alone can become infected or as part of an infection that involves other pelvic organs, called pelvic inflammatory disease (PID). (See Chapter 15.)
- Cysts and tumors: Usually benign, these ovarian cysts and tumors don't produce symptoms and are discovered only through a pelvic exam or ultrasound. Many cysts are perfectly normal—in fact, during the first half of the menstrual cycle, every woman has three to nine follicular cysts on her ovary. If you don't, then you're considered sterile. Occasionally, one or more of these egg-containing cysts misbehaves or malfunctions and then symptoms such as pain or bleeding may occur.
- Polycystic ovary syndrome (PCOS): A condition in which many small cysts form on the ovaries. It is associated with a lack of ovulation and irregular periods (and infertility).

If your doctor suspects an ovarian problem, there are several diagnostic choices:

- Examination: Your doctor will first give you a complete physical and pelvic exam.

- Ultrasound: If there's a chance of an ovarian cyst or tumor, you may need to undergo an ultrasound scan, which uses high-frequency sound waves to produce a detailed image of the pelvic organs.
- Laparoscopy: The organs can be visualized directly by means of laparoscopy, a surgical procedure in which a special viewing instrument is inserted into the abdominal cavity while the patient is under general anesthesia.

Ovarian infections

Ovarian infections are most frequently caused by STDs. If diagnostic tests reveal an ovarian infection, your doctor will prescribe an antibiotic.

Ovarian cysts

Ovarian cysts are fluid-filled sacs on the surface or within an ovary. Some ovarian cysts occur when a follicle continues to grow and fill with fluid long after the egg has been released. Although most benign ovarian cysts disappear after a few menstrual cycles, some grow large enough to cause discomfort.

Many ovarian cysts and tumors don't produce any symptoms and are detected during a routine pelvic exam, an ultrasound scan or unrelated surgery. Sometimes the growths disrupt the production of ovarian hormones, causing irregular bleeding or an increase in body hair, or they press on the bladder, leading to more frequent urination. If a cyst or tumor ruptures or twists as it attaches to the ovary, it can cause significant abdominal pain. If the growth is large, the ovary is twisted, or there is abnormal hormone production, you may notice the following symptoms:

- Abdominal fullness or heaviness
- Pressure on the rectum or bladder
- A longer, shorter, absent or irregular menstrual cycle
- Pelvic pain (a constant dull aching that may radiate to the lower back and thighs) during sex or before or after menstruation

When a growth does produce symptoms, they may be similar to ovarian cancer, PID, ectopic pregnancy, or endometriosis. Appendicitis or other problems related to the gastrointestinal tract can also produce similar symptoms. For these reasons, you should always have your doctor diagnose any suspected ovary problem.

Tests your doctor might perform

The first test will probably be a vaginal ultrasound, which is the most accurate way to visualize your ovaries by introducing a small instrument into the vagina to bounce sound waves off your uterus, fallopian tubes, and ovaries. This allows your doctor to determine the size of the cyst and whether or not it's filled with fluid. This can help determine the type of cyst you have; certain types of ovarian cysts make fairly reliable patterns. Unfortunately, ultrasound can't provide a definite diagnosis of whether or not the cyst is malignant, so if the ultrasound shows solid areas within a cyst, surgery will be needed to remove and biopsy it.

Treating ovarian cysts

Treating ovarian cysts is often unnecessary; they tend to disappear on their own. If you're under 40 and your ovarian cyst is soft and smaller than two inches in diameter, your doctor may suggest that you delay surgery for one or two menstrual cycles to see whether the cyst disappears spontaneously. Some doctors prescribe birth control pills to women with a suspected ovarian cyst in the belief that hormones in the pills will help the cyst regress, thus eliminating the need for surgery. Of you're over age 40, your doctor may recommend prompt surgery to rule out the possibility of cancer.

New treatment methods allow your gynecologist to remove a cyst through small incisions in your abdomen in an outpatient technique called laparoscopic surgery. Using a telescope placed through the navel and small instruments near the pubic bone, the doctor cuts through the thinned ovarian tissue, gently peeling the cyst away from inside the ovary. The cyst fluid is then removed with a suction device. The cyst, which now looks like a deflated balloon, can easily be removed through the small laparoscopy incision.

Polycystic ovarian syndrome

Despite its name, PCOS is not a single disease, nor should it be confused with single ovarian cysts. This often overlooked condition affecting millions of women is not only one of the most common causes of infertility, but a disease that has far-reaching effects on a woman's overall health, as well.

PCOS occurs when egg follicles get trapped just under the surface of the ovary and, unable to release their eggs, form into multiple small cysts. This multiple cyst condition may be associated with obesity, infertility, and excessive body hair. However, since many women with PCOS are not obese or hairy, absence of these signs does not necessarily mean a woman doesn't have the condition.

There are several theories as to what causes PCOS. Some doctors believe that it is caused by

Unofficially... First identified more than 60 years ago, PCOS is the most common endocrine disorder and a leading cause of infertility among more than three million women of childbearing age. Specialists are still learning more about diagnosis and treatment every day.

overproduction of male hormones; others suspect that PCOS occurs when insulin resistance reaches the point where it affects biochemical functions in the ovary, preventing the ovary from releasing the eggs.

Symptoms include

- Feeling of fullness or pressure on one side of the abdomen (very rare).
- Sharp abdominal pain (very rare).
- Irregular vaginal bleeding.
- Acne.
- Absent menstrual periods.
- Increase in facial or body hair.
- Irregularities in bowel movements or urination (very rare).

For years, many physicians did not understand the full scope of PCOS and thought it was just a cause of infertilty; today, experts realize PCOS effects far more than reproduction.

What causes PCOS?

What doctors now realize is that PCOS is not one simple disease, but actually a set of reproductive and metabolic disorders probably caused by one or more genetic flaws. Many women with PCOS have an elevated level of male hormones (particularly testosterone) and rarely ovulate. They may complain of irregular periods, infertility, obesity, male-pattern hair growth or loss and acne. Exactly why male hormones begin to rise in these women remains unclear.

Normally, the pituitary gland in the brain secretes two hormones that stimulate ovulation; the hormone that triggers ovulation also prompts the ovaries to produce progesterone, which is converted into testosterone and then into estrogen. But

Bright Idea
PCOS appears to be an inherited condition. If you have the symptoms of PCOS and you have a family history of the condition, your doctor should consider this diagnosis.

testosterone production goes awry in women with PCOS and the resulting excess of male hormones disrupts the entire hormonal cascade leading to ovulation, preventing the formation of a dominant follicle. As time passes, the ovary becomes filled with unreleased cysts.

More recently, researchers have discovered that most (although not all) women with PCOS are also resistant to their own insulin, the hormone that helps cells absorb sugar from the bloodstream. As their blood sugar levels start to climb, they start to gain weight; as insulin resistance and body weight rise, the pancreas churns out even more insulin, which causes the ovaries to produce even more testosterone. The potential long-term consequences of this deadly chain reaction include diabetes, high blood pressure, heart disease, and stroke.

Of course, not all women with PCOS have all these problems. Some do not have excessive testosterone levels but do have severe insulin problems, while others suffer the reverse. It's because of this diversity that doctors suspect they may not be dealing with one disorder, but many. There is still much to understand about this condition.

Current PCOS treatments

Recent attention to PCOS during the past five years has led to more research and better treatments that focus on insulin resistance, a key part of the syndrome. In fact, it's the insulin resistance that makes PCOS a potential long-term health threat, boosting the risk of diabetes, high blood pressure and heart disease. In addition, the chronic lack of ovulation leads to chronic estrogen stimulation of the uterine lining, which increases the risk of endometrial cancer.

Watch Out!
Girls who have irregular menstrual cycles are more likely to have multiple ovarian cysts than girls with normal periods, according to researchers at the Medical Centre Free University in Amsterdam.

Traditional treatments for PCOS include an oral contraceptive to lower androgen levels and establish monthly menstruation, combined with a drug to block the action of androgens and thus address the problem of excess hair and acne.

Today's more modern approach focuses on new drugs that help cells use insulin more efficiently. Although these prescription drugs were developed for diabetics, studies show they also ease a wide range of PCOS symptoms in some women, including infertility. Metformin (Glucophage) reverses some of the physical and metabolic consequences of PCOS, but experts caution that this drug isn't the answer for all women with this syndrome, especially those who want to get pregnant, due to the lack of data about how safe these drugs are for a developing fetus. Experts note that larger, long-term studies of these drugs have not been completed.

On the horizon...

Scientists are now studying other insulin-sensitizing agents that may be even more effective in treating PCOS. A new drug under investigation called D-chiro-inositol, which can be found naturally in fruits and vegetables, helps the body better use insulin and subsequently promotes ovulation and boosts overall health, according to researchers at Virginia Commonwealth University in Richmond. The drug, under development by INSMED Pharmaceuticals, Inc. of Richmond, is not yet available, but findings suggest that insulin resistance in PCOS may be related to a deficiency in D-chiro-inositol, which can be cured by administering this drug.

Other experts—who are now close to identifying one gene—hope they will soon discover the genetic

Unofficially...
A number of small studies have shown that common diabetes drugs can bring about normal menstrual cycles in women with PCOS, according to research published in the June 25, 1998 issue of the *New England Journal of Medicine*.

roots of the syndrome, revealing the cause of the condition, who is susceptible, and better ways to treat it.

Just the facts

- If you're not menopausal and your period suddenly stops, odds are you're either pregnant, you've lost weight, or you're exercising too much.

- Today, experts suspect PMS may be caused or influenced by neurotransmitters, genetics, and diet.

- Progesterone pills are no better than placebos in treating PMS; antidepressants do appear to work more effectively.

- Many fibroids may simply be left alone and monitored.

- Mild endometriosis may not need surgery, but severe disease may require hysterectomy and oophorectomy.

- Polycystic ovarian syndrome (PCOS) is an under diagnosed, complex problem affecting millions of American women and can lead to several significant health risks including obesity, coronary artery disease, and stroke.

Bright Idea
To get the best available care, experts recommend you find a doctor who understands PCOS. Contact the Polycystic Ovarian Syndrome Association, Inc. at www.pcosupport.org for details. Hershey Medical Center has an ongoing study of PCOS; call the center at 717/531-8521 to enroll for evaluation and possible treatment.

GET THE SCOOP ON...
Newest birth control methods ▪ Birth control no-nos ▪ Testing infertility ▪ Infertility lifestyle risks ▪ Fertility killers

Fertility and Infertility

Having a child . . . not having a child—today, it's a choice whether a woman and her partner want a child to be part of their lives. Before safe and reliable birth control was introduced in this country, that choice just wasn't available. Careful family planning is a key to enjoying good physical and emotional health throughout your childbearing years. It's an important choice—some women prefer not to interfere with conception because of religious beliefs or their own desires But most women in the United States prefer to plan the number of children they have.

On the other hand, five million American women who desperately want children can't conceive—or if they conceive, can't carry a baby to term. The drive to become parents is strong in the United States today, as baby boomer women approach the end of their fertile years and more than 15 percent of all American women have received some type of infertility service.

Birth control
It's a sure bet that out of the variety of safe and affordable birth control methods on the market

Watch Out!
The only birth control method that will protect you from STDs is latex or polyurethane male and female condoms used in conjunction with spermicide.

today, an American woman can find one especially tailored to her health status, her pocketbook, her independence, how often she has sex, and how many partners she has had.

Methods you can count on

Effective birth control methods include

- Hormonal methods: Hormone implants, injections and oral contraceptives work by interfering with ovulation, conception, or implantation.

- Barrier methods: Condoms, diaphragms, cervical caps, and sponges work by physically preventing sperm from moving through your reproductive system and fertilizing an egg.

- Intrauterine devices: An IUD is a physical device that is inserted into a woman's uterus to prevent pregnancy. They seem to work by creating a hostile intrauterine environment that kills sperm before they can reach the tubes; the IUD does cause abortion of a fertilized egg.

- Natural family planning: Avoiding sex on the days of your menstrual cycle when you are most likely to get pregnant (from five days before ovulation up to and including the day of ovulation).

Methods that don't work

Before reviewing all the possible choices, it's important to make sure you know which methods you shouldn't rely on as a means of birth control:

- Sex during your period: It may seem safe, but in fact there's still a slim chance you can get pregnant during this time.

- Douching after sex: You can't destroy all the sperm by douching; in fact, you may instead force them higher into the uterus.

- Urinating after sex: Urine and sperm travel through two separate passages in your body, so urinating won't have any affect on sperm traveling up your vagina.
- Washing after sex: No matter how fast you think you can wash, sperm are already swimming madly through the cervix, where they won't be destroyed by washing.
- Early withdrawal: Even if the penis is removed before ejaculation, there is usually some sperm in the pre-ejaculatory liquid (the penis doesn't even need to be inside the vagina for some sperm to make it through the cervix and fertilize an egg). In fact, as many as 50 percent of the sperm are contained in the clear fluid that is released just before actual ejaculation.

Natural birth control methods

Another form of birth control that does not use devices or pills is natural birth control. Basically this means not having sex on the days of your menstrual cycle when you are most likely to get pregnant. Because sperm may live in your reproductive tract for up to seven days—and the egg remains fertile for about 12 hours—you can still get pregnant from five days before ovulation up to and including the day of ovulation. In order to figure out when you're fertile, you can use a method based on your menstrual cycle, changes in cervical mucus or changes in body temperature. Most natural family planning advocates now use some form of urine testing to help determine ovulation. Even so, the failure rate runs around 20 percent.

There are several ways to predict your fertile times:

- The "rhythm" or calendar method predicts your fertile days based on previous menstrual cycles. However, because your cycles may not be regular, it's best not to rely on this method alone.

- The basal body temperature method involves taking and charting your body temperature the same way every day. The fraction of a degree temperature rise signals an egg has been released. However, it's important to realize that your temperature may change in response to emotional or physical stress. If you're going to use this method, you should chart your temperature for at least three months before relying on this method.

- You can use the cervical mucous method to estimate when ovulation takes place. The hormones of the menstrual cycle cause changes in the quality and quantity of your mucous secretions in the cervix just before and during ovulation. Your health care provider can teach you to recognize your own pattern. (This is also called the ovulation method.)

Barrier methods

Barrier methods of birth control physically stop sperm from getting into the uterus (and the spermicide used with many of these barriers also kill sperm). When used with spermicide, barrier methods are among the safest and cheapest ways to prevent pregnancy—and they can also help reduce your risk of being infected with certain STDs, pelvic inflammatory disease (PID—an infection of the fallopian tubes or uterus that is a major cause of infertility in women), and, perhaps, even cervical cancer.

Bright Idea
If you don't like the taste, feel, or smell of spermicide, try switching brands or choosing one of the tasteless, odorless versions now available.

However, if you don't use them consistently and correctly, barrier methods have a relatively high failure rate. You need to put a good amount of effort into practicing these methods, and most of them require your partner to cooperate.

Spermicide

Vaginal spermicide is inserted into the vagina where it kills sperm on contact; it's most effective when combined with a barrier method of birth control (such as a diaphragm or condom). When it comes to choosing a vaginal spermicide, you've got lots to pick from, including foam, cream, jelly, film, suppository or tablets.

While all products contain a sperm-killing chemical, you've got to follow package instructions, because some products require you to wait 10 minutes or more after inserting the spermicide before having sex. Once you've inserted it, one dose of spermicide is usually effective for one hour; for repeated intercourse, you've got to apply more spermicide. After sex, you must keep the spermicide in place for at least six to eight hours to ensure that all sperm are killed (this means you can't douche or rinse the vagina during this time). The failure rate is between 6 and 8 percent.

Condom: His and hers

Condoms (both male and female versions) are latex or polyurethane barriers to sperm; the male version fits over the erect penis; the female variety is inserted into the vagina, covering the cervix inside and the lips of the vagina outside.

Condoms (both his and hers) can be used only once. Some have spermicide added (usually nonoxynol-9 in the United States) to kill sperm,

Unofficially...
According to a 1996 Food and Drug Administration advisory committee panel, some vaginal spermicide containing nonoxynol-9 may reduce the risk of gonorrhea and chlamydia transmission.

although spermicide doesn't seem to provide more contraceptive protection beyond that provided by the condom alone. Because condoms act as mechanical barriers, they prevent direct vaginal contact with semen, infectious genital secretions and genital lesions and discharges.

Other than not having sex at all, the use of latex condoms is the most effective way to lower the risk of infection from the virus that causes AIDS and other HIV-related illnesses, as well as other STDs. Most condoms are made from latex rubber (hence their nickname), except for polyurethane condoms, which have been marketed in the United States since 1994. This type of condom may be used to protect against STD infection by those allergic to latex.

A small percentage of condoms are made from lamb intestines (lambskin condoms). Unlike latex or polyurethane condoms, lambskin condoms don't always prevent STDs because they're porous and may permit passage of viruses like HIV, hepatitis B, and herpes.

Some condoms are prelubricated, but these lubricants don't provide more birth control or STD protection. Non-oil-based lubricants (such as water or K-Y jelly), can be used with latex or lambskin condoms, but oil-based lubricants, such as petroleum jelly (Vaseline), lotions, or massage or baby oil, should not be used because they can weaken the condom material.

Used alone, the male condom has an expected failure rate of 2 percent and a typical failure rate of 12 percent (mostly because it can slip or break during withdrawal). Used with spermicide, the failure rate can be reduced almost to zero. When using a male condom, your partner needs to immediately withdraw after climax, since the penis shrinks slightly afterward and can slip out of the condom.

Watch Out!
Don't use a female condom together with a male condom, because they may not both stay in place.

Female condoms, approved by the Food and Drug Administration (FDA) in 1993, are sold under the brand names Femidom and Reality. Less likely to slip or burst than the male version, the female condom is a lubricated polyurethane sheath with a closed flexible ring at one end and a larger open ring at the other. You insert the closed ring into the vagina, fitting it over the cervix, leaving the open end hanging outside the vagina where it partially covers the labia. You must carefully remove it after sex, and insert another each time you have sex. If used correctly, the female condom seems to be as effective as the diaphragm or cervical cap.

Diaphragm

Available by prescription only and sized by a health professional to achieve a proper fit, the diaphragm has a dual mechanism to prevent pregnancy. A dome-shaped rubber disk with a flexible rim covers the cervix so sperm can't reach the uterus, while the spermicide applied to the diaphragm before insertion kills sperm. The spermicide you use may be enough to help prevent the spread of certain STDs, but it doesn't guarantee your safety against all of them.

The diaphragm protects for six hours; after that, (or, for repeated intercourse, within this period), you should insert fresh spermicide into the vagina with the diaphragm still in place. While you need to leave it in for at least six hours after last having intercourse, you shouldn't leave it there for longer than 24 hours because of the risk of toxic shock syndrome (TSS), a rare but potentially fatal infection (see Chapter 15). Used consistently and correctly, the diaphragm carries a failure rate of about 6 percent, but the typical failure rate is more like 18 percent.

Remember to check the fit of your diaphragm:

- At your annual gynecological exam
- Whenever you gain or lose 10 pounds or more
- After an abortion
- After a miscarriage
- After a full-term pregnancy

Cervical cap

The cap is a soft rubber cup about the size of a thimble, with a round rim; it's sized by a health professional to fit snugly around the cervix. It's available by prescription only and, like the diaphragm, is used with spermicide (although you don't need to use as much). The spermicide you use may be enough to help prevent the spread of certain STDs, but it doesn't guarantee your safety.

It protects for 48 hours and for multiple acts of intercourse within this time. Wearing it for more than 48 hours is not recommended because of the risk, though low, of TSS. Also, with prolonged use of two or more days, the cap may cause an unpleasant vaginal odor or discharge in some women.

The cervical cap is basically a smaller version of the diaphragm, and fits over the cervix and is held in place by suction. However, because it can be difficult to insert and doesn't fit all women, it's a less popular method than the diaphragm. On the other hand, it can be left in place longer than the diaphragm and can be used to collect menstrual blood.

The sponge: It's back!

The sponge, a donut-shaped polyurethane device containing the spermicide nonoxynol-9, is inserted into the vagina to cover the cervix, much like a diaphragm. A woven polyester loop is attached for easy removal. The sponge is a low cost, nonprescription product that protects for multiple acts of sex for 24 hours. You need to leave it in place for at least six hours after sex for contraceptive protection, but no more than 30 hours after insertion because of the slight risk of TSS (see Chapter 15).

Once so popular a form of birth control it became a famous joke on the TV comedy *Seinfeld* ("Are you sponge worthy?"), the Today brand sponge was taken off the market in 1995 for financial, not health, reasons. The sole manufacturer (Whitehall Laboratories of Madison, NJ) had decided it would cost too much to correct manufacturing problems the FDA had discovered at the old factory where the sponge was made. (The FDA stressed that there never was any problem with Today's safety, just with the factory.)

Some 116,000 American women had been using Today in 1995 when its manufacturer stopped production, making it the most popular choice among methods that didn't require a doctor's visit. The only other woman-controlled, nonprescription choices were spermicide and the female condom; unlike those options, the sponge could be inserted up to 24 hours before sex and didn't require new applications for repeated intercourse.

With its low risk of side effects, the sponge was attractive to women who didn't want to have to be fitted by a doctor, who had problems with prescribed hormonal contraceptives, or who enjoyed its ease of insertion.

Competing sponges were sold in France, Canada, and a few other countries, but once Today was off the U.S. market, no contraceptive sponge had been sold in this country until 1999, when the sponge was brought back by Allendale Pharmaceuticals of New Jersey. Because the FDA never revoked Today's approval, getting it back on the market was a quick process.

The failure rate for the sponge is about the same as for other barrier methods; in women who have had children, there is a 9 percent failure rate for "perfect use" and 28 percent "typical use"; for women who have never had a child those rates are 6 percent and 18 percent, respectively.

Intrauterine device

An IUD is a T-shaped device inserted into the uterus by a health care professional. Today, there are only two types of IUDs produced and sold in the United States: The Paragard Copper T 380A and the Progestasert Progesterone T. The Paragard IUD can remain in place for 10 years, while the Progestasert IUD must be replaced every year.

During the 1970s, the Dalkon Shield IUD was taken off the market because it was associated with a high incidence of pelvic infections and infertility, and some deaths. Today, serious complications from IUDs are rare. Other side effects can include perforation of the uterus, abnormal bleeding, and cramps. Complications occur most often during and immediately after insertion.

It's not entirely clear how IUDs prevent pregnancy. They seem to work by creating a hostile intrauterine environment that kills sperm before they can reach the tubes; the IUD does not seem to cause abortion of a fertilized egg. However, IUDs prevent only uterine pregnancy (not ectopic pregnancy) because their mechanism of action appears to be the creation of a nonviable environment for the fertilized egg. They do nothing to stop the implantation of an ectopic pregnancy in a fallopian tube.

IUDs have one of the lowest failure rates of any contraceptive method. In the population for which the IUD is appropriate (those in a mutually monogamous, stable relationship who aren't at a high risk of infection), the IUD is a very safe and very effective method of contraception. It has an expected failure rate of between one and two percent, depending on the type, and a typical failure rate of about 3 percent. Still, menstrual cramps and excessive bleeding lead a sizable minority of women to have their IUDs removed during their first year of use.

Hormonal contraception

Hormones: either you love them or you hate them! Given in the form of injections, pills, or implants, hormones can interfere with normal ovulation, conception, and implantation very effectively. Unfortunately, they also have a range of side effects:

- Headaches
- Weight changes
- Nausea and vomiting
- Depression
- Menstrual irregularities
- Thrombophlebitis

Despite these problems, which only occur in a few patients, for many women the benefits of hormonal methods (they are the most easy to use and among the most effective) make them a popular choice. Implants and injections in particular can be a good choice since they are estrogen free and easy to use (you don't have to remember to take a pill each day).

The Pill

Oral contraceptives have been on the market for more than 35 years and are the most popular form of reversible birth control in the United States. The Pill works by suppressing ovulation (the monthly release of an egg from the ovaries) as a result of the combined actions of the hormones estrogen and progestin. If you remember to take the Pill every day as directed, you have an extremely low chance of becoming pregnant. However, the Pill's effectiveness may be reduced if you're taking some medications (such as certain antacids, the sedative phenobarbitol, antiseizure medications Dilantin and Tegretol, the antifungal medication griseofulvin, and a few antibiotics), so be sure to tell your doctor you're on the Pill when prescribed medications.

In the past, versions of the Pill with high doses of estrogen made this type of contraception dangerous for women over age 35; newer, safer forms are now highly effective and reasonably safe for most non-smoking, low-risk women up to age 45 or until menopause. The Pill has been used for generations in some countries such as Sweden. To date, no long-term adverse effects have been found. In addition, long-term use of the Pill (more than seven years) halves the risk of developing cancer of the ovary or cancer of the uterine lining and decreases the risk of osteoporosis.

Besides preventing pregnancy, the Pill offers additional benefits. The Pill can

- Make menstrual periods more regular.
- Protect against PID.

Bright Idea
If you forget to take one Pill, no backup method is needed, but if you miss two pills in the first two weeks, take two pills each of the next two days and use backup contraception for a week. If two pills are missed in the third week, or if more than two pills are missed at any time, use a backup method for a week and start a new pack of pills.

- Protect against ovarian, endometrial, and some breast cancers.

Birth control pills are safe for most women (safer even than delivering a baby). While current low-estrogen pills have fewer risks associated with them than earlier versions, however, there are some risks for some women. For this reason, consult with your doctor before making the decision to take the Pill. The Pill may contribute to high blood pressure, blood clots, and blockage of the arteries. One of the biggest questions has been whether the Pill increases the risk of breast cancer in past and current pill users. An international study published in the September 1996 journal *Contraception* concluded that women's risk of breast cancer 10 years after going off birth control pills was no higher than that of women who had never used the Pill. During Pill use and for the first 10 years after stopping the Pill, women's risk of breast cancer was only slightly higher in Pill users than non-Pill users. Most health experts advise the following women not to take the Pill:

- Women with a history of blood clots
- Women with a personal history of breast or uterine cancer; however, most women with family histories of breast cancer aren't at increased risk and may be helped
- Women with heart disease
- Smokers over age 45

Some women object to the Pill not because of health concerns but because of side effects, which include nausea, headache, breast tenderness, weight gain, irregular bleeding, and depression. While the problems may subside after a few months, some women experience continued problems.

Unofficially...
Despite years of trying, scientists haven't been able to come up with a hormonal contraception for men, mostly because the sperm ejaculated today were produced 75 to 90 days ago. Taking a pill today, therefore, won't have any effect for three months.

Another type of oral contraceptive, called the mini pill, is taken daily, but contains only the hormone progestin, with no estrogen. The mini pill works by reducing and thickening cervical mucus to prevent sperm from reaching the egg. The mini pill also keeps the uterine lining from thickening, which prevents a fertilized egg from implanting in the uterus.

Because they lack estrogen, these pills are slightly less effective than combined oral contraceptives. Mini pills can decrease menstrual bleeding and cramps, as well as the risk of endometrial and ovarian cancers and PID. Because they contain no estrogen, mini pills don't present the risk of blood clots associated with estrogen in combined pills. They are a good option for breastfeeding women because the progestin-only Pill won't interfer with milk production, as can sometimes happen with oral contraceptives containing estrogen. Side effects of the mini pill include menstrual cycle changes, weight gain, and breast tenderness.

Watch Out! Call your doctor if you're taking the mini pill and you notice abdominal pain. It could be caused by an ectopic pregnancy or an ovarian cyst. Remember—if you take the mini pill late (even by as little as three hours), you increase your chance of becoming pregnant.

Contraceptive implants

One of the newest types of birth control options you have is the contraceptive implant—small, matchstick-sized tubes containing a progestin (levonorgestrel), inserted just under the skin of your arm. Once in place, the implants release a small amount of hormone that can prevent pregnancy for at least five years, blocking ovulation and thickening cervical mucus. Other than vasectomies, the implants are probably the most effective method of contraception available. Once the implants are removed, you can become pregnant again.

The implants can be inserted during an office visit. First, your doctor will numb your skin with local anesthetic, then imbed the tubes under the skin in your upper arm. They must be surgically removed (which may be difficult).

Some women may experience inflammation or infection at the site of the implant. Other side effects include menstrual cycle changes, and breast tenderness. Some experts believe that the implants may also cause a loss of bone mass, but this has not yet been shown to occur.

While implants are very effective, they can cause all of the side effects typically related to other hormonal types of birth control. Some symptoms are more serious, however; call your doctor if you notice

- Arm pain.
- Pus or bleeding at the insertion site (which could signal an infection).
- Expulsion of the implant.
- Delayed menstrual periods after having regular periods for a long time.

You shouldn't use implants if you

- Are (or might be) pregnant.
- Have unexplained unusual vaginal bleeding.
- Take antiseizure drugs.
- Take the antibiotic rifampin.
- Have blood clots in your veins.
- Are obese (the implants don't work as well in obese women).
- Have had pulmonary embolism (blood clots in your lungs) or liver disease.

Birth control injections

If having implants inserted into your arm makes you queasy, you might want to consider hormone

Unofficially...
The six-rod Norplant implant provides protection for up to five years (or until it is removed), while the two-rod Norplant 2 (not yet available in the U.S.) protects for up to three years. Norplant failures are rare, but are higher with increased body weight.

injections instead. These injections, which are considered to be safe and effective, involve a long-acting type of progesterone that is injected into your body every 12 weeks. The method uses a progestin that is normally injected into the buttocks (it's not too painful).

The injections work by preventing ovulation; when taken as scheduled, this type of birth control is over 99 percent effective and completely reversible once the hormone is eliminated from your body. (You should schedule a shot within five days of the start of your menstrual period to get full protection from pregnancy right from the beginning.) You should not have the injections if you are (or might be) pregnant, or you've had unexplained unusual vaginal bleeding at any time in the past three months. Also, you shouldn't have the injections if you have blood clots or have had a pulmonary embolus.

Once you've taken the injections for several cycles, you actually have a bit more protection (a few weeks longer than three months); this gives you a "safety net" if you can't get to the doctor right away for your next shot. However, once you've gotten the injection, there is no way to become fertile again until it wears off. It may take up to a year for fertility to be restored after using DepoProvera (especially in very thin women).

Because the injections aren't metabolized in the liver, you can avoid some of the side effects commonly found with pills, but you may still experience

- Nervousness.
- Decreased sex drive.
- Depression.
- Acne.

Watch Out!
Even if the area where you received the shot hurts, don't massage the area—you may interfere with the effectiveness of the injection!

- Dizziness.
- Weight gain.

Call your doctor if you
- Bleed excessively.
- Have severe headaches.
- Are depressed.

Birth control interactions

If you're using birth control methods that include hormones (birth control pills, hormone injections or hormone implants), you need to know that they can affect other medications or lab test results. If you are using one of these methods, be sure to tell any doctor who is going to prescribe medicine for you.

If you're using the Pill, the estrogen and progestin in the drug can affect your liver function. If you take the Pill together with other drugs that are metabolized by the liver, you may have higher blood levels of the medications and more toxic side effects than other people. These effects might be strongest with use of pills with large amounts of progestin.

Sterilization

Surgical sterilization is a contraceptive option intended for people who don't want children in the future. It's considered permanent because reversal requires major surgery that is often unsuccessful. In general, vasectomy is less expensive and less risky than female sterilization, and less effective (failure rate is about one in 100).

If one of a couple has been sterilized and now is considering reversal, the other partner should be examined for infertility before the reversal operation is attempted.

Unofficially...
Women don't need their husband's or partner's permission to be sterilized, but having the procedure without talking about it can cause problems in a relationship.

Female sterilization

In female sterilization, the doctor blocks the fallopian tubes with various surgical techniques so the egg can't travel to the uterus. Sterilization is usually done under general anesthesia with laparoscopy using electrodessication of a segment of each tube (or applying special clips to the tubes). This prevents the egg released each month by an ovary from coming in contact with sperm.

Female sterilization, known as tubal coagulation, can also be done under local anesthesia. If you are interested in this procedure, be sure to select a gynecologist experienced in doing this procedure under local anesthesia.

Your doctor will introduce gas into your abdomen to push the intestines away from the uterus and fallopian tubes, and then insert a lighted tube (laparoscope) through the same incision. Next, instruments are introduced through the laparoscope (or a smaller second incision at the pubic hairline). Your doctor then seals the fallopian tubes using one of these methods:

- Tubal ligation: Also known as "tying the tubes," your doctor will tie surgical sutures around the fallopian tubes in two places, removing the section between the ties (this is frequently performed during a mini-laparotomy).

- Electrocoagulation/electrodessication: Your doctor burns the walls of the fallopian tubes with electrical energy so that the two parts of the tubes are blocked.

- Mechanical blocks: Your doctor will place clips or bands to block and crush the fallopian tubes.

Complications are rare but may include infection or damage to the bowel or blood vessels, or reactions to general anesthesia. Some studies suggest that sterilization may cause changes in a woman's menstrual cycle or lead to abdominal pain later.

Male sterilization

In male sterilization (vasectomy), a doctor seals, ties, or cuts the vas deferens (the tube that carries the sperm from the testicles to the penis). Just as laparoscopy and mini-laparotomy, vasectomy is a quick operation (usually taking less than 30 minutes), with only minor possible postsurgical complications, such as bleeding or infection.

A man can have sex a few days after surgery, but there may still be some mature sperm in the reproductive tract, so pregnancy could still result. Typically, a man should ejaculate 15 times after a vasectomy before he's deemed infertile. It's best to use some sort of back-up birth control method until a doctor can verify two consecutive sperm counts of zero.

Some studies have suggested a man who's had a vasectomy is more likely to get prostate cancer than one who hasn't, but more research is needed.

Emergency contraception: The "morning after" pill

Emergency contraception refers to the birth control method you can use to prevent pregnancy after you've had unprotected sex or after your method of birth control has failed (if the condom breaks, for example).

Doctors sometimes prescribe higher doses of combined oral contraceptives for use as "morning after" pills, to be taken within 72 hours of unprotected intercourse to prevent the possibly fertilized egg from reaching the uterus. While there's no guarantee, the morning after pill probably cuts your chances of getting pregnant by 90 to 95 percent.

The morning-after pill has been officially recognized as safe and effective by the FDA as of February 1997. Scientists aren't sure exactly how it works, but they suspect that the large doses of hormones prevent the lining of the uterus from getting thick enough to allow an egg to implant or that they interfere with ovulation, in some way, slowing the way the egg travels through the fallopian tube.

On the down side, the larger dose of hormones may cause side effects similar to (but stronger than) those you'd experience after a regular dose of birth control pills. Your next period may be late (or early) because of the pills, but if you don't have a period within three weeks of treatment you need to contact your doctor to make sure you're not pregnant.

For more information about emergency contraception or to find a referral for a local source, call 888/NOT-2-LATE or check the web opr.princeton.edu/ed.

Watch Out!
If you get so sick that you throw up, you may lose the pills before they can work. Your doctor may suggest you take another dose in this event.

When birth control fails...

No birth control devices are 100 percent foolproof—and too many times, people don't use the methods correctly or consistently. If you do have an unwanted pregnancy, you have the choice of ending the pregnancy or carrying the baby to term. The sooner you make a decision, the better for yourself (if you decide to terminate), and the better for both you and the fetus if you decide to continue the pregnancy.

If you decide to terminate, you should seek help from an experienced abortion provider, since the earlier you end a pregnancy, the less dangerous it is. (However, surgical abortions should never be done before eight weeks because of the increased risk of not being able to adequately empty the uterus, causing a failed abortion.) Nevertheless, at all stages, surgical abortion is safer than delivery at term when done by an experienced physician. Although abortion is currently legal in the United States, some states do have mandatory waiting periods, some require parental involvement for minors, and some require that your doctor show you graphic material designed to discourage abortion.

RU-486 (mifepristone)

Medical abortions use drugs to end the pregnancy. Abortions using the "French abortion pill" (mifepristone, or RU-486) are only available at limited settings in the United States, although wider FDA approval is expected. Unlike surgical abortion, which is often not done before the seventh or eighth week of gestation, medical abortion can be used earlier—as soon as pregnancy is determined.

The drugs are antiprogestins that block the action of natural progesterone; without progesterone's effects, the uterine lining softens and breaks down, leading to menstruation. This is most effective when used in the first weeks after fertilization and implantation, when progesterone is being produced mostly by the ovaries. As pregnancy proceeds, the placenta takes over progesterone's role, and the antiprogestins are less effective.

In Europe, the process is this:

1. Between 49 and 63 days after the first day of the last menstrual period, you would swallow the drug and stay in the clinic for an hour.
2. Two days later you return to the clinic for an oral dose of prostaglandin (which boosts uterine contractions).

3. After staying at the clinic for four hours wearing a sanitary pad, most women experience a shedding of the uterine lining, passing the fertilized egg or embryo. (The process continues for a day.)

4. You would then return to the clinic two weeks later for a follow-up visit.

About 4 percent of women don't abort and require a surgical abortion.

Surgical abortion

This is the only type of abortion currently available in the United States; in some states, it's very hard to obtain. Abortion services are offered in hospitals and clinics, and usually are done before 12 weeks of gestation. After 11 to 12 weeks, complication rates escalate, although they never get as high as delivering a baby at term.

The most common technique is to use suction to remove the uterine contents; if the pregnancy is beyond 15 weeks, the process is more complicated because of the size of the fetus. After a surgical abortion, women will experience light to medium bleeding over five to seven days and cramps. Most doctors recommend not having sex until the cervix has closed (usually when the bleeding stops).

Watch Out! After an abortion, call your doctor immediately if you notice heavy bleeding or any signs of infection (fever and chills).

Infertility: Cause and effect

Infertility is defined as the inability to conceive a child despite trying for two years (one year if the couple is older). If you have been trying to get pregnant only for a few months, you may just need to keep trying. You know you want to have sex as close to the time of ovulation as possible in order to get pregnant, but how can you tell when that is?

The simple, inexpensive way of finding out the approximate time of the month you ovulate is to take your basal temperature every morning and record it on a chart. You can buy a basal body thermometer at your drug store. Save all your charts so you can review them with your doctor (three or four months of charting should be good enough). If you don't want to mess with taking your temperature every day, there are other ways to detect when you're ovulating:

- Buy an ovulation-predictor urine test at your drug store.
- Note twinges in your lower abdomen (your ovaries are on the right and left sides of your lower abdomen) at ovulation.
- Check for clear, stretchy vaginal discharge at your fertile time.
- Ask your doctor to request an ultrasound or appropriate blood tests to determine ovulation.

Even cheaper—and possibly better—is just to have sex no closer than every 48 hours during days 10 through 20 of your cycle (closer than 48 hours lowers the sperm count). It is not necessary to come any closer than 24 hours of the moment of ovulation.

However, if you've been trying for a year without success, you're one of the 5.3 million Americans (9 percent of the reproductive age population) considered to be infertile. It's not just a "woman's problem," however; of the 80 percent of cases with a diagnosed cause, about half are based at least partially on male problems (referred to as "male factor infertility").

Is it him...

Male sperm production problems can exist from birth or develop later as a result of severe medical illnesses, including mumps and some STDs, or from a severe testicle injury, tumor or other problem. Inability to ejaculate normally can prevent conception, too, and can be caused by many factors, including diabetes, surgery of the prostate gland or urethra, blood pressure medication, or impotence.

...or is it her?

The other half of infertility cases are linked to female factors, most of which involve ovulation problems—if you can't ovulate, your eggs won't be available for fertilization. You should suspect a problem with ovulation if you have irregular menstrual periods or you don't menstruate at all. Simple lifestyle factors (stress, diet, or athletic training) can affect a woman's hormonal balance. Much less often, a hormonal imbalance might be caused by a serious medical problem, such as a pituitary gland tumor. You also might have a fertility problem if your fallopian tubes are blocked at one or both ends so the egg can't get into the uterus. Blockage may result from PID, surgery for an ectopic pregnancy or endometriosis (the abnormal presence of uterine lining cells in other pelvic organs).

Factors other than physical

While most cases of infertility are caused by physical problems, there are a host of other factors that can influence your fertility success:

- Substance abuse: Even one glass of wine a month can lower your odds of getting pregnant by as much as 50 percent, because alcohol boosts prolactin levels, which can interfere with ovulation; occasionally, levels of prolactin rise so high, hyperprolactinemia ("too much prolactin") can result, making a woman essentially infertile until the prolactin level drops.

Bright Idea
Most physicians advise you not to worry about infertility unless you've been trying unsuccessfully to conceive for at least one year. However, if you're over age 30, or you have a history of PID, painful periods, miscarriage, irregular cycles, or if your partner has a known low sperm count, you may want to seek help sooner.

- **Coffee:** Caffeine may interfere with fertility; drinking both coffee and alcohol can lower your fertility by 74 percent.
- **Marijuana:** Some studies suggest that men who smoke marijuana have lower sperm counts.
- **Bacterial vaginal infection:** A bacterial infection in your vagina can kill sperm; ask your doctor if you should have a cervical culture before trying to conceive.
- **Smoking:** toxins in smoke can lower sperm count or slow down the sperm's motility; it may take smokers up to seven months longer to conceive than nonsmokers.
- **Weight:** Women who weigh 30 percent more or less than their ideal body weight may have irregular periods and thus, more problems conceiving (very thin women may stop ovulating altogether).
- **Stress:** Severe life stress can interfere with your menstrual cycle, which can make it harder to get pregnant.
- **Overheating:** For healthy sperm, the testes should be five degrees cooler than a man's body temperature, so your partner should avoid hot tubs, saunas, and steam rooms if you're trying to conceive.
- **Herbs:** Taking large doses of echinacea, ginkgo biloba, or St. John's wort over a long period of time damages hamster sperm, according to a recent report in *Fertility and Sterility*. More studies need to be done with humans to see if the risk is real.
- **Environmental toxins:** Pesticides, chemicals, and lead may be to blame for some cases of infertility.

Unofficially...
In one recent Danish study, women who drank fewer than five alcoholic beverages a week were twice as likely to conceive within six months as women who drank more than 10 drinks a week.

Are you infertile?

If you're having trouble getting pregnant, the first thing you and your partner should do is consult a family doctor or gynecologist to rule out basic health problems that may be causing the problem. Most gynecologists can start an infertility workup including semen analysis, checking for ovulation, and looking for blocked tubes. If these are discovered, then referral to the appropriate infertility expert can be done. Most gynecologists can and should be able to start treatment of anovulation.

When you are referred to an infertility specialist:

1. Make sure all your test results (if any have already been performed; see the "Infertility Tests" section below) are sent to the specialist.

2. Call to see that the test results have arrived before your scheduled appointment.

3. If you have suspected tubal or uterine problems and a hysterosalpingogram has been done, ask the X-ray department or radiologist's office for the actual X-ray films; you can take them to your appointment with the specialist so he or she can review them with you.

Finding a fertility specialist

Fertility specialist is the popular term for a physician who treats infertility problems, but it's not a licensed medical specialty—a doctor can't become a "board-certified fertility specialist" because there is no postgraduate board-certification course in the country for specialists in fertility. This means that any doctor (even a Ph.D.) can call himself or herself a "fertility specialist," whether or not the person is qualified to treat fertility problems. Instead, an infertility specialist in this country is called a reproductive endocrinologist, which is a bona fide area of specialty; these experts are licensed and credentialed to handle all forms of infertility.

Unfortunately, some gynecologists decide to become self-styled infertility specialists having no more specialized training in the matter than a well-trained recent graduate. Never go to any fertility specialist until you are familiar with the person's credentials.

While your ob/gyn is the best place to start in diagnosing your infertility problem, most aren't expert in infertility treatment. Ob/gyn residency programs usually include only a few weeks of infertility training, without much emphasis on the endocrinology and physiology that contribute to female and male infertility. And rarely is time devoted to understanding ways to help couples deal with the emotional component of infertility.

Instead, if you need a fertility specialist who concentrates on female infertility, look for a reproductive endocrinologist (a gynecologist who specializes in reproductive endocrinology), and who is qualified to manage a female fertility workup. A fertility expert specializing in male infertility is usually a urologist or an andrologist (an M.D. or Ph.D. who specializes in male fertility and in assisted reproductive technologies). Many urologists are also andrologists.

To become board-certified in reproductive endocrinology, a doctor must first become board-certified in obstetrics/gynecology and then

- Attend a two- or three-year fellowship in reproductive endocrinology.
- Pass a written exam on the topic.
- Complete a two-year practice experience in reproductive endocrinology.

- Pass a three-hour oral exam in reproductive endocrinology.

Some doctors have completed all but the oral examination and are still undergoing their practice experience in reproductive endocrinology. These doctors are board-eligible in reproductive endocrinology. Many ob/gyns advertise themselves as specialists in "obstetrics, gynecology, and infertility," but these doctors are seldom, if ever, reproductive endocrinologists.

Urologists with a subspecialty in andrology are the most highly qualified doctors to handle all aspects of male factor infertility. These doctors have completed a two-year fellowship and passed an examination to become a board-certified andrologist.

Choosing a good doctor

Infertility can cause feelings of frustration and helplessness. One way to ease some of these feelings is by finding a good specialist and taking an active role in your own medical care so that you can regain some sense of control and feel the satisfaction of actively participating in the decisions that will affect the course of your infertility treatment. Two ways to find a good specialist who is board-certified in reproductive endocrinology are to

- Look in the *Directory of Medical Specialists* published by Who's Who (available at most public libraries); it lists all ob/gyns and their training.
- Contact the infertility organization RESOLVE (see Appendix A) to obtain their 700-member physician referral list, including geographic area, medical training, special expertise, and interests. Or call the ob/gyn department at your nearest medical school.

What to ask your doctor

Once you've found a specialist you think you and your partner can be comfortable with, make an appointment to discuss your case—and be sure to ask the following basic questions:

- What's the fee structure?
- Are there payment plans?
- Is there a call-in time for questions?
- Do you have weekend and holiday hours for lab and ultrasound services?
- What's the availability of procedures performed on weekends?
- With which hospitals are you associated?
- If assisted reproductive technology is needed, what is the take-home-a-live-baby rate?

What to expect on your first visit

Most infertility specialists will want to see you and your partner together at the first appointment to review what's been done and what tests are still needed. This is a good time to establish a solid doctor-patient relationship. Remember, infertility is a couple problem—both of you need to cope with the stress, frustration, and sadness of your reproductive problems. It's essential that your doctor recognize these emotional issues and include both of you in discussions on how to pursue treatment.

If your problem is a "male factor" problem, your doctor may refer your partner to a urologist who specializes in infertility, or to an andrologist (a subspecialty in urology). In either case, it's essential that there is good communication among all doctors involved in your infertility care. Don't assume that the doctors themselves will make this happen.

Ask your doctor to send reports to the other participating doctors, and request that they communicate with each other—and you—frequently.

Infertility tests

A medical evaluation may determine the cause of your infertility. But if a medical and sexual history doesn't reveal an obvious problem (like improperly timed sex or absence of ovulation), specific tests may be needed.

For you, the first step in testing is to determine if you are ovulating each month. This can be done by charting changes in morning body temperature, by using an FDA-approved home ovulation test kit (which is available over the counter), or by examining cervical mucus, which undergoes a series of hormone-induced changes throughout the menstrual cycle.

Your doctor can check your ovulation in the office with simple blood tests for hormone levels or ultrasound tests of the ovaries. If you are ovulating, further testing will need to be done. Common female tests include

- Postcoital test (this should never take the place of a complete semen analysis, and is felt to be of little use at all these days).
- Laparoscopy: An outpatient surgical examination of female organs for endometriosis, tubal health, or pelvic scarring, using a miniature light-transmitting tube inserted into the abdomen through a one-inch incision below the navel while under general anesthesia.
- Endometrial biopsy: An examination of a small shred of uterine lining to check the quality of the uterine lining.

If you haven't had these tests done, ask your doctor about them. It's useless to proceed with treatment unless you have ruled out all the possibilities. Keep in mind hat all these tests aren't always done; evaluation depends on your own history, exam findings and results of prior tests.

Getting a second opinion (or changing doctors)

As the patient, it's your job to evaluate the care you're getting. Educating yourself about infertility is a good way to do this. It may be time to change doctors if

- Your doctor doesn't seem to have a treatment plan or wants to continue the same treatment that has been used for three to four cycles without success.

- Communication is poor; you feel reluctant to ask questions or you feel like your concerns are quickly dismissed.

- The doctor seems confused about your case; you have to remind him or her that various tests have already been done.

- The obstetrical part of your doctor's practice seems to affect the amount of quality time your doctor can spend with his or her infertility patients.

- Hormonal treatments aren't being carefully monitored.

Unexplained infertility

The results from the fertility tests will likely determine the treatments that are recommended, but 80 to 90 percent of infertility cases are treated with

Bright Idea
If you're thinking of making a transition from a gynecologist to a fertility specialist, you may want to do this before a diagnostic laparoscopy is scheduled.

drugs or surgery. Unfortunately though, after all the infertility tests have been done, there will still be between 10 and 15 percent of all infertile couples who will never discover the reason for their inability to conceive or carry a baby to term.

Of those infertile couples who are given a diagnosis of unexplained infertility, about 20 percent will become pregnant each year for three years. The rest just aren't successful. However, even in the case of unexplained infertility, fertility drugs and a number of assisted reproductive technologies (ART) may eventually lead to a pregnancy.

Fertility drugs

If you aren't ovulating, drugs or hormones can induce ovulation artificially. Therapy with the fertility drug Clomid or with a more potent hormone stimulator—Pergonal, Metrodin, Humegon, or Fertinex—is often recommended for women with ovulation problems. The benefits of each drug and the side effects (which can be minor or serious but are always rare), should be discussed with your doctor. Multiple births occur in 10 to 20 percent of births resulting from fertility drug use.

Other drugs—used under very limited circumstances—include Parlodel (bromocriptine mesylate), if you have high levels of the hormone prolactin, or a hormone pump that releases gonadotropins necessary for ovulation.

Between 80 and 90 percent of women using these methods will start ovulating, but the pregnancy rate is lower, depending on what other factors are present that may be affecting your infertility.

Note that it's quite common for women taking fertility drugs to experience depression, which can sometimes be quite severe. Infertility itself can be a

Unofficially...
A recent Harvard University study found that women undergoing fertility treatments showed depression levels equal to women facing treatment for cancer or AIDS.

depressing condition for many couples. In addition, fertility drugs trigger hormonal changes that can cause depression by interfering with estrogen (a natural antidepressant). If you're experiencing severe symptoms of depression, you should discuss your feelings with your doctor.

Surgery

If drugs aren't the answer, surgery to repair damage to your ovaries, fallopian tubes, or uterus may be recommended—but this is major surgery, so it's recommended only if there is a good chance of restoring fertility.

Artificial insemination

If your partner has a problem with sperm production, artificial insemination by a donor may help you conceive. With this method, your reproductive endocrinologist will place sperm from a selected donor into your uterus. Costs vary, but the procedure alone will set you back about $120, not including any other lab tests or sperm procurement. The success rate for this procedure varies depending on the reason that you're not able to conceive.

Bright Idea
If your partner has a few healthy sperm, it may be possible to use his sperm in artificial insemination after special washings and concentrating treatments.

Sperm banks

A sperm bank maintains frozen sperm donated by healthy men, which are then screened for diseases and made available for implantation. In the United States, donating sperm is a commercial enterprise and donors are paid for their donations. (This is not the case in most other countries, where sperm donation is viewed much like giving blood—as an altruistic service that you can perform to help others.)

Today, there are more than 400 sperm banks in the United States, some of which are state-licensed and regulated; however, throughout the country, complying with licensing regulations and standards is still fairly voluntary. Current sperm-bank standards require initial and interval testing for at least some infectious diseases, including AIDS, syphilis, and hepatitis B and C. Donors also should be tested occasionally for chlamydia and gonorrhea. Because a donor's sperm could be infected with a disease such as AIDS or hepatitis, most banks freeze and quarantine sperm for six months while the donor undergoes repeated testing for these diseases. The semen is released when the tests are negative for at least 180 days after donation. Sperm banks guarantee a minimum number of live sperm per specimen.

Most sperm banks charge a registration fee or require a physician referral. Prepared semen costs between $100 and $250, depending on the geographic location of the bank, the quantity of semen in each vial and (among banks that reveal detailed characteristics) the popularity of the donor.

All reputable, ethical reproductive endocrinologists have a relationship with a sperm bank that meets all of the above criteria. If yours doesn't, get a new reproductive endocrinologist.

The process...

Before ordering sperm, a woman should get a physical exam and lab tests to rule out pregnancy-related risks, as well as genetic health risks for a child. Many banks recommend testing for immunity to rubella (German measles), a Pap smear, and a culture for chlamydia. Some banks may require testing for AIDS, syphilis, and gonorrhea.

Most sperm banks can deliver sperm anywhere from a few days to a few weeks, depending on their own requirements; it's possible to send sperm directly to the home, but some banks will only ship to a physician.

Selecting a donor

You can select a donor after reviewing donor characteristics (the amount of donor information available to you varies from one bank to another). Some sperm banks offer just a brief physical description and a medical history, whereas others provide detailed information featuring donor hobbies, IQ, awards, education, personality, occupation, and reasons for becoming a donor.

By 1980, at least one "superbaby" sperm bank had been established in order to allow Nobel Prize winners to sell their sperm. Twelve years later, two more sperm banks in California began to specialize in selling the sperm of "gifted" men. One bank, the Repository for Germinal Choice, affiliated with the Foundation for the Advancement of Man, provides detailed descriptions of each donor for approved applicants.

Confidentiality

In the past, all sperm banks kept information about donors confidential, with the implication that being paid for sperm severed all rights the donor might otherwise have had to any offspring. Recently, a few, more progressive, sperm banks have begun to release information about the donors to children born as a result of donor insemination, once they reach 18.

The Sperm Bank of California in Berkeley was the first bank to offer this service, releasing the name, address, phone number, social security number, driver's license number, and hometown of donors. This "sunshine" policy is still fairly unusual in the United States, although fertility experts believe it may become more common over time. In Sweden, this "open donor identity" has been mandatory since 1989.

Offspring limits

Many sperm banks also limit the number of children who can be born as a result of insemination from one donor. This is done to reduce the chance of closely related biological children inadvertently marrying. While there is no legal requirement, most banks set a limit of five children born per state and another five out of state. (It's possible, however, that the same donor may provide semen to another sperm bank, thus exceeding the recommended limit.)

Assistive reproductive technology: The latest

If drugs, surgery and artificial insemination don't work for you, there's still hope. New, more complex ART procedures, including in vitro fertilization, have been available since the birth 18 years ago of Louise Brown, the world's first "test-tube baby."

How do you decide where to go for assistive reproductive technology? The Society for Assisted Reproductive Technology (SART), an organization of ART providers affiliated with the American Society for Reproductive Medicine (ASRM), has been collecting data and publishing annual reports of pregnancy success rates for fertility clinics in the United States and Canada since 1989. In 1992, Congress passed the Fertility Clinic Success Rate and Certification Act, which requires the Centers for Disease Control and Prevention (CDC) to publish pregnancy success rates for fertility clinics in the

Unofficially...
To guard against the marriage of closely related biological children, some countries, such as England and Sweden, maintain a central registry that limits the total number of children from one donor's semen.

United States. The 1996 report of pregnancy success rates (released in 1999) is the second to be issued under the law.

In vitro fertilization (IVF)

IVF makes it possible to combine sperm and eggs in a lab to produce a baby that is genetically related to one or both partners. IVF is often used when a woman's fallopian tubes are blocked. This is how it's done:

1. Medication stimulates your ovaries to produce multiple eggs.
2. Once mature, the eggs are suctioned from the ovaries and placed in a lab culture dish with your partner's sperm for fertilization.
3. The dish is then placed in an incubator.
4. About two days later, three to five embryos are transferred to the woman's uterus. Within 11 to 14 days, a blood test can tell you whether you're pregnant. If the woman does not become pregnant, she may try again in the next cycle.

While IVF doesn't have an encouraging success rate, remember that in normal fertile couples, only 55 percent of all pregnancies result in a live birth. With IVF, about 23 percent of all IVF pregnancies will end in a live birth (that figure drops to less than 10 percent in women over age 40). (The rate of miscarriage in IVF pregnancies is higher than in the general population as well; 25 to 30 percent of all IVF pregnancies end in first trimester miscarriage.)

If you haven't conceived after four completed IVF tries, it's probably time to look at alternatives. The average cost of one IVF cycle in the United States (including drugs, doctor, and clinic fees) is about $7,800. Fees paid to sperm donors range between $25 and $75; fees paid to egg donors range between $1,500 and $3,000.

Gamete intrafallopian transfer

Gamete intrafallopian transfer (GIFT) is a type of ART similar to IVF (but about half as expensive and requiring about a third of the time) that is used if you have at least one normal fallopian tube. Instead of fertilizing the eggs in a lab, three to five of your mature eggs along with donor sperm are mixed in a syringe and placed in the fallopian tube for fertilization inside your body. A general anesthetic is necessary, which can make recovery uncomfortable.

The entire procedure takes about an hour, and it carries a slightly higher success rate than IVF (pregnancy rate is about 35 percent), but it also carries the same risks and stresses as IVF. A maximum of four GIFT cycles is recommended.

Zygote intrafallopian transfer

Zygote intrafallopian transfer (ZIFT, or tubal embryo transfer) is a hybrid of IVF and GIFT. Basically, ZIFT is the same thing as GIFT except that the eggs are fertilized in the lab but not cultured into embryos; instead, the fertilized egg and sperm are transferred in an undivided state (called a "zygote"). In ZIFT, the transfer of the sperm and egg is done 18 to 52 hours after the egg is retrieved. Either laparoscopy or an ultrasound-guided transvaginal procedure is used to transfer the zygotes into the fallopian tube.

Donor egg IVF

You may prefer IVF with a donor egg if, for example, you have impaired ovaries or carry a genetic disease that can be transferred to your offspring. Eggs are donated by another healthy woman and fertilized in the lab with your partner's sperm before being transferred to your uterus.

Women who get pregnant with donor eggs have a higher rate of miscarriage and a higher implantation failure rate (probably because of a lesser capacity to maintain a pregnancy). ART with egg donoration among women with premature ovarian failure is the most successful treatment for infertility—success rates are as high as 50 percent. The price of a donor egg cycle is about equal to the price of adoption: $14,000 to $20,000.

Frozen embryos
Embryos are most often frozen when more eggs are retrieved in one cycle than can safely be transferred to the woman's uterus after fertilization. Rather than throw them out, most clinics fertilize and freeze them for transfer in later cycles.

There are a variety of techniques that involve freezing embryos so that you can sustain your fertility if you're at risk for ovarian failure or if you want to try repeated IVFs. With this method, you can have your eggs harvested and fertilized and then have the embryo frozen to be transferred at a later date. The pregnancy rate with two or three embryos transferred is about 15 to 25 percent and the odds go up with each repeated transfer. This technique is useful if you don't get pregnant on the first cycle or if you want another baby in the future.

Just the facts
- The newest birth control methods involve hormonal implants and injections, female condoms and the contraceptive sponge.

- Newer, safer forms of the pill are highly effective and reasonably safe for most nonsmoking women up to age 45.
- Infertility is diagnosed if you are unable to become pregnant after trying for a year.
- Most cases of infertility are successfully treated using drugs or hormones.
- Assisted reproductive technologies are the most modern ways to treat infertile couples and include in vitro fertilization, gamete intrafallopian transfer, and zygote intrafallopian transfer.

GET THE SCOOP ON...
Choosing a health practitioner ▪ Evaluating screening tests ▪ Having a healthy baby

Pregnancy

Pregnancy is a time of change and anticipation. If you've just learned that you're expecting, you've got nine months to experience the joys and tribulations of pregnancy. If your pregnancy is a little further along, you've already had a taste of what expecting a baby entails.

Pregnancy tests: Are they reliable?

Detecting pregnancy early makes it possible for you to take the best possible care of yourself—and your baby. If you think you may be pregnant, you'll want to verify your suspicions as soon as possible. You can buy a home pregnancy test at any drugstore—there are many brands of these home tests, but they all diagnose pregnancy by detecting a hormone called human chorionic gonadotropin (hCG). Home tests can detect the hormone as early as a day or two after a missed period, and they yield results in just minutes. (Make sure you read the instructions before performing the test, and then follow the directions carefully.)

Because home pregnancy tests are more often correct when they indicate a positive than a negative result, if you do a home test and get a negative

Unofficially...
Decades ago, pregnancy tests were downright deadly to female rabbits, which were injected with urine from a woman who was thought to be pregnant. The rabbit was then killed; if the rabbit's ovaries had matured and developed blood spots from the urine, the woman was pregnant. Today, more humane means of testing have been developed and rabbits are no longer sacrificed.

result, it's a good idea to retake the test in a few days (some brands are sold with two tests to a box), or go see a doctor or lab for another test.

Your doctor will use either a urine or blood test to determine pregnancy. The urine test detects the presence of hCG, just as with the at-home tests. If the test is done in a doctor's office, you'll probably get the results before you leave, but results from lab tests usually need to be phoned in to the doctor's office, and then relayed to you. The blood test is extremely reliable and can detect pregnancy very early after conception by measuring the exact amount of hCG found in the blood. This can give a rough idea of gestational age, but it can't detect pregnancy before implantation, which occurs about seven days after conception.

Choosing a practitioner who's right for you

Congratulations—you're pregnant! The first important decision you'll need to make is choosing what type of health care provider you'll use to see you through the pregnancy. It's extremely important to get good care early on, since regular prenatal visits are vital to having a healthy baby. You, your partner, and your practitioner will work as a team to make sure your pregnancy is successful. There are many types of practitioners available today to oversee your pregnancy, labor, and the birth of your baby. Each is described in the sections that follow.

Obstetrician/gynecologist

You're probably most familiar with the ob/gyn who holds either an M.D. or doctor of osteopathy (D.O.) degree. The distinction between M.D.s and D.O.s is vanishing. An ob/gyn has completed at least four years of specialized training in obstetrics and gynecological medicine after medical school. Many are board certified in these areas after passing the American Board of Obstetrics and Gynecology exams. An ob/gyn also may be a fellow of the American College of Obstetricians and Gynecologists (FACOG); a doctor can only become a fellow after being board certified in ob/gyn.

Perinatologist

This is an obstetrician with specialized training in handling high-risk pregnancies (sometimes called a maternal-fetal medicine specialist). If you're pregnant with five or six babies, you might want to think about working with a perinatologist; generally, you should be referred from another physician. Most perinatologists don't primarily handle pregnancies on their own; rather they work in conjunction with a general ob/gyn for management of a high risk pregnancy. In addition, they perform advanced ultrasounds and invasive procedures such as amniocentesis. Women who may benefit from seeing a perinatologist include those with diabetes, high blood pressure, or other pregnancy complications. Often, a perinatologist is used as a consultant by an ob/gyn or midwife.

Family physician

Also called a "family practitioner," this person is an M.D. with specialty training in family medicine, including obstetrics. The family physician is an updated version of the old-time general practitioner, and can serve as an internist, ob/gyn, and pediatrician, all rolled into one. Some family practitioners actively practice obstetrics and are competent to handle low-risk pregnancies; others have no interest or desire to deliver babies.

Other care providers

There are several categories of birth care providers, ranging from nurse midwives to birthing assistants (doulas). Most work independently, but others work together with an obstetrician as part of a team.

- Certified nurse midwife (CNM): Licensed health care practitioners educated in the two disciplines of nursing and midwifery, CNMs provide primary care to women of childbearing age. They can offer prenatal care, labor and delivery care, care after birth, gynecological exams, newborn care, assistance with family planning decisions, preconception care, menopausal management, and counseling in health maintenance and disease prevention. CNMs are certified by the American College of Nurse Midwives, the official professional organization. The minimal academic entry level degree in most states is a master's degree (67 percent of CNMs and certified midwives [CMs, see below] have master's degrees). CNMs attend births mainly in hospitals, but can also be found in birthing centers and at home. For more information about education and training of nurse midwives, check out www.midwife.org.

- Lay midwife: The North American Registry of Midwives recently began credentialing midwives who are not registered nurses, called "certified midwives." Also known as a "lay midwife," the CMs have midwifery training but no nursing degree. Training and the exams necessary for licensing vary from state to state (some states don't license midwives). NARM's Web site is www.mana.org.

- Labor assistant: Also called a "doula," this health care provider is trained and experienced in childbirth to provide physical, emotional, and informational support to women and their partners during labor and birth. Doulas can offer help and advice on comfort measures such as breathing, relaxation, movement, and positioning; help families gather information about the course of their labor and their options; provide continuous emotional reassurance and comfort; and specialize in non-medical skills. Doulas can't diagnose medical conditions, offer second opinions, or give medical advice; instead, they help the woman have a safe and satisfying childbirth as the woman defines it. A doula should not be confused with a nurse midwife, who actively handles labor and delivery. The Doulas of North America Web site is found at www.dona.com.

Watch Out!
If you choose a midwife as your primary or secondary practitioner, make sure you get details about her credentials. Be sure whomever you choose has access to a doctor to help if necessary during labor and birth.

So many choices...

Although all of these health care practitioners share a common goal of seeing you through pregnancy, labor, and delivery, their philosophies, attitudes, and methods may vary a great deal. It's very important to find a practitioner with whom you feel at ease, and who shares your basic attitudes toward pregnancy and birth. Work with your partner to find someone with whom you both feel comfortable—remember, it's your pregnancy.

Where to find a practitioner

There are several ways to find out about doctors and other health care professionals available in your area:

- Referral: If your health care provider doesn't do deliveries, ask for a referral—remember that doctors normally recommend others with similar attitudes and philosophies.

- Ask friends: Poll your friends who are pregnant or have recently had babies, asking about their practitioners' attitudes and philosophies. (Keep in mind, however, that somebody your friend thinks is perfect might not be a good fit for you.)
- Internet: Lots of hospitals maintain their own web sites these days; many of these web sites list doctors by their areas of specialty. Many physicians and practices also have their own web sites these days. Or check out www.obgyn.net.
- Hospital staff: If a local hospital has a good reputation, ask a staff member to give you the names of the facility's obstetricians and midwives.
- Birthing center: If you're interested in a birthing center and there's one nearby, ask for some references (this is especially helpful if you're interested in a midwife).
- Teaching hospital: If you're moving to a new area and want to find a physician, call the closest teaching hospital and ask to speak with the chief resident in the specialty you're looking for.

Interviewing a health practitioner

Once you have some names and details about practitioners in your area, it's time to schedule an appointment with the ones you're most interested in. Think of these appointments as your opportunity to interview your potential doctor or midwife, and don't be afraid to ask questions. While it's highly unlikely that you, your partner and your health care provider will agree 100 percent on everything, it's important to share basic philosophies concerning pregnancy, labor, and delivery. Of course, it's not

Bright Idea
Check out www.babycenter.com/health/search, which offers a "Find a Health Care Provider" service. The American College of Nurse Midwives Web site has a "Find a Midwife" service, too: www.midwife.org/find.

unreasonable to be charged for this visit, so be prepared to pay. In addition, your attitude at the visit is essential; remember, you and the provider are on the same side. Don't be confrontational. Be sure you find out the practitioner's attitudes concerning

- Your role during pregnancy, labor, and birth. Will your practitioner encourage you to play an active role, or prefer that you sit back and let him or her run the show?
- Birthing options (birthing rooms, birthing beds, family-centered care and so on).
- The use of pain management available at your chosen birthing facility, and the health care provider's attitude toward pain management.
- Cesarean sections (some practitioners are much quicker to perform C-sections than others).
- Ask about the practitioner's attitude toward intervention during birth: "Could you tell me the circumstances under which you would use the following: internal monitoring, vacuums, and episiotomies?"
- How much of your labor you should (or would like to) do at home.
- Getting out of bed during labor and/or laboring in water.
- Who will cover for your practitioner if he or she is not available when you are ready to deliver.
- During how much of your labor will the practitioner actually be there for?
- Can your partner cut the cord or help catch the baby?
- If a C-section is necessary, can your partner be in the operating room?

- The use of cameras or video cameras in the birthing room. (This is a new controversy; some hospitals are now forbidding videotaping during births. Find out the policy beforehand.)

You and the practitioner you choose will be working together over the next nine months to make sure you deliver a healthy baby. It's important to feel confident about your choice so you'll be inclined to listen carefully to him or her and try hard to follow his or her recommendations. Don't try to tie the practitioner's hands in advance. It's important to realize that there is no right answer to a lot of these questions, and it's often difficult to predict what will happen in your labor. C-sections, forceps, vacuum—all may become necessary very quickly.

The birth site: The inside scoop

Choosing a practitioner isn't the only thing you've got to consider; you'll also need to decide where you want to have your baby. While nearly 99 percent of all American babies are born in hospitals, more and more women are choosing to give birth at home or in birthing centers.

In colonial times, birth was a social event; relatives and neighbors would join with one or more midwives as the mother labored and birthed her baby. This was a time when the mother's mortality rates were 1 in 100. It wasn't until the beginning of the 1900s that doctors began attending deliveries in women's homes. By the 1940s, most women in the United States were having their children in hospitals—and the mortality rate dropped to 1 in 10,000.

Where you choose to have a baby isn't only a matter of which you'd prefer, however; other factors affecting where you'll have your baby include

- Whether or not you think you're going to want anesthesia.
- Where your practitioner chooses to practices, or where he or she has hospital privileges.
- Whether or not you're at risk for complications during pregnancy and delivery.
- Your preferences: Do you prefer a medical setting or your own bed as the birth place?
- The type of medical insurance you have and the cost of care.

The hospital

There are many advantages to having your baby in a hospital. First, it's the place best equipped to handle any medical complications that may crop up during labor and delivery. Specialized skills, experienced personnel, and any necessary equipment or supplies ensure the best possible care for you and your baby. In addition, most hospitals offer more options for your labor and delivery today than ever before, so make sure you find out what's available in your hospital. If you're thinking about giving birth in a hospital, ask your practitioner about these options:

- Birthing rooms: More homelike, comfortable, and private than the traditional delivery room, birthing rooms allow a woman to labor, deliver, and experience a recovery period all in the same setting. Check with your hospital to see how many birthing rooms there are, and what happens if they're all in use when you begin labor.
- Rooming in: With this option, your baby stays with you in your room instead of returning to the nursery between visits and feedings. Rooming in is intended to enhance the important early bonding between baby and parents,

and to give you more experience handling your baby before taking him or her home. The disadvantage to rooming in is that you might not get as much rest as you would if your baby was spending time in the nursery. Ask about the flexibility of your hospital's rooming in policy. If you decide you need to rest, will you be able to send your baby to the nursery?

- Mother-baby care: Also called "family-centered maternity care," this option provides one nurse to each mother and baby. The baby stays with the mother (at least during the day, and often at night, too), while the nurse assists with things like feeding and bathing.

- The nursery: Birthing is hard work, so don't feel that you're a bad mother if you want to skip rooming in and have your baby returned to the nursery so you can get some much-needed rest. You'll have more than your share of late nights with your baby once you get home.

The birthing center

A birthing center separate from a hospital may seem like an innovation, but birthing centers aren't some newfangled idea popularized by baby boomers looking for novelties. The first birthing center in the United States was opened during the 1940s in New Mexico as an option for women who couldn't afford to have their babies in hospitals.

While many women without much money or any insurance still prefer birthing centers, centers are becoming more popular with women searching for an alternative to the sterile atmosphere of the average hospital delivery room.

Birthing centers must be licensed by the Commission for the Accreditation of Freestanding

Birth Centers, and normally are staffed by certified nurse midwives who work together with obstetricians should a problem arise.

Generally, staff at these centers consider birth to be a natural process, not a medical procedure, and natural childbirth is encouraged. While most practitioners agree that birthing centers are safe for women with low-risk pregnancies, most experts believe that women with high-risk pregnancies should give birth in a hospital. However, even low-risk women can occasionally experience a serious emergency. It's important to ask the question: How would I feel if my baby or I suffered a rare but life-threatening complication that could have been avoided in a hospital?"

If you and your partner are considering a birthing center, be sure to ask these questions:

- Is the center accredited?
- Who staffs the center, and what are their credentials?
- What type of specialized equipment is available at the birth center, should any be necessary?
- What backup is available in case of an emergency?
- What transportation is available in case you need to get to a hospital?
- What hospital would you be taken to and how long would it take to get there?
- What's the policy regarding pain medication?
- How long would you stay in the birthing center after birth?
- What insurance is accepted by the birthing center and what costs are involved?

Bright Idea
For more information about birthing centers, send a self-addressed, stamped envelope to the National Association of Childbearing Centers, RD 1, Box 1, Perkiomenville, PA 18074.

Home births

While home births have always been popular in certain rural areas of the country and among some religious groups, the idea is gaining popularity among more and more American women who, for one reason or another, prefer not to give birth in a hospital. While the idea of having your baby in the comfort and familiarity of your own home might sound appealing, there are also some risks associated with the practice.

Bright Idea
For more information on home birth, contact Informed Homebirth and Parenting, P.O. Box 3675, Ann Arbor, MI 48106. Or, call the center at 313/662-6857.

The primary disadvantage of a home birth is the lack of immediate medical backup in case of an emergency. Some doctors and licensed nurse midwives won't agree to do a home birth because of the risks involved, and some insurance companies won't cover the cost of a home birth. Women who are considered "high-risk" may not want to consider having their babies at home.

Regardless of where you decide to have your baby, the most important thing is a safe labor and delivery. You'll need to get all the information you can, and consider all the advantages and disadvantages of these birthing options before making your decision.

Your first prenatal visit

At your first prenatal visit, your practitioner will probably determine your due date. Purely by arbitrary convention, health care providers calculate an average pregnancy as lasting 280 days, counting from the first day of the last period. To calculate your due date:

- Determine the first day of your last period.
- Count backward three months to find out the month in which you'll have your baby.

- Now add seven to the day of the month that your last period began. That's your due date.

This method works 85 percent of the time if you have regular periods 28 days apart.

Remember that only 5 percent of all babies are born on their due dates; delivery within a week or two either way is considered normal. If you make the mistake of assuming you'll begin labor on your due date, it can be psychologically difficult to have to wait for labor to start—and remember, first babies are notoriously "late." It's best to assume your baby will appear a week beyond your due date; that way, you can be pleasantly surprised if you go into labor before that time.

At each visit (usually once a month), your practitioner will probably check your weight, your blood pressure, and test your urine for sugar and protein. He or she will look for any signs of swelling in your hands and feet (which could indicate a serious condition called pre-eclampsia), and check your legs for indications of varicose veins. Be prepared with any questions and concerns.

Screening tests: do you need them?

Once you know that you're definitely pregnant, most practitioners will want you to take at least a few diagnostic tests to make sure your baby is healthy and developing normally. Some tests (such as urinalysis) are routine and may be done at every checkup; others (such as amniocentesis), are recommended only in some cases.

Basic tests

There are a range of basic tests that most practitioners consider for many women, including

Unofficially...
A baby's heartbeat can be detected with extremely sensitive devices at as early as six weeks' gestation; normally, it can be seen with ultrasound at about 10 to 12 weeks, and heard at about 18 to 20 weeks with a stethoscope.

- Blood tests: The blood test checks for your blood group and Rh factor; screens for a range of conditions including anemia, hepatitis, syphilis; and checks for immunity to diseases such as rubella (German measles). Depending on the state, AIDS testing frequently requires the woman's specific written consent.
- Cervical cultures: This test checks for infection with gonorrhea and chlamydia.
- Genetic tests: If you're at risk for genetic conditions, you may be tested for sickle-cell anemia, Tay-Sachs disease, or cystic fibrosis.
- Chromosomal or chorionic villus sampling (CVS) tests to rule out chromosomal problems (for example, if mom is older than 35).
- Pap smear: A smear will help rule out cervical cancer and other conditions.
- Diabetes screening: This is done especially for women who are gaining weight too fast, have a family history of diabetes, or have previously delivered a very large baby (nine pounds or larger). It's done at 28 weeks and is recommended for all pregnant women by some, and only for those for those who have risk factors by others. Risk factors include age 25 or older, family history of diabetes, previous large baby, previous stillbirth, or weight over 200 (some say 250) pounds.

Ultrasound: how many, how often

There's nothing like watching a video of your baby while he or she is still floating around inside the womb. But there is a difference between screening and diagnostic ultrasounds. Most studies have shown little value of screening (that is, doing ultrasound on all pregnancies). As a diagnostic test, however, ultrasound is the most valuable diagnostic advance in obstetrics this century.

Ultrasound uses high-frequency sound waves to form pictures of the fetus that appear on a computer screen. Ultrasound is used to

- Verify due date.
- Determine the cause of bleeding.
- Check health, growth, and position of the fetus.
- Assess placental health.
- Check for fetal anomalies and verify general health.
- Measure amount of amniotic fluid.

Generally, your health care provider may order one ultrasound in the first trimester (before 12 weeks) and one ultrasound in the second trimester (at approximately 22 to 24 weeks).

Ultrasound is not always covered by insurance. Because "everyone" has an ultrasound, too often women assume insurance automatically covers it. Ultrasound must be deemed medically necessary to be covered.

Alpha-fetoprotein (AFP) test

This simple blood test carries no risk to the fetus since it simply measures the levels of AFP in your blood. Most women are offered the AFP test (it's optional) to identify if the baby is at higher-than-average risk for certain serious birth defects. Your practitioner should give you thorough counseling regarding the implications of this test.

Neural tube defects are among the most common and severe problems associated with high AFP levels. In about 2,500 babies in this country, the neural tube (part of the developing brain and spinal cord) doesn't close properly during the fourth week after conception, leading to birth defects, such as spina bifida (the improper formation of the spinal column so that part of the lower spine is open; this may affect various functions such as walking, urinating, and defecating). Low AFP levels are sometimes associated with chromosomal abnormalities such as Down syndrome, but this test isn't as accurate in detecting these problems. Most chromosomal defects other than Down syndrome are not identified by enhanced AFP screening, nor can the test definitely diagnose or rule out Down syndrome, as can amniocentesis or CVS.

The test is most often done between 15 and 18 weeks after the last menstrual period, and the results are usually available within a week. If the AFP levels are abnormal, the test may be repeated, but in most cases an abnormal result doesn't mean the fetus is abnormal—it just identifies those at higher risk. Further testing is needed to confirm a problem.

As many as 100 out of every 1,000 women who take the test have an abnormal result, but only about 10 of these 100 women will have a fetus with a birth defect. For the others, the abnormal AFP level just means the fetus is either a few weeks older or younger than first thought. A multiple pregnancy also can lead to an elevated reading.

Triple screening

Most women today are offered an enhanced AFP test called "triple screening," which measures AFP and two pregnancy hormones called estriol and hCG (discussed above). This test appears to detect at least 60 percent of Down syndrome cases, compared to about 30 percent with AFP screening alone. A computer calculates the risk of Down syndrome based on the levels of these three substances plus the woman's age and certain other factors.

The main purpose of the triple screen is to determine which women under age 35 are at risk for having a child with Down syndrome. About 80 percent of Down syndrome children come from women who are under 35 and wouldn't be offered an amniocentesis based on age alone. This is because, while the risk is lower in women under 35, the number of women having babies under that age is much greater than the number over the age of 35.

Remember the triple screen never specifically points to the presence of Down syndrome; rather, it takes maternal age, presence or absence of diabetes, maternal weight, race, and the results of the three tests run as the triple screen and determines a statistical risk for that particular pregnancy. That risk may be as low as 1 in 10,000, but it is never 0 in 10,000.

Amniocentesis: Not for everyone

This test (performed at 16 weeks) checks out cells shed by the fetus into the amniotic fluid. Your doctor will insert a long, thin needle through your abdomen to extract fluid from the womb (often guided by ultrasound to avoid nicking the baby). Amniocentesis can reliably identify the sex of the fetus and indicate problems such as Down syndrome or Tay-Sachs disease. Results take 10 days to two weeks. However, the test may be done as early as 12 weeks to spot chromosomal anomalies and as late as nine months, depending on many factors.

While considered to be safe in most cases, it can cause cramps, leakage of amniotic fluid, and vaginal bleeding and may boost the risk of miscarriage by between 0.5 and one percent. While some experts believe it's not a test that should be automatically offered to every woman, any woman of any age may have an amniocentesis simply by asking.

Chorionic villus sampling (CVS)

This prenatal test, which can diagnose or rule out certain birth defects, is a slightly earlier alternative to amniocentesis. It has slightly different complications and risks. It's usually performed between 10 and 12 weeks after your last menstrual period, it's not routinely offered to every pregnant woman because of the slight risk of miscarriage and other complications. Because some babies were born with missing or shortened fingers or toes when the test was performed before the tenth week, CVS is now performed only after this date. You may decide to have the test if your baby is at higher risk of chromosomal problems or genetic birth defects.

During the test, the practitioner extracts a small piece of the chorionic villi (CV), a part of the placenta, by inserting a catheter or needle into the womb via the cervix. Basically, CVS is a biopsy of the placenta; placenta chromosomes are usually (but not always) the same as fetus chromosomes. Preliminary results are often available within 24 hours, with the final results at 7 to 10 days.

One woman in three has some bleeding or spotting after CVS, and one in five have cramps after the procedure. More than 95 percent of high-risk women who have the test find that their babies don't have any disorders.

CVS versus amniocentesis

Some women prefer CVS to amniocentesis, because test results are available sooner than for amniocentesis. On the other hand, some women prefer amniocentesis to CVS because

Watch Out!
CVS is usually not a good idea if you've had any vaginal bleeding or spotting, or if you have a family history of neural-tube defects (the test can't screen for these). Also, the less experienced a practitioner is with CVS, the higher the risk of CVS-related pregnancy loss, according to studies.

- Studies suggest amniocentesis has a slightly lower risk of miscarriage (less than 1 in 200, compared to the risk for CVS of between 1 and 2 in 100; the risk may rise to about 5 in 100 for a woman with an abnormal uterus).
- While CVS is very accurate in ruling out certain chromosomal defects and specific genetic problems, it's more likely than amniocentesis to give inconclusive results.

How you'll look, what you'll feel

You're about to experience some wonderful (and maybe not so wonderful) changes over the next nine months. Here's some insight into what you may be feeling, how you can expect to look and what your baby will look like during the course of your pregnancy.

First trimester

You won't look much different during the first month of your pregnancy. Your menstrual period will probably stop (that may have been the first clue that you're pregnant!), but you may experience spotting or light bleeding, together with significant fatigue.

During the first trimester, you'll probably notice that your breasts may be swollen and tender, and you may feel bloated. Morning sickness can occur at any time during your pregnancy (and not just in the morning), but it usually appears during the first trimester and then disappears by the third month. Morning sickness rarely is a serious problem, but if it's severe you should discuss it with your practitioner.

By the second month, your heart starts pumping more blood and the function of many of your organs (even your skin) is changing. You may be visiting the bathroom constantly to urinate, or you may

Bright Idea
To help control nausea, eat small amounts of healthy food at frequent intervals, nibble a few dry crackers (such as saltines) right before getting up, and avoid foods and smells that make you feel sick. Many women swear by acupressure wrist bands (available at any drug store).

be constipated. By the end of the first trimester, you'll start to put on weight and your clothing will probably feel tight. You may notice veins on your breasts and other areas, and you might be feeling hungrier, especially if symptoms of morning sickness have diminished.

What your baby looks like

By the end of the first (post ovulation) month your baby is a tiny embryo, smaller than a grain of rice, with a head, a trunk tiny buds that will later become arms and legs, a developing digestive system, and a tiny heart that has begun beating. By the end of the second month, your baby has grown to an inch, with a beginning nervous system. All major internal organs have begun to appear, the heart is pumping blood and facial features are visible. There are arms and legs and the beginnings of fingers and toes. By the end of the first trimester, your baby is about four inches long and weighs a bit more than an ounce. The heart is forming its four chambers, major blood vessels are nearly complete and ears and eyelids have appeared.

How you may feel

During the first three months, you'll probably experience mood swings much like those associated with PMS. You might feel elated one moment and then sad and tearful the next, for no apparent reason. This is a time of great ambivalence in terms of your emotions—ambiguity is de riguer. The realization of a profound impending life stage change is unnerving for many women and takes enormous adjustment.

Second trimester

In the beginning of the second trimester, you'll probably have a better appetite than you did during the first few months. Odds are, your nausea and vomiting will stop by now. You may notice the beginnings of hemorrhoids, but probably don't have to urinate as frequently. Your abdomen will be enlarging, and breast changes will continue. Your nipples and areola (the dark area around the nipple) might darken, and you may notice a dark line running from your navel to the top of your pubic hair. This is called the "linea nigra," and usually disappears or fades after delivery. You also might develop chloasma (the "mask of pregnancy"), dark patches on your face that become darker in the sun. (Relax! This fades away once the baby comes.)

If you're very slender or have had other children, you might be able to feel some fetal movement by the end of the fourth month; however, it's not unusual to feel no movement at this stage. You should feel movements by the end of 20 weeks, however.

As you near the end of the second trimester, the skin on your abdomen starts to stretch and grow taut. You're probably experiencing a vaginal discharge, which will continue and grow heavier for the rest of your pregnancy. This is normal, but itching or a fishy odor is not and should be evaluated by your health care provider. Constipation may continue, and you might experience nasal congestion, nosebleeds, bleeding gums when brushing your teeth, leg cramps, and backaches. There may also be changes in your lovemaking: Orgasm for some women becomes easier; others find it more difficult to attain. Weight gain begins to pick up to a pound a week in the sixth month.

Your practitioner also may listen for the baby's heartbeat, and check the size of your uterus to see if the growth of the uterus is appropriate for the anticipated due date.

What your baby looks like

By the end of 16 weeks, your baby is six to seven inches long, with a bit of fuzzy hair, tooth buds, eyebrows and skin. By now, your baby is sleeping and waking, sucking, swallowing, and passing urine. By 22 weeks, your baby is about 10 inches long and weighs between a half and one pound. He or she is now covered with downy hair called lanugo.

By the end of the second trimester (28 weeks), your baby is about 12 inches long, and weighs between a pound and a pound and a half. The skin is thin and has no underlying fat. Finger and toe prints are visible. If your baby were born now, he or she could survive with special, intensive care. The survival rate, after 8 to 12 weeks in the Neonatal Intensive Care Unit at a cost of about $3,000 per day, is about 90 percent. About 90 percent of those survivors will have no evidence of neurological damage by one year of age. How many of them have behavior or academic problems in school is unknown. The mother's uterus is still the best incubator known.

Unofficially...
You may want to start talking to or playing music for your baby, since at 28 weeks he or she can hear and data show that the number of brain cells your baby has reaches the critical mass necessary to begin cognition.

How you may feel

You're probably feeling truly pregnant by this time, which is very reassuring to some women and anxiety provoking to others—but all these feelings are normal. In general, the second trimester is when most pregnant women feel wonderful, although some women may still be moody and might have trouble concentrating or may even become forgetful (so-called "pregnancy dementia"). As you near the end of the second trimester, your mood swings may even out, although you still might feel anxious about your pregnancy and any absentmindedness may continue.

Third trimester

Braxton-Hicks contractions (painless contractions as the uterus hardens briefly) might have already started (they can begin as early as 16 weeks). However, whether contractions are painless or not is of no significance to the development of premature labor. Any woman who has four contractions (painless or painful) per hour for two hours in a row should contact her health care provider immediately.

During the third trimester, you may notice stretch marks on your breasts and abdomen. Your breasts have enlarged and may leak some colostrum, the substance that precedes breast milk. You may have difficulty sleeping because it's hard to get comfortable, and you may still suffer with leg cramps, backache, and a stuffy nose. You might feel short of breath as the uterus begins to push against the bottom of your diaphragm, and you'll probably need to urinate more frequently—you may even leak some urine.

In your last month, you'll still feel your baby moving, but his or her movements will be less intense because there is less room to move around. Your navel may protrude as your skin gets increasingly tight across your abdomen. Your cervix is softening in preparation for childbirth, and your ankles might swell. Weight gain usually levels off.

Your practitioner will probably want to see you more often during your last trimester. In addition to the other checks, he or she will probably estimate the weight of your baby, and may do an internal examination of your cervix.

What your baby looks like

Your baby is growing rapidly now; he or she should be about 15 inches long and weigh between two and

Bright Idea
Tensing the muscles around your vagina and anus for 10-second intervals may help stop urine leakage, and will also help prevent incontinence after delivery. When you consciously stop the flow of urine by tensing the muscles, you are performing a "Kegel exercise."

Unofficially...
The best sleeping position during pregnancy is on your left side, with one leg crossed over the other and a pillow between them. Side sleeping maximizes the flow of blood and nutrients to your baby.

a half and three pounds at about 32 weeks. Bones are starting to harden, and your baby may open his or her eyes, suck a thumb, hiccup, and cry. Your baby can respond to stimuli, such as sound and light; if he or she is born during this final three months, he or she will have a better chance of surviving, but may still require intensive care.

By the end of the eighth month, your baby is about 17 inches long and weighs between four and five pounds. He or she may move into the head-down position, getting ready for birth. The growth of the brain at this time is very rapid, and most of the baby's systems are developed, with the exception of the lungs, which might still be immature.

As you approach labor and delivery, your baby is gaining weight very rapidly—about a half pound each week, so that by delivery your baby will be about 20 inches long and weigh between six and nine pounds. As birth nears, your baby drops lower into the abdomen and curls up.

How you may feel

Many women dream about having their babies by now—and don't be surprised if it's in the form of a nightmare about something going wrong; this is completely normal. You may be nervous about the labor and delivery, or about what kind of mother you'll be.

If you have nightmares, try a session with a clinical hypnotist. Some women get relief from nightmares after just a few gentle suggestions from a hypnotic therapist. Talk to your practitioner about a referral to a mental health care specialist with experience in hypnosis.

As you near the end of your third trimester, you may find yourself getting more absentminded than ever and worrying about the labor, delivery, health of your baby, and the changes about to occur in your life. You may have alternating bursts of energy and fatigue, of elation and anxiety. You're probably napping during the day because you're finding it very hard to sleep well at night. You probably feel impatient and somewhat confined.

How to have a healthy baby

Pregnancy is a time for caution and good sense, but not a time for fear. The best way to have a healthy baby is to

- Exercise regularly.
- Get early prenatal care.
- Eat a well-balanced diet (including vitamins).
- Avoid alcohol, cigarettes, and illegal drugs.
- Avoid X-rays, hot tubs, and saunas.
- Avoid infections.

Eat a good diet

There are few things that will affect your baby's growth and development more than your diet. Studies have shown repeatedly that babies are born healthier when their mothers get proper nutrition during pregnancy. This is why it's so important that you pay attention to what you eat, and make sure you get all the nutrients that you—and your baby—need.

Never eat raw fish, such as sushi, or raw shellfish when you're pregnant. Contaminated raw seafood can cause serious harm to you and your unborn child. Thoroughly wash all produce (even if you grew it yourself without pesticides). Because of the risk of listeria bacteria (a risk that is rising in this country), avoid deli meats (such as hot dogs and sausages), raw meat, and soft cheeses.

Unofficially...
If you exercise, you may be able to head off miscarrying a baby with normal chromosomes. According to Columbia University researchers, jogging, swimming, and other regular aerobic exercise lowered the miscarriage risk by 40 percent.

Watch Out! Food poisoning is more dangerous if you're pregnant because it can affect your baby. Follow guidelines about handling and storing food, and, if you suspect food poisoning, contact your health practitioner immediately.

While it's true you're eating for two now, this doesn't mean you can eat an entire box of Ho-Hos with impunity! Your weight will be an issue throughout your pregnancy: You don't want to gain too little weight, but you don't want to gain too much, either. It's no picnic trying to shed the weight you've gained during pregnancy, so remember that the more you gain, the more you'll eventually have to lose once your baby comes.

That said, the amount of weight gained should vary depending on the habits of the woman prior to pregnancy. An underweight woman should probably gain 35 to 40 pounds, while an overweight woman should gain no more than about 15 pounds. There is evidence that there is no benefit to gaining any more weight once you have reached a total weight of 200 pounds. On the other hand, weight loss by anyone is not good during pregnancy and should be avoided.

If you've gained 25 pounds by delivery time, about 10 or 11 pounds will actually be the baby, placenta, and amniotic fluid. The rest of the weight will be distributed as follows: three pounds in the breasts and uterus, four pounds of maternal blood, two to three pounds of tissue fluid, and four to five pounds of maternal fat.

It's important to remember that a reasonable weight gain is normal and is necessary for the health of your baby. You should not think about jeopardizing your baby's well-being by trying to diet. Gaining weight during pregnancy does not mean you are getting fat. It means your baby is growing and is healthy. In the U.S., it is recommended that pregnant women should consume an extra 300 calories per day above the nonpregnant need. In Canada, the recommendation is no additional calories for the first 20 weeks and then 500 additional calories per day for the last 20 weeks.

Drink up!

You need extra fluids during pregnancy, so don't forget to drink at least eight glasses of liquids a day. Certainly some of this should be water, but you can count milk, fruit juice, and naturally decaffeinated coffee and tea. Get in the habit of carrying a bottle of water with you. You'll be surprised at how much more you'll drink if it's easy to get to. Extra fluids during pregnancy will help flush toxins from your body, minimize the chance of constipation (a common problem), improve your skin, and reduce swelling. They're necessary for your baby, too.

Vitamin supplements

Pregnancy requires increased amounts of nearly every vitamin and mineral. This makes it difficult to always get the pregnancy recommended dietary allowance (RDA) from the food you eat, even if your diet is good. Iron and folic acid are especially important during pregnancy. Experts believe that folic acid may help prevent some birth defects, while iron is necessary to develop good red blood cells. Calcium, which helps your baby to develop strong bones and teeth, is another important mineral for pregnant women.

Recent studies have shown that up to 70 percent of neural-tube defects can be prevented if women consume folic acid (a B vitamin) before and during the early weeks of pregnancy. All women of childbearing age should consume 0.4 mg of folic acid each day prior to conception and during the first months of pregnancy. Since it's hard to get enough folic acid through diet alone, taking a daily multivitamin can make up the difference. There are many foods that are being supplemented with folic acid/folate, from OJ to cereals. It's recommended that you get half your RDA from natural sources (such as leafy green vegetables) and half from a supplement. The trick here is to get sufficient folic acid before you get pregnant—that's where the research shows a big leap in folic acid's preventative benefits.

Your doctor will probably recommend a special prenatal vitamin/mineral supplement to make sure you get enough vitamins and minerals—but don't feel that by taking your supplements you are free to gorge yourself on junk food. Remember: Vitamins don't let you off the "healthy eating" hook. A poor diet enhanced by supplements is still a poor diet.

If you choose an over-the-counter prenatal vitamin, be careful about what you take. Your supplement should contain no more than 4,000 IU (international units, the standard of measurement for certain vitamins) of vitamin A, and no more than the pregnancy RDA of vitamins A, D, E, and K. Excessive amounts of water-soluble vitamins such as vitamin C will be excreted in urine. If you buy an over-the-counter supplement, ask your pharmacist or practitioner which brand is best.

Exercise during pregnancy

If running a mile before breakfast is your idea of fun, don't stop just because you're pregnant. Many practitioners think that women in good physical shape who maintain top condition during pregnancy will have an easier labor, delivery, and recovery than will couch potatoes.

If you're not so fit, start exercising slowly. If you've never exercised before, starting a new exercise program now may not be a good idea. Otherwise, you can exercise for 20 minutes of moderate exercise, three or four times a week—walking probably is the best and easiest way to start. Begin at a comfortable pace and gradually increase. Swimming is the best exercise for pregnant women (especially during the third trimester) because the water supports the pregnant uterus.

Be certain to talk to your doctor or midwife about exercise, and don't overdo it. Even seasoned athletes need to use caution during pregnancy; you require more oxygen, your heart pumps more blood and your joints and ligaments relax and spread.

Although most exercise is considered safe, you should avoid some activities (such skiing, volleyball, jumping jacks, horseback riding, rock climbing, and scuba diving). Common sense is your best guide. Avoid extreme sports (such as motorcycle riding or bike racing) during pregnancy.

Use caution exerting yourself in hot weather, and be alert to signs of heat stroke, which can be extremely dangerous to you and your baby. If you become dizzy, nauseous, extremely fatigued or short of breath, or experience blurred vision, stop exercising immediately and get some help. Likewise, stop exercising right away if you notice pain in your chest or abdomen, or vaginal bleeding. Your heart rate should not exceed 140 beats per minute during pregnancy. A heart rate in excess of this could trigger dangerous conditions for you and your baby.

Be sure to drink plenty of water before and during exercise, even if you don't feel thirsty. By the time you do feel thirsty, you're already experiencing a level of dehydration, and your energy level will decrease significantly.

Unofficially...
Women who exercise vigorously before pregnancy are more likely to carry their babies to full term, compared with women who exercise less or not at all, according to a studies published in the October 1998 issue of the *American Journal of Public Health.*

What to avoid during pregnancy

Because you want to give your baby the best start possible, there are certain things you *must not* do during pregnancy, and there are others that require a degree of caution. Avoid the following:

- Alcoholic beverages
- Cigarettes and other tobacco products
- "Recreational" drugs (including marijuana—one joint of marijuana has the same effect as smoking 10 cigarettes, producing the same amount of tars and carbon monoxide)
- Hot tubs and saunas: In the first few weeks of pregnancy such heat increases the risk of neural tube defects; later on it may increase the risk of pre-term labor

Others you need to use with caution:

- Caffeine
- Artificial sweeteners
- Prescribed drugs
- Exposure to potentially harmful substances
- Exposure to infections

Alcohol

Everyone agrees that severe alcohol abuse during pregnancy is harmful to the unborn. What is much more controversial is whether an occasional glass of beer or wine is permissible. Some health care providers believe it's okay, others strongly recommend against it.

Remember that when you drink alcohol, your baby drinks it, too. Although it's not been proven that one or two drinks will hurt your baby, there's no known "safe" level of alcohol use during pregnancy.

The March of Dimes, the American College of Obstetrics-Gynecology, the American Association of Family Practitioners, and the American Academy of Pediatrics all recommend avoiding alcohol altogether during pregnancy. What many experts say is this: In most cases, an occasional glass of wine or beer will not hurt the baby after the first trimester, but since there is the *potential* for harm, the safest course is to avoid all alcohol.

What is known for sure is that too much alcohol during pregnancy causes a number of birth defects, classified collectively as fetal alcohol syndrome (FAS). Even moderate drinking during pregnancy can lead to a milder form of the condition known as fetal alcohol effect (FAE), which causes some (but not all) of the problems associated with FAS.

Fetal alcohol syndrome is one of the most common causes of mental retardation. Among the prevalent characteristics found in FAS (some of which are found in FAE) are

- Abnormally small head and brain.
- Small, wide-spaced eyes.
- Short, upturned nose.
- Flat cheeks.
- Malformations of joints, arms, and legs.
- Abnormal organs (especially the heart).
- Small length and low weight at birth.

Later in childhood, babies with FAS may have

- Poor coordination.
- Hyperactivity.
- Short attention span.
- Extreme nervousness.
- Behavioral problems.

Bright Idea
Information on how to stop smoking is available from the American Cancer Society: 800/ACS-2345; the American Heart Association: 800/AHA-USA1; and the American Lung Association: 800/LUNG-USA.

Cigarettes

Women who smoke during pregnancy are at higher risk of having a miscarriage or a stillborn baby. Infants whose mothers smoked during pregnancy are more prone to sudden infant death syndrome (SIDS) than those whose mothers did not use tobacco; the increased risk of SIDS is about four times higher.

Smoking doubles the incidence of low birth weight, the leading cause of infant death during the first month of life. It also doubles the incidence of unexplained stillbirth.

If another member of the household smokes and the pregnant woman does not, the effect of the smoke is cut in half, but it still impacts the baby. If one member of the household smokes after the child goes home, the incidence of asthma, admission to the hospital for pneumonia, and SIDS are doubled over children in nonsmoking households.

Recreational drugs

Recreational drugs will put your baby at severe risk for a range of health problems and birth defects. If you're using drugs and can't stop, it's urgent that you tell your health practitioner. He or she can help you get the treatment you need. Most obstetricians are prepared to handle these situations so you should be as honest as possible with your health care provider.

Caffeine

Caffeine is a drug, and its use during pregnancy is controversial. Research indicates that small amounts of caffeine during pregnancy are not harmful, so you needn't cut out your morning cup of coffee if you don't want to. But be prudent, and remember that juices and water are more refreshing and healthier for you than coffee and soda. After all, would you feed a one-year-old a cup of coffee for breakfast? Remember that when you drink coffee, your unborn child is drinking it, too. Keep in mind that a host of other substances also contain caffeine, including chocolate, soda, tea, and certain pain relievers.

Watch Out!
If you're trying to cut down on caffeine, don't simply substitute herbal teas. Some herbs may have an adverse effect on your baby. Make your own 100 percent safe "herbal" tea by adding lemon slices and cloves, or orange slices and a cinnamon stick to hot water.

Artificial sweeteners

Artificial sweeteners are found in more than 1,500 common products in your grocery store. The use of artificial sweeteners during pregnancy is controversial, but because some research has suggested that these products may cause fetal brain damage, many health practitioners tell pregnant women to avoid them or limit their use. Be sure to read the labels of products you buy. You may be surprised at some foods (certain types of yogurt, club soda, and so on) that contain artificial sweeteners.

Prescription and over-the-counter medicines

Some medicines are safe to take during pregnancy, and some are not. If you take any medicine regularly, make sure your practitioner knows about it—in any event, you should try to avoid taking medicine whenever possible. It's best to have discussed this with your practitioner prior to pregnancy since most drugs have their worst effect in the first 8 to 12 weeks of pregnancy. Some of the most common groups of over-the-counter medications (safe and unsafe) are listed below:

- Pain relievers: Use only acetaminophen (Tylenol, Panadol, etc.), unless your doctor advises you differently. Aspirin and ibuprofen (Advil, Motrin IB, Nuprin, and so on) could harm your baby.

- Antacids: Generally considered safe to use (lots of calcium!); Tums may be the best source of calcium supplementation. They are flavored and five a day for life will provide you with the best bones you can get when you enter menopause.

- Laxatives: Generally considered safe, but it's better to avoid constipation with fiber-rich foods, plenty of fluids, and exercise. Metamucil is a good constipation preventative; it's flavored and one tablespoon at bedtime works wonders. Some laxatives may stimulate uterine contractions, however, so always check with your practitioner before taking any.

- Cold medicines: Some of these (such as Actifed, Sudafed, or Co-Tylenol) are considered safe. Whenever possible, however, avoid taking medicine, and treat your symptoms instead with non-drug remedies such as chicken soup, hot water with lemon, or a humidifier.

Hot tubs and saunas

It's not clear, but some experts believe that an internal body temperature of more than 104 degrees Fahrenheit increases the chance of some birth defects, especially early in the pregnancy. It's possible for your body temperature to reach 104 degrees if you linger in a hot tub or sauna, so if you must indulge, don't soak for more than 10 minutes at a time.

Travel

Always use a lap belt when you travel in a car, because car accidents are the most common cause of death among pregnant women. No matter how short the trip, buckle up. When buckling your lap belt, place the bottom part of the belt below your abdomen, across the tops of your thighs. The shoulder harness should go between your breasts, and to the side of your belly.

Air travel usually is fine if you've had no problems with your pregnancy and aren't close to your due date. Check with your health practitioner before taking any long trips, especially if you plan to travel outside the United States. Also check with the airline (some airlines have restrictions on flying in late pregnancy).

Chemical exposure

You don't need to worry about everyday household cleaners if you use them carefully and according to the package instructions, but be sure you never mix ammonia and chlorine-based products—it causes highly toxic fumes. Protect yourself by wearing rubber gloves when working with household products, and avoid working in small areas with poor ventilation. Avoid oven cleaners and dry cleaning solvents, which contain caustic fumes.

Problems: Not likely, but possible

If it seems like you're encountering one problem after another—nosebleeds, bleeding gums, dry eyes, blotchy skin, constipation, heartburn, varicose veins and backache—don't despair. These are common conditions in pregnancy caused by the rapid changes occurring within your body. Your joints are loosening, your heart is working harder, you've got an increased blood supply and your organs are being compacted as your baby grows. Take good care of yourself, and trust that these conditions will disappear after your baby is born. Of course, contact your doctor or midwife immediately if you suspect your

Watch Out!
If you have clothing dry-cleaned, hang them outside or in a well-ventilated area for a couple of days before bringing them into your closet. This dissipates the fumes from the chemicals used in dry-cleaning.

Unofficially... Infants conceived between 18 and 23 months after the birth of an elder sibling are at lowest risk of problems such as low birth weight or small size, according to scientists at the Centers for Disease Control and Prevention. Shorter and longer times between conceptions carry higher risk.

symptoms indicate something other than a normal pregnancy condition. While fairly unlikely, there are a few more serious things to keep in mind.

Pre-term labor

One of the most frightening things that can occur in a pregnancy is premature labor (pre-term or early labor). The severity of the situation depends on how far along you are in the pregnancy. Basically, pre-term birth occurs when your baby is born three weeks or more before the due date. It's best for your baby to be born sometime around 40 weeks of pregnancy so that his or her organs have enough time to mature and function well. When babies are born pre-term, they have a much higher risk of having health problems throughout their life. They may not be able to suck or to digest well, their livers often cannot function properly, and they may have breathing problems.

You need to understand your risks for pre-term labor. These include smoking, drug abuse, infection, chronic illness (such as high blood pressure, diabetes, or kidney disease), fibroids, multiple fetuses, or an "incompetent cervix"—a weak cervix that opens on its own. Women who have had other premature deliveries are also at higher risk.

Fortunately, there are many simple things you can do that may help prevent pre-term labor:

- See your health care provider for a pre-pregnancy visit.
- Get early and regular prenatal care.
- Understand which activities might be contributing to the symptoms of pre-term labor.
- Look at how you can change your daily activities to reduce or avoid pre-term symptoms.

Most causes of pre-term labor are unknown. If you feel you may be having contractions, call your health care provider immediately. The earlier the diagnosis and treatment, the better chance of stopping labor. If labor has begun and your baby is not under stress, your doctor will probably prescribe bed rest, which improves the blood flow to the baby. Try to lie on your side so that the baby does not press on veins leading to the heart. Your doctor may also prescribe medication to stop labor, called tocolytics. These can be very effective if given early.

Preeclampsia: Can you avoid it?

Preeclampsia is a condition that occurs in between 5 and 7 percent of pregnancies that can lead either to separation of the placenta or to eclampsia (a life-threatening seizure condition for mother and child).

It's most common in first pregnancies, in women under age 20 and over 40, and in those with a family history of related conditions, such as diabetes or kidney problems. It's treated with bed rest and medication to lower blood pressure. Symptoms include

- Headache.
- Nausea/vomiting.
- Abdominal pain.
- Seeing shooting stars.

Abruptio placentae

In abruptio placentae, there is a partial or complete separation of the placenta from the uterus before the baby is born. It's a very serious condition, since the placenta brings your baby nourishment and oxygen and removes waste products. The incidence of this complication varies, but averages nearly one in 150 deliveries.

Some studies suggest that at least 30 percent of unborn babies whose mothers develop this dangerous condition will die, while those who survive are at risk for serious neurological defects.

Although the exact cause is unknown, the condition is associated with a number of conditions:

- High blood pressure during pregnancy
- Diabetes mellitus
- Smoking
- Drinking alcohol
- Cocaine use
- Abdominal trauma

Since separation of the placenta can also cause severe hemorrhaging in the mother, it used to be a significant cause of maternal death, but improved obstetrical care and emergency services have decreased this danger substantially.

Unfortunately, some women may not experience obvious symptoms. Treatment varies from bed rest to immediate delivery, often by cesarean section. If you experience any of the following symptoms, get immediate emergency medical treatment:

- Heavy vaginal bleeding
- Premature labor
- Uterine tenderness
- Lower back pain

Bleeding

You shouldn't dismiss vaginal bleeding at any time during pregnancy, but it typically occurs during the first trimester in one of four pregnancies. Despite its frequency, you should report bleeding that occurs at any time during your pregnancy. Bleeding in the first trimester can sometimes signal miscarriage, while bleeding at the end may indicate abruptio placentae (see above) or placenta previa (a condition in which the placenta covers the cervix, usually resulting in cesarean section delivery; see below).

Bleeding during pregnancy doesn't necessarily mean you'll lose the baby; about half of women who experience bleeding during pregnancy go on to have normal deliveries and healthy babies. Light, brownish bleeding without cramping very early in pregnancy, for example, could be caused by the embryo implanting in your uterus; this bleeding may occur around the time you would have had your next period. Even bright red blood may not indicate a serious problem, since this can sometimes occur when part of the placenta briefly pulls away from the uterus and then falls back into place, or when the lining of the uterus swells and sheds without damage to the baby.

Still, you should call your clinician right away if you notice bleeding during your pregnancy. If your health care provider can't see you immediately, lie flat with pillows beneath your hips and legs so they are higher than your shoulders, and don't take any medication or alcohol. Show any clots that you pass to your doctor.

Placenta previa
In a very small number of pregnancies (about 0.5 percent) the placenta implants itself in the lower part of the uterus, partially or completely covering the opening of the cervix. If this happens, your baby must be delivered by cesarean section to avoid massive, even fatal hemorrhage. The condition can lead to prematurity, intrauterine growth restriction, and a much higher chance of fetal death shortly before and after birth.

Fortunately, this condition is usually detected by an ultrasound scan. The primary symptom is sudden, painless vaginal bleeding late in pregnancy (usually around the 30th week). Blood flow may be so heavy that it stains your clothing or bed with bright red blood. Such bleeding may be very dangerous to the baby—if profuse enough, the baby can die, as can the mother. This kind of bleeding warrants a 911 call.

If you're 35 to 37 weeks or more pregnant, your obstetrician will probably perform a Cesarean section. If bleeding occurs before this time, you'll be hospitalized and put on complete bed rest until it stops. You'll also be given blood tests for anemia and blood matching, in case you need a transfusion. Once bleeding stops, you may be able to go home, but will be advised to rest and to avoid sex and travel.

Doctors don't know what causes placenta previa, but the risk rises if you

- Are over age 35.
- Are carrying more than one baby.
- Smoke.
- Had placenta previa in an earlier pregnancy.
- Had a previous Cesarean section that left a low, transverse scar.

Ectopic pregnancy

Another concern among women during early pregnancy is the possibility of ectopic pregnancy. This is when the fetus becomes implanted outside the uterus, usually in the fallopian tubes (although it's also possible for the fetus to implant in other sites such as the ovaries or in the abdomen). Ectopic pregnancies are often referred to as tubal pregnancies. Signs of an ectopic pregnancy include

- Cramplike pain and tenderness in the lower abdomen; may start on one side and then spread.
- Light bleeding or spotting.
- Vomiting (although this can easily be mistaken for morning sickness).
- Feeling of rectal pressure.
- Shoulder pain.

If you experience any of these symptoms, call your doctor immediately. Prompt medical help is necessary to save your life. An ectopic pregnancy is an emergency that needs to be treated surgically. It is important to remove the developing embryo before the fallopian tube bursts. Hemorrhage from a ruptured ectopic pregnancy is a leading cause of maternal death (fortunately, it's rare in this country, with all the modern diagnostic care).

Infections

There are many infectious diseases that may cause serious harm to your unborn child. They include

- Chicken pox: Contracting this disease during the first three or four months of pregnancy carries a 5 percent risk of fetal damage; the earlier in pregnancy, the higher the risk of fetal problems. However, if you have chicken pox and deliver within five days or so, there is a fairly high chance that your baby could become infected, and chicken pox in a newborn may be fatal.
- Chlamydia: Some (not all) studies have linked this infection to a higher risk for premature birth, low birth weight or premature ruptured membranes. It can also cause an eye infection

in the baby if present at the time of a vaginal delivery, which is why state laws mandate that all newborns get antibiotic drops in the eyes shortly after birth.

- Cytomegalovirus: This viral infection may not produce symptoms in the mother, but can harm the fetus. While most affected babies are born perfectly normal, about 10 percent are born sick. Of these, 20 to 30 percent may die.
- Fifth disease: Up to 2.5 percent of pregnant women who contract this viral disease that affects red blood cells have spontaneous abortions or stillbirths, but most babies born to infected women are healthy.
- Genital herpes: A first-time episode of herpes in a pregnant woman is much more serious than a recurrent episode in a previously infected woman; women with active lesions at delivery should have a cesarean section to prevent the baby from being infected as it moves through the birth canal.
- German measles (rubella): One of the most serious infections a pregnant woman can encounter, this disease can cause 85 percent of women to miscarry if contracted during the first trimester. (The risk drops to between 10 and 24 percent during 14 to 16 weeks; after 20 weeks, the risk is close to zero.)
- Gonorrhea: Untreated gonorrhea during pregnancy can cause uterine infection, premature birth, low birth weight, or an infection in the amniotic fluid, and may lead to eye infections.
- Group B strep: This microbe is a normal bacterium found in the genital urinary track of

many women, but it can be transmitted to some babies under certain circumstances during childbirth. Of these babies, a small percentage become very ill and may even die. As a result, the Center for Disease Control now recommends that all women either be screened at 35 to 37 weeks for the presence of the bacteria in their vaginas and rectums or be given antibiotics during labor if there is fever or their water is broken for longer than 18 hours. If your practitioner screens you for the bacteria at 35 to 37 weeks and the test comes back positive, this means you carry the bacteria; you'll be offered antibiotics throughout your pregnancy and IV antibiotics while you're in labor. It's important to remember that if you carry the bacteria it doesn't mean you have an infection; it simply means you carry the bacteria and can pass it to your baby during childbirth.

- Hepatitis B: An infected mother can transmit this virus during the last three months of pregnancy; if you have the infection, your baby may breastfeed after receiving HBIG and the first dose of the hepatitis B vaccine.

- AIDS: A mother infected with HIV or AIDS can pass the infection on to her unborn child; medication during pregnancy can offer significant protection to the fetus. Cesarean section prior to the onset of labor has also been shown to decrease the chances of the baby being infected with HIV. The infection also can be transmitted via breastfeeding.

- Japanese encephalitis: Women who are infected during the first two trimesters may miscarry.

- Listeriosis: A baby infected with listeria bacteria in the womb may be born prematurely, have low birth weight and be very sick with breathing problems, blood poisoning, or meningitis. Half of these babies die even if promptly treated. This infection also carries an increased risk of miscarriage.

- Lyme disease: It's possible for the spirochete to cross the placenta and harm the fetus, although most babies born to infected women are normal. An infected mother does have a higher risk of miscarriage or stillbirth.

- Syphilis: An untreated pregnant woman can pass the infection to her unborn baby at any stage of the disease; the bacteria can cross the placenta and enter the baby's blood. Congenital syphilis can lead to serious illness, birth defects, and death, and it's becoming more common.

- Toxoplasmosis: A blood infection that is most severe if it occurs during the first three months; complications include miscarriage, premature birth, and poor growth in the womb. If it occurs in later pregnancy, it can also lead to mental retardation. Fortunately, toxoplasmosis is very rare in the United States.

Watch Out! Stay away from your cat's litter box while you're pregnant; cat feces sometimes contain a parasite that can cause a blood infection called toxoplasmosis. This can cause blindness, deafness, or mental retardation in your baby.

Are all birthing classes equal?

Get some recommendations from your doctor or midwife and line up a partner (you're not required to attend classes with your baby's father). If you're single or for some reason the baby's father isn't going to be present at the birth, you may use anyone you want as your birth partner.

Birthing classes are the perfect opportunity to share concerns with other pregnant couples, learn about childbirth options, potential problems, and techniques, and get your partner increasingly involved with your pregnancy. There are many types of classes, so be sure to ask what is available before signing up. Also, make sure you agree with the philosophy of the instructor and that the atmosphere of the classes is one of support, not confrontation.

For more information about childbirth classes and childbirth education philosophies, try these sources:

- International Childbirth Education Association, P.O. Box 20048, Minneapolis, MN 55420-0048; 612/854-8660; www.icea.org
- Aspo/Lamaze, Suite 300, 1200 19th St., N.W., Washington, D.C. 20036-2412; 800/368-4404; www.lamaze-childbirth.com
- Bradley: American Academy of Husband-Coached Childbirth, P.O. Box 5224, Sherman Oaks, CA 91413; 800/423-2397; in California: 800/42-BIRTH; www.bradleybirth.com
- The Read Natural Childbirth Foundation, P.O. Box 956, San Rafael, CA 94915; 415/456-3143

Just the Facts

- Screening tests can help determine the health of your baby—but understand the risks and the benefits of each test before you take it. But remember: No test can detect all abnormalities or guarantee a perfect baby.
- Home births aren't a good option for women with high-risk pregnancies.
- Women who exercise vigorously before getting pregnant are more likely to carry their babies to term. However, you should not begin an

exercise program for the first time during pregnancy without first consulting your practitioner.

- You should try your best not to drink caffeine or alcohol, smoke cigarettes, use artificial sweeteners, or take over-the-counter drugs during pregnancy.

GET THE SCOOP ON...
What to expect at the hospital ▪ Pain relievers ▪
The three stages of labor ▪ Induced labor ▪
Cesarean sections ▪ Miscarriage and stillbirths

Childbirth

You've made it through the past nine months of pregnancy—and now comes the moment you've been waiting for... labor and delivery! The nursery is painted, the crib is assembled and the mattress is covered with the matching sheet and comforter. You've bought diapers, bottles, powder and a half dozen of those funny little sleepers. Nine months seem like a long, long time—until they're over. Before you know it, your due date is here and you're ready to deliver your baby.

Labor: A woman's fears

Some women fear it, others look forward to it—but odds are, you spend a lot of your nine months wondering exactly what labor and delivery will be like. Anxiety and fear are normal. Talk to your doctor and to other women who have had babies. Remember that women have been having babies since time began, and the procedure today is safer and more comfortable than ever before. Here are some common concerns:

- The pain: By the time you're ready to have a baby, you've probably heard some pretty scary stories from women who seem to revel in the gory details. What's worse is that no woman seems to be able to remember accurately how the pain really felt, or communicate those feelings to you. Talk with your practitioner and come up with a plan for painkillers. Don't make the mistake of ruling out medication completely, even if you want a natural birth. Use the methods of relaxing and managing pain that you'll learn in childbirth classes, and work with your partner to come up with a plan for handling pain.

- Strangers will be watching: The only strangers who may be in your birthing room are hospital or birthing facility personnel who are trained and experienced in childbirth. They've seen about everything there is to see concerning the business of childbirth, and they're not judging your "performance."

- Unplanned bowel movements during labor: This is a common (but usually unvoiced) concern. It's not unusual for some feces to be expelled during the pushing stage of labor, and it's nothing to worry about. If this happens, it will be quickly cleaned up and hardly noticed. Everyone will be focused on the impending birth.

- Getting to the hospital in time: Not making it to the hospital is extremely rare, especially with a first baby. You nearly always have plenty of time.

- If something goes wrong: This fear is universal. Unfortunately, babies sometimes die before or after birth, and a few are born with birth defects. However, the number is relatively small, and, odds are, your baby will be just fine. Talk to

Timesaver
Be prudent about calling the doctor after your labor begins. Have your bags packed ahead of time, and when it's time, get to the hospital! (And if your doctor hasn't discussed when to go to the hospital with you, bring it up no later than at 28 weeks.)

your partner about your fears, as well as members of your childbirth class, other family members, and your practitioner.

Pain control: The real deal

You and your practitioner definitely should discuss the options for pain medication well before your labor starts. While contraction-relaxation control exercises and breathing techniques that you learned in prenatal classes help you cope with the pain of childbirth, sometimes you can't completely avoid using pain medication. Some of the possibilities to find out about are discussed in the following sections.

Tranquilizers, sedatives, and narcotics

Tranquilizers don't specifically relieve pain, but they can make your pain more manageable by easing your anxiety. Some women even find they can doze during the early part of labor with the aid of these medications. Narcotics provide pain relief, but they can have some side effects, such as nausea and vomiting, itching, and dizziness. They also can affect a baby's breathing at birth, so they can't be used too close to delivery. While they won't always stop pain completely, they do lessen it. Narcotics frequently used as obstetrical analgesics include Nubain, Demerol, morphine, and Stadol, and are usually given intravenously or as an injection into a muscle. However, these narcotics aren't usually used too close to delivery because they can cause respiratory depression in the baby.

Local anesthetics

A local anesthetic is injected into tissue to numb the surrounding area. It's usually used before an episiotomy (an incision in the perineum, the area between the vagina and anus, to make the vaginal opening larger to accommodate the baby's head), or before repairing a tear in the perineum.

A pudendal block numbs the vulva for delivery. It delivers rapid relief, has no ill effects on the baby, and is done easily, but it (and local injections) have no effect on the pain of labor. This is an excellent form of anesthesia for delivery and can be given when the baby's head is far down on the birth canal.

Regionals: Epidurals and spinal blocks

Your doctor may inject regional anesthetics into the space surrounding the dura, which is the sac containing the spinal fluid and the spinal cord. These anesthetics are getting more and more popular for pain control during labor. They can provide almost total pain relief, while allowing you to be awake as your baby is born. In some hospitals, 80 percent of labors are conducted under epidural. What makes epidurals especially helpful is that they also can be used as anesthesia if a C-section if needed. Epidurals are associated with the same side effects as spinals.

A spinal block is injected into the spinal fluid at the lower back and is used to provide relief from the pain of contractions (or even for a C-section). A saddle block is a form of spinal block in which only the area that would touch a saddle is blocked, and it only numbs the perineum. It's used only for the very last stages of pushing and episiotomy and is rarely used today.

Spinals and epidurals carry some potential side effects:

- Low blood pressure during delivery
- Postdelivery headache

- Temporary impairment of bladder function
- Convulsions or infection (this side effect is rare)

Epidural anesthesia is injected through a catheter in the space between the sheath surrounding the spinal cord and the bony vertebrae of your spine, numbing your body from the waist down. An epidural takes 15 to 20 minutes to work, and the catheter will be left in your back throughout labor in case you need more anesthesia. It provides complete pain relief in 85 percent of women, partial relief in 12 percent, and no relief for an unfortunate 3 percent. It can also be used for Cesarean delieveries.

One of the major benefits of epidural is that it can block certain areas of the body. For example, if given appropriately, it can numb the area from one or two inches above the navel to one to two inches below—this is all that is needed for labor. As labor progresses and the baby's head enters the pelvis, the anesthesiologist can boost the anesthesia of the area below the navel, as needed. If a Cesarean is necessary, anesthesia of the area above the navel can be increased.

Potential side effects (that are still exceedingly rare) include

- Diminished ability to push.
- May cause low blood pressure.
- Severe postpartum headache.
- Difficulty urinating or walking after delivery.
- Abnormally high fever.
- Prolonged labor.
- Slower infant heartbeat.

Get the answers to your questions before your labor begins

Long before your labor starts, you should talk to your practitioner about when to call him or her, once your labor begins. Should you call if your membranes rupture (your "water breaks") but you haven't started contractions? Should you wait until your contractions are 10 minutes apart? Five minutes?

At the initial visit, you should already have discussed any concerns and questions you have regarding labor and delivery. Discuss whether you're going to breastfeed or use a bottle, and talk about potential concerns—if you want to walk around during delivery or avoid an episiotomy. And remember, you and your doctor are both on the same side.

Labor: Is this the real thing?

It's not called "labor" for nothing—it's hard work. But it's something to manage, not to fear. Don't be surprised if you get 10 different stories about labor from 10 different women; all labors are different (even the same woman usually experiences labor several different ways).

Nobody knows exactly how labor begins. We do know that when it's time for you to deliver, your body produces prostaglandins (chemical signals that shorten, soften and dilate the cervix). These signals trigger uterine contractions to become stronger, and the contractions trigger production of more prostaglandins. Voila! Labor begins. We don't fully understand, however, what causes the body to begin producing prostaglandins. Somehow, your body knows when it's time for your baby to be born. Most experts today believe that some signal from the baby triggers the onset of labor.

There are three stages of labor:

- First stage: The onset of labor until complete dilatation of the cervix. This first stage is divided into the latent and active phases. The latent phase (up to 4 to 5 cm dilated) lasts an average of 14 hours in a first labor and six hours in subsequent labors. The active phase starts at about 4 to 5 cm dilated and will progress at an average rate of 1.5 cm per hour in first labors and 2.5 cm per hour in subsequent labors.

- Second stage: From when the cervix is completely dilated until the baby is delivered. It takes between two and three hours in first labors and 1.5 to 2.5 hours in subsequent labors.

- Third stage: This lasts from delivery of the baby until the delivery of the placenta. This can normally take up to 30 minutes.

Latent labor is the longest and least intense; active labor is shorter, but the contractions are more intense and that second stage (pushing) is hard work.

Signs of labor

Don't rush off to the hospital as soon as you think labor is beginning and your contractions start. Try to relax and do something to divert your attention. Read a book, watch television, try to sleep, take a warm shower, chat with your partner or have a light snack. Many women remain at home for the entire latent stage of labor, preferring familiar surroundings to the hospital or birthing center. However, if the membranes have ruptured, most physicians will want their patients in the hospital. Cords can prolapse after membranes rupture.

Unofficially...
Many women experience a burst of energy shortly before the onset of labor and with it, a need to put things in order at home. Called the "nesting instinct," it's not uncommon to get an urge to straighten closets and cabinets, or dust the baseboards.

Here's how to tell labor is beginning or imminent:

- Lightening: As your due date gets close, you'll notice that your baby has "dropped"—this is called "lightening," and it means he or she is getting ready to be born. Some women are immediately aware when this happens, and others hardly notice it at all. In first pregnancies, this usually occurs about four weeks prior to labor. If it hasn't happened by the onset of labor (in first pregnancies), there is a 50 percent chance that a Cesarean will be needed.

- Effacement: Your cervix thins outs (or effaces) as your body prepares for birth. The cervix changes from about an inch in thickness to the thickness of paper, but since you can't see in there yourself, you won't know this unless your practitioner does a pelvic exam and tells you.

- Dilation: In preparation for birth, your cervix opens up (or dilates) from 0 to 10 cm. This also can be detected during a pelvic exam, which some practitioners do and others don't.

- Bloody show: A bit of bleeding is often the first real sign of impending labor. It's caused by the loss of the mucus plug that blocked the cervix during pregnancy to bar bacteria. The plug looks like a thick discharge or stringy mucus, and can be clear or tinged with blood. While it can be a sign that labor is imminent, it also can appear days before labor actually begins. Some women never have any bloody show.

- Rupture of membranes: You may have heard it described as "breaking of waters." It occurs when the amniotic sac breaks or starts leaking, releasing the fluid that has surrounded your baby during pregnancy. It can be just a trickle, a flow or a tsunami, but most women don't experience it at all because their membranes rupture during labor, rather than before. Always call your practitioner if your water breaks before labor begins, since you risk infection if you don't begin labor within 24 hours of rupture. If labor doesn't start within 24 hours, your practitioner might induce labor.

- Nausea or diarrhea: These are common conditions at the beginning of labor and may be attributed to increased amounts of prostaglandin in the body.

Watch Out!
If your membranes rupture, tell your doctor IMMEDIATELY. Don't do anything that could bring bacteria into your vagina: Avoid baths, don't use tampons, don't have sex, and don't try to feel inside your vagina.

Contractions

One of the best signs that labor has begun is the beginning of labor pains. However, you've probably been experiencing Braxton-Hicks contractions for some time, as your uterus prepares for childbirth. These probably have gotten stronger as you've moved toward your due date, and may even have been painful. Often, it's hard to tell if contractions indicate labor has really begun, or if you're just experiencing strong Braxton-Hicks contractions.

There are several things you can try to determine if your contractions are warm-ups, or the real thing:

- Time them: Measure the time from the beginning of one pain to the beginning of the next. If they develop a regular pattern and start coming closer together, it's likely it's true labor. The pains of false labor come irregularly.

- Duration: Measure how long each contraction lasts. True labor pains should last about 15 to 30 seconds when they first start, and get progressively longer. False contractions will have a set pattern.

- Exercise: Change positions or take a walk, because false contractions often stop if you get some exercise. Real contractions will continue even if you stand on your head.

- Location of pain: If the pain from the contractions is only in your lower abdomen and groin, chances are they're not the real thing. Real contractions will hurt in your lower back and spread to your abdomen. The pain also may move down to your legs.

- Try the water test: Drink four glasses of water and lie on your left side, counting your contractions for one hour. If they remain constant at five minutes or less apart then you are probably in early labor. If contractions space out, become irregular (some 5 minutes, some 8 minutes, some 10 minutes), or lose their intensity, you are experiencing false labor.

It's sometimes impossible to tell whether it's false labor or not. It's better to err on the side of caution—your practitioner won't be upset with you if your labor turns out to be false, so if you get to the hospital for nothing, consider it valuable experience for the next time.

When to call the doctor

Your practitioner probably has given you guidelines on when to call: Some suggest when contractions are 10 minutes apart, others 8, still others 5. No matter how far apart your contractions are, call your practitioner if your water breaks or if your contractions are becoming extremely strong and painful.

It's better to be cautious than to risk waiting too long. Always call your practitioner if something seems to be wrong.

What to take with you to the hospital

If you're someone who habitually packs five suitcases for a weekend jaunt, try to rein yourself in when packing for the hospital or birthing center. Remember, you'll probably be there just a short time, and hospital and birthing center rooms don't have a lot of space for your personal items. Besides, you're going to have to bring it all home again and get someone to put it away for you. Here's a list of what you do need to take:

- Bathrobe
- Nightgown or pajamas, if you prefer your own to the hospital's
- Warm socks (several pair) to wear during labor
- Telephone credit card
- List of phone numbers of people to contact
- Camera or video camera, if you desire and you're allowed
- A tape or CD player with your favorite music, if you want
- Glasses (you'll probably need to remove your contacts)
- A watch for timing contractions
- Popsicles: they're better than drinking ginger ale and much tastier than ice chips
- Hard candy for you to suck on and a snack for your partner
- Toiletries (throw in Dad's toothbrush, too)

- A nursing bra, if you're breastfeeding; a supportive bra, if you're not
- Underwear
- Something to read
- Loose clothing to wear home (you won't fit into your pre-pregnancy clothes just yet)
- An outfit for your baby to wear home (don't forget a hat and blanket)
- A car seat (check with the hospital; some facilities offer one cheap or for free)

What to expect at the hospital

Your practitioner may tell you to come to the office once you've called, or to go directly to the hospital or birthing center. If you're delivering in the hospital, here's what you can expect to happen:

- You should already have figured out which entrance to use—go there.
- Have the driver let you out as close to the entrance as possible.
- Check in at admissions (you should have already filled out your admissions forms ahead of time).
- You'll then be taken to a labor or birthing room and prepared for childbirth.

Bright Idea
Most hospitals require you to pre-register, making the admission procedure much faster once you arrive. Check with your hospital.

Hospital prep

Hospital preparation varies from hospital to hospital and from doctor to doctor. You should have already talked with your practitioner ahead of time about things such as intravenous setups and fetal monitoring. If not, you can voice your opinion at the hospital (but it may or may not be honored, depending on policy).

This is not the time, however, to start a fight with your practitioner or the attending nurse. If something is not exactly to your liking, try to remember that you and your practitioner are working toward a common goal: the safe delivery of your baby. You don't want to waste precious energy on things that don't really matter.

Nowadays, dads are usually allowed in the labor and delivery rooms, but your partner might be asked to leave the room while you're admitted and prepared for childbirth. This is a good time for him to make a few quick phone calls, grab a snack, or check on things at home or at work.

The next step...

At the hospital, you're likely to be given a pelvic exam to see how dilated and effaced your cervix is. Your practitioner may rupture your membranes at this point, if they have not ruptured on their own. Try to take a few minutes mentally to review the breathing and relaxation techniques you learned in childbirth class, and try to remember that, in a relatively short time, you'll be holding your baby.

If your labor is induced

For one reason or another, your practitioner might decide to induce labor. You should discuss induced labor with your practitioner well before you're ready to deliver. Labor is induced because of concerns for the baby or the mother, and may include

- Post-term pregnancy.
- Pregnancy-induced or chronic high blood pressure.
- Diabetes mellitus.

- Previous stillbirth.
- Intrauterine growth restriction.
- Premature rupture of membranes.
- Abruptio placenta (separation of the placenta from the wall of the uterus), if the baby can tolerate the labor.

Your doctor won't induce labor if you have placenta previa (when the placenta implants itself over the mouth of the cervix so that it is delivered before the baby, cutting off oxygen supply), or an unusual presentation of the baby that would make vaginal delivery hazardous or impossible. It also isn't appropriate if your baby's head is too big to fit through your pelvis, or if you have a genital infection (such as herpes or gonorrhea). Many obstetricians also think inducing labor is not a good idea if you have more than one baby, there is fetal distress, or you have an unusually distended uterus.

To induce labor, your doctor will give you oxytocin (Pitocin), a synthetic version of a labor-inducing hormone made by your body that stimulates uterine contractions and causes contractions that are often stronger and more frequent than those occurring naturally. Mothers who have labor induced are somewhat more apt to need a Cesarean section than those who go into labor naturally, most likely because of the reason the labor was induced in the first place. Prostaglandin gel or a preparation of prostaglandin called cervadil may also be used. Misoprostol (Cytotec) a prostaglandin derivative may also be used orally or intravaginally. These new induction agents can be employed in certain circumstances and do a slow, less painful and more efficient job than Pitocin.

Latent phase of first stage of labor

The latent stage of labor might be half over before you know it's begun. During this stage, your cervix opens to three centimeters and effacement takes place. This can occur over a period of days or weeks, or it can happen quickly. Contractions, once they start, will be mild to moderate, lasting about 30 to 45 seconds, and come between 5 and 20 minutes apart.

Active phase of first stage of labor

During the active stage, your contractions will be closer together (usually every three to four minutes), they'll last longer (40 to 60 seconds) and they'll be stronger. You'll feel the contraction start, reach a peak and subside, only to be followed by another one starting up. Your cervix will dilate to seven centimeters during this stage. If you haven't yet gone to the hospital or birthing center, you probably will get there early in this stage.

You'll likely be concentrating very hard on what's happening and be unable to think about much else. If you can, walk around a bit, or at least change your position from time to time. Try to remember to urinate, even if you feel like you don't need to. You'll probably be getting tired now, so try to rest between contractions as much as possible. (It may be hard, but you'll need your energy for pushing.)

If you're thirsty, ask for a drink or some ice chips to suck on. If the pain is intense and you want some relief, tell the attendant. Many times, the attendant will ask you to wait for 15 minutes or a half hour, then re-evaluate whether you still need medication.

Keep your partner and the attendant informed about how you're feeling. When you reach the point

Unofficially...
Traditionally, no progress for two hours of labor (active phase of first stage) with adequate contractions was considered to be an indication for a C-section, but a new study at the University of Alabama suggests that if you continue with labor for another two hours with adequate contractions, you can deliver vaginally.

Bright Idea
Despite childbirth classes and all that practicing, some women find breathing exercises to be distracting, annoying, or just too hard. Don't feel that you're going to flunk "Labor 101" if you don't use them. It's your choice. Your baby is coming, either way.

where you can't talk during a contraction, you can begin your breathing exercises. Your partner can help you. If you're experiencing back pain, it might help to have your partner rub your back, or exert pressure against the area where it hurts. The entire process for a woman having her first birth is between 12 to 15 hours on the average.

Second stage of labor

The second stage of labor is intense and demanding—but, fortunately, it normally doesn't last too long. This stage of labor is when your cervix dilates from 4 cm to the full 10 cm. Your contractions come one after another and are at their strongest now. They can last up to a minute, only to be followed by another one before you've had any rest at all. The last three centimeters is called "transition" and contractions may be incredibly intense.

This stage of labor can be extremely painful, so it's best to be prepared. The pain doesn't mean something's wrong—the birth canal is stretching, and that's going to hurt. Some women find the contractions nearly unbearable. You might be nauseated, or even vomit. Your legs might shake, or you might get cramps; you might even get hiccups.

Have your partner help you as much as possible: Ask your partner to rub your back, massage your legs give you ice chips, and monitor your contractions to tell you when they've peaked. If you haven't had any medication for pain, and you feel that you want something now, go ahead and ask. As long as the dose of medication is not excessive, it can also be given late without causing serious respiratory depression in your newborn.

It may still be possible to get an epidural or spinal anesthetic. However, at this point, you need to concentrate on your labor, either with or without pain medication. Think about each contraction as it comes, and don't dwell on one that has passed, or worry about those still to come.

Transitional labor can be scary. You may be in great pain and sure that something has gone terribly wrong. You might even worry that you're going to die. Your anxiety might express itself as anger (many women in labor have gotten really cranky with their partners), or you might scream and cry.

If you do lose control, it's not the end of the world. Your body knows what to do. But try to stay in charge by telling yourself that you're capable and you'll get through it. Keep foremost in your mind that as bad as this stage of labor seems, it means it's almost over. Your baby soon will be here.

Pushing

Pushing is a natural, often overwhelming, need for a woman about to have a baby. Your practitioner will try to keep you from pushing until your cervix has fully dilated, because pushing before that time can actually slow delivery. If you're told not to push yet, try blowing out short puffs of air, which might help delay the urge. Usually, the urge to push doesn't come until the baby's head is about one-third to one-half of the way down the birth canal. The urge is caused by the baby's head pushing on the rectum. In fact, the most effective push is when you are straining as if you were constipated and have to have a bowel movement.

As soon as your practitioner gives you the go ahead, take a deep breath and push. Pushing is most effective during a contraction, when your uterus is already working to get your baby born. Try to push for 10 seconds, then get a quick breath and keep pushing. Try to push through as much as the contraction as you can.

The truth is that pushing hurts. The baby's head is straining against your vagina and perineum, and the result is burning and pain. The good thing about pushing is that, despite the pain, you know you're helping to get your baby out. Many women feel exhilarated and energized, knowing the end is near and feeling they have some control.

This is also a point when many mothers "lose it," believing the baby is never going to come out. It can be a scary part of the delivery, since you can really feel like you're not ever going to finish.

It's important to keep pushing as long as you can through a contraction. The baby will move a little bit back up the birth canal after each contraction. You can minimize this by pushing effectively through the contractions.

At last—A baby!

As your baby moves down the birth canal, your baby twists his or her head to one side, with chin on chest. Typically, the back of the head (a baby's widest part), leads the way, as the baby strains to get out. Soon the back of the head will emerge, followed by the forehead and then the face. When the head emerges, it's called "crowning," and usually it's the last really hard part of delivery. After the baby's head has emerged, the rest of its body should slip out easily.

What happens now?

There's a lot of work done just after your baby is born to ensure your baby's breathing properly and doesn't need any special care. As soon as his or her head emerges, your practitioner will clear fluid from the nose and mouth. Once your baby's fully emerged, he or she will be given some help with breathing, if necessary.

Nurses or midwives will check heart rate and circulation and note your baby's color. Apgar scores are checked at one minute and five minutes after birth.

Usually, attendants (or maybe your partner) will clamp and cut the umbilical cord before you hold your baby for the first time. Some practitioners prefer not to cut the cord until the placenta has been delivered.

An attendant will place an ID bracelet on your baby's wrist and ankle (and usually mom's wrist, too) and give him or her eye drops to prevent the possibility of chlamydia or gonorrhea being passed from you to the baby, which could cause blindness. An injection of vitamin K will ensure your baby's blood coagulates properly. When your baby reaches the nursery, he or she will be given a full physical examination to check for any abnormalities.

Unofficially...
Developed in 1953 by Dr. Virginia Apgar, the Apgar test serves as a quick evaluation of a newborn's health: Color, pulse, reflexes, muscle tone, and breathing are scored from 0 to 2 in each category. Many doctors downplay the scores, saying they're not always an accurate indicator of a newborn's health.

The afterbirth

While your baby is being attended to, you'll continue to have mild contractions, although you may not even notice them. These are necessary to separate the placenta (afterbirth) from the uterine wall and move it downward so it can be expelled. Your practitioner will ask you to push to help expel the placenta, which he or she will examine to make sure it's intact, with none left in the uterus. After the delivery of the placenta, the health care provider will inspect the cervix and vagina to make sure there are no lacerations. Your practitioner will stitch you if you've had an episiotomy, or if you've had a tear in your perineum. You'll be given a local anesthetic before stitching.

Cesarean birth

You probably don't think it really matters how your baby comes into this world, as long as he or she arrives safe and sound. Some experts and insurers, however, worry about the ever-increasing rate of C-sections in this country. In fact, C-sections are done more often than gall bladder removals or tonsillectomies.

Is a C-section necessary?

The national rate for C-sections reached about 24 percent (up from 4 percent in 1965), but is now starting to decline again. Many doctors privately believe that at least some C-sections are done because of the fear of litigation (especially in the case of breech presentations). Some C-sections are planned, but most are done unexpectedly because of problems during labor. Your doctor might choose a Cesarean because of any one of the following reasons:

- Repeat operations: It used to be automatic that a woman who had a Cesarean once would need another for the next child. Repeats do account for one-third of all C-sections, but today, more and more women are given the option of trying a vaginal delivery after having had a Cesarean.
- Labor not progressing: One of the most common reasons for Cesarean deliveries is when labor slows down drastically or stops.
- Fetal distress: If the baby becomes distressed (such as not getting enough oxygen), a cesarean may be indicated.
- The baby won't fit: Sometimes a baby just won't fit through the pelvis.
- Breech: If the baby doesn't enter the birth canal head first (called the "breech position"), a Cesarean birth might be necessary.

- Maternal risk: If you have a condition such as heart disease you may need to have a Cesarean to avoid further risk.

- Multiple births: When there's more than one baby, there's a good chance that one will be in an unfavorable position and a Cesarean birth will be necessary.

- An emergency: Emergencies sometimes occur during labor, and quick action must be taken to ensure the safety of the mother and baby. Cesarean birth is often the fastest and safest option.

What to expect

Some women get upset when they find out they need a Cesarean, but if your practitioner thinks it's necessary, you've got to assume it's the best thing for your baby and for you.

There are several steps that will be taken before your delivery. First, you'll be prepared for an operation. This procedure varies among hospitals, but may include shaving any hair on your abdomen and part of your pubic area, and a scrub with an antiseptic wash. Your doctor and an anesthesiologist will discuss with you what type of anesthesia you'll receive. An attending nurse will insert an intravenous catheter in your hand or arm, put a cuff on your arm to monitor your blood pressure, attach devices to monitor your heart and your oxygen level and insert a urinary catheter. You probably will be given either an epidural or a spinal block so you will be awake and alert during the operation (you may already have an epidural needle in place). General anesthesia is used in less than 20 percent of Cesarean births—usually only in emergency situations.

Moneysaver
For an interesting look on the ethics of C-sections, check out *Just Take It Out!: The Ethics and Economics of Cesarean Section and Hysterectomy*, by D. Campbell Walters (Topiary Publishing).

Two incisions are necessary for Cesarean birth: One in the abdomen, and one in the uterus. There are several options for each of these cuts. Your doctor will decide which to use, depending on the situation and the urgency of the birth; these days, 99% of the time both cuts are horizontal (the "bikini incision").

After the baby is pulled out through the incisions, the birth is complete. As soon as the baby is delivered, the doctor will remove the placenta from your uterus and begin stitching you up. This stitching can require some time, but you'll probably be feeling drowsy and hardly notice what's happening. (Many doctors today use staples instead of stitches to close the skin.) Start to finish, most C-sections take only about 30 minutes.

After a Cesarean birth

After the operation, you'll be taken to a recovery room, where your vital signs will be monitored as the anesthesia wears off. You'll continue to be monitored closely for 24 hours, and given pain relief as the anesthesia wears off. Get up as soon as possible, even though it hurts the first time you get out of bed. You'll probably be asked to take short walks starting about eight hours after the operation to help your circulation, prevent fluid buildup in the lungs and promote healing.

If your recovery is uneventful, you should be able to have your baby with you and you may be able to begin breastfeeding. In fact, some doctors will allow you to breastfeed your baby in the operating room during closure of the abdomen; ask if this is possible. If you do breastfeed, you'll probably notice some contractions as you do, which may be quite painful. Although you may want to practice relaxation techniques or coordinate your pain medication with breastfeeding, you shouldn't be overly concerned. These contractions are nature's way of controlling bleeding.

You'll probably stay in the hospital for two or three days following your Cesarean, if there are no problems. If you are eating, having bowel movements, are infection-free, are walking around, and have help to take care of the baby, you are ready to go home. Once you get home, you'll need extra rest for four to six weeks as your body heals.

You can start doing breathing exercises the first day in the hospital. Then each day, you can gradually find small exercises to do to get back into shape. Don't return to your previous exercise routine unless your doctor says it's okay. Overdoing it will only slow your recovery. By the end of two weeks, you may be feeling well, although you're still dealing with some pain. Most women don't have any pain six weeks after a C-section. After this period, you can usually resume most activities (some doctors let you drive after two weeks, others ask that you wait the entire six weeks).

Bright Idea
Try wearing an elastic belly support when you get home from the hospital after a C-section. During the first few days, it can make lying on your side and rolling over in bed much less painful.

Vaginal birth after C-section

If you've already had one C-section, you may still be able to have a vaginal birth this time around. Discuss the "VBAC" (vaginal birth after cesarean) option with your doctor. A history of more than two C-sections, however, will usually rule out the possibility of vaginal birth from here on out because of the risk of rupturing the earlier incision.

If there's a problem

Losing a baby, or having a baby with a health problem, is every woman's nightmare. Unfortunately, in a few cases, the nightmare comes true.

Miscarriage

A miscarriage is the spontaneous loss of an embryo or fetus. If it occurs after 20 weeks, it's considered to be a stillbirth. Medically known as a "spontaneous abortion," miscarriage is relatively common, occurring in about 20 percent of recognized pregnancies and it's especially common during the first few weeks of pregnancy. (As many as 45 percent of all pregnancies end in miscarriage, but many of these women never knew they were pregnant.)

Many times, the cause of a miscarriage is simply not known. The problem is more common after age 35. One prior miscarriage does not increase the risk of a subsequent one and two doesn't increase the risk much, either; it's only after three or more miscarriages without having had a live birth that the subsequent risk of miscarriage goes up significantly; even then, however, about one-half of women will have a live birth.

Between 35 and 50 percent of miscarriages during the first two months of pregnancy are caused by serious genetic defects in the fetus. Other causes include

- Problems with the uterus or cervix.
- Hormonal imbalances.
- Viral and bacterial infections.
- Recreational drug and alcohol use.
- Exposure to environmental toxins such as arsenic, lead, and formaldehyde.

Whatever the reason, miscarriages can be emotionally devastating. The good news is that most women who miscarry eventually go on to have a subsequent normal pregnancy. Even a woman who has had four consecutive miscarriages still has a 60 percent chance for a successful pregnancy the fifth time.

Watch Out!
Pregnant women who spend time with young children have an increased risk of infection with parvovirus B19, which has been linked previously to an increased risk of miscarriage, according to Danish researchers. The rate of miscarriage among women infected with parvovirus B19 during pregnancy ranges between 1 and 9 percent.

Contact your doctor if you notice any of these signs during the first trimester (up until 12 to 13 weeks), which could be symptoms of miscarriage:

- Bleeding (heavy): Sometimes bleeding from the vagina follows a brownish discharge.
- Lower back pain.
- Disappearance of morning sickness, breast enlargement, and other pregnancy symptoms.

While these symptoms could indicate the possibility of a miscarriage, their presence does not necessarily mean you will miscarry; many women who have some bleeding go on to have healthy babies. Bleeding especially doesn't always indicate the onset of miscarriage.

If you suspect you may be miscarrying, call your practitioner immediately. Don't have sexual intercourse or take part in strenuous activities. If the bleeding and pain stop, you will probably have a normal pregnancy.

While medical treatment can't stop an impending pregnancy loss, you may need a dilation and curettage (D&C) to cleanse the uterus of retained tissues if the miscarriage isn't complete. Your doctor will advise you how long to wait before you try for another pregnancy (usually two or three menstrual cycles).

Stillbirth

The death of a fetus between the 20th week (5th month) of pregnancy and birth is a stillbirth, not a miscarriage. According to statistics, there are 7.3 stillbirths for every 1,000 live births, according to the Centers for Disease Control. Sadly, about half the time there is no known cause. For the rest, stillbirths may be related to genetics, birth defects,

Bright Idea
A 1991 study found that using a computer terminal does not increase the risk of miscarriage, although many experts do recommend using special monitor screens.

infections, problems with either the placenta or the umbilical cord.

The umbilical cord is the baby's lifeline, providing nourishment and oxygen, and rarely a problem with the cord can be fatal to the baby. As the baby moves around in the placenta, the cord may kink or knot, interfering with the flow of oxygen and food. Or the cord problem may not occur until the baby moves down the birth canal, when it can be squeezed or wrapped around the baby's neck, causing suffocation. A "prolapsed cord" occurs when the cord comes out of the vagina before the baby, obstructing the flow of blood and oxygen. (A prolapsed cord is a true accident that will probably not happen again in future pregnancies.)

Stillbirth also may be caused by problems in the placenta—either placenta abruptio or placenta previa. Implantation site is really a matter of chance. Maternal factors such as age, smoking, high blood pressure, and previously scarred uterus are risk factors for placenta previa or abruptio. A previous placenta previa or abruptio does increase the chance of it happening again in a subsequent pregnancy, especially if the same risk factors are present.

There are many signs that something may be amiss with a pregnancy. You may notice vaginal bleeding, or cramps and stabbing pains in the pelvis, lower back, or abdomen. Or you may realize that your baby hasn't moved for more than 24 hours. When you bring your concerns to your practitioner, he or she will assess the movement and heartbeat of the fetus.

Whatever the reason, stillbirths can be one of the most emotionally wrenching experiences you can have, especially if you went into labor not realizing there was a problem. The good news is that most women who have a stillborn child eventually go on to have a subsequent normal delivery.

Birth defects

Birth defects are abnormal conditions, ranging from heart defects to bone deformities to imbalances of body chemistry, and may be minor to severe. Some may cause debilitating disease, physical or mental disability, or early death. About 3 percent of all pregnancies include some type of birth defect, but most are fairly minor (such as an extra finger). Serious birth defects, the leading cause of infant death, occur in one of every 75 to 100 births.

Sometimes there is nothing that anyone can do to prevent a birth defect—it can happen to anyone's child. You may have had regular prenatal care, eaten well, avoided cigarettes, alcoholic beverages and drugs—and still have an affected child. Birth defects may be inherited or be caused by a problem in the womb (resulting from an infection, for example); they also may be caused by environmental factors, such as worksite chemicals or pollutants. Scientists don't yet know the cause of many of the 3,000 different birth defects, but we do know how to help prevent or correct some of them.

If you discover your child has a birth defect, you may feel shock, fear, anger, and self-pity. You'll need to talk about your feelings with your partner, your health care provider, a minister, or other counselor. Other parents of affected children can be especially understanding and supportive. Right from the beginning, be open with friends, neighbors, and family members about your child's condition. Speaking openly of your child with love will help put others at ease so they can accept your child just the way he or she is.

Watch Out!
Pregnant women who are exposed to organic solvents on the job are at much higher risk of giving birth to a child with birth defects, according to researchers at the University of Toronto. Your employer is required by law (when asked) to supply you with a list of all chemical exposures on the job.

While most birth defects can't be completely corrected, many can be treated to some degree. Surgery after birth is now commonplace for cleft lip and palate, clubfoot, heart malformations, bowel obstructions, and many other conditions. Chemical regulation by drugs, hormones, vitamins, and dietary supplementation or restriction can be effective.

In addition to birth defects, unborn babies are subject to a wide range of health conditions which may be treatable before birth. These include

- Drugs to reverse fetal heart failure.
- Transfusions to counteract severe Rh blood disease.
- Hormone and vitamin therapy to correct metabolic problems.
- Prenatal surgery (still experimental) to correct internal malformations.

In the future, gene therapy (replacement of faulty or missing genes with new ones) may give some children a second chance for a life nearly free of disabilities. Genes involved in high cholesterol, alcoholism, cystic fibrosis, anemia, and many more problems have been identified. The first human gene therapy trials began in 1990 and there are about 50 projects now under way.

Intrauterine growth restriction

Each year in the U.S., about 90,000 babies are born too small (growth restricted). These are infants whose weight is below the 10th percentile for gestational age (small for gestational age). However, this isn't the same thing as a low birth-weight newborn. A low birth-weight baby weighs less than five pounds at birth, but may still be the right size for the gestational age if birth was premature. Thus, a birth weight less than five pounds in a pre-term (less than 37 weeks gestation) newborn may be an appropriate weight for gestational age.

Newborns who experienced early and continuous growth restriction in utero often catch up quickly and easily if the growth problem was caused by the mother's high blood pressure, for example—once the baby is born and out of the less-than-optimal environment. Some, however, never fully catch up. These infants may be less alert and responsive during the newborn period than other full-term babies are, and may be more irritable and fussy, or overly sensitive. Being smaller than normal is also associated with an increased risk of infant death or childhood health problems.

There are several causes for growth restriction, although in about one in three cases, no special risk factor can be found:

- Smoking, and alcohol and drug use
- Pregnancy-induced high blood pressure
- Chronic health problems in the mother
- Multiple births
- Placenta problems
- Chromosomal abnormalities
- Poor nutrition

Ultrasound can help your practitioner evaluate your baby's growth during pregnancy. Your practitioner will also measure the height of your uterus at each prenatal visit. If any sign of growth restriction is found, you may be asked to have more ultrasounds or more frequent office visits to monitor the situation. Screening tests of various types may also be done to try to determine why your baby is growing so slowly. You'll be advised to rest and get good nutrition.

An orange with hair...

Your baby has arrived, and you're sure he or she will be the most beautiful thing you've ever seen. Well, your baby may be—but probably not the very first time you see him or her, so be prepared!

If you think labor and delivery were hard work for you, imagine what your baby had to go through. It's no picnic, being squeezed down that tiny, dark birth canal into the bright lights of the delivery room. Shortly after birth, most likely your baby will bear little resemblance to one of those pink, round, smiling babies on the magazine covers. Your baby's head was squeezed and compressed as he or she came through the birth canal, and he or she may well look more like a conehead than the baby you expected. Your baby may have a bump on the scalp from pressing against your cervix before it was fully dilated, or the head might be bruised from the pressure. That tiny nose might be flattened, also from pressure in the birth canal. Don't worry. In a few days your baby's head will lose its pointed appearance, and the bump will disappear. Your baby will be as beautiful as you imagined.

Your baby's skin may appear blue when he or she first emerges, and his or her hands and feet a blue-gray color. Don't panic. This is the normal color of a baby in the uterus, and it will disappear once your baby starts breathing well on his or her own. Babies born to nonwhite parents may have a particularly poor color just after birth, but as the blood gets more oxygen, the color will improve. You'll probably notice better color first in your baby's tongue and lips. A baby's skin, especially if he or she is premature, can be covered with vernix (the waxy, cheesy coating that protected the baby's skin in the uterus). This will be cleaned off.

Your baby may be born almost completely bald or may have a full head of hair—but don't get excited either way. All babies eventually lose their newborn hair and grow a new crop, often of a different color and texture. In addition to the hair on his or her head, your baby may still be covered with very fine hair (lanugo) on his or her shoulders, back and part of his or her face. This is usually gone by the end of the baby's first week.

Nothing is as it seems, and this holds true for eye color, too. Don't assume that your baby's eyes will remain the color they are at birth. They probably won't be their true color for six to nine months. Caucasian babies are usually born with blue eyes, and non-Caucasians with brown. The eyes might be puffy at birth, often caused by the eye ointment given to your baby to prevent infection. This can look like a discharge in the baby's eyes but it's perfectly normal.

Holding your baby

Many practitioners think it's a good idea for you to hold your baby as soon as possible after birth, and many encourage you to let the baby try to nurse. Place your baby on your chest and enjoy the closeness.

But don't panic if, for some reason, you feel you don't want to hold your baby right away. You might be too tired, or you might even feel resentment toward the baby if you had a long, difficult labor and delivery. Tell your practitioner. This doesn't mean you're a bad mother, or that people in the delivery room will think you're awful. You'll have plenty of time to hold your baby after you get a nap and feel better.

Unofficially...
Swollen genitals and breasts are common in both boy and girl babies, triggered by maternal hormones. These conditions disappear in about 10 days and don't harm the baby.

Feeding your baby

Normally, you can try breastfeeding your baby as soon as you hold him or her for the first time. If your baby agrees to try nursing (some are too tired to bother), go ahead and nurse. At this point, your breasts are producing a type of pre-milk called colostrum that contains many important antibodies (things which will help your baby fight off everyday germs and infections). Your milk won't come in for three or four days, at which time your breasts may become engorged, making them swollen, hard, and quite painful.

Breastfeeding has gone in and out of fashion during this century, but it's now widely regarded to be the healthiest, most natural way to feed your baby. Breast milk is the perfect food for babies, and the breast is the easiest means to allow them to eat. Breastfeeding creates intimacy between you and your baby, is convenient—and it's free! Talk to your practitioner about the benefits of breastfeeding, and express any concerns you have. Together, you can decide what's best for you and your baby.

Your hospital stay

Watch Out! Some hospitals give babies sugar water in the nursery, but some practitioners don't think this is a good idea, fearing it satisfies the baby's appetite, making him or her less interested in nursing.

With the advent of managed care, hospital stays following childbirth have gotten shorter and shorter over the past decade. It's quite common to be in the hospital for only 18 to 24 hours after your baby is born vaginally, if there are no complications. Following a C-section, the average hospital stay is three to four days. Federal law that became effective in 1998 allows a woman a two-day stay after a vaginal delivery and a four-day stay after a Cesarean. Not all women need to stay this long, but, if you want to, you can.

Whatever the length of your stay, learn as much as you can from the nurses about bathing, feeding, diapering, and dressing your baby. You'll also learn about child safety and what to do in the case of an emergency.

Taking your baby home

The most dangerous part of childbirth is the drive home—you and your baby are more likely to meet with harm on the road than in labor or delivery. A rear-facing infant car seat in the back seat is required by law, and many hospitals will not release your baby unless you confirm that you have an infant seat installed. Never ride in a car with your baby in your arms or on your lap.

Once home, you might be tempted to fill your house with friends and family so you can show off your baby. Lots of people will want to stop and see your family's new addition. Be firm! You're still recovering from childbirth; it's a good idea instead to rest and let your baby get acquainted with his or her immediate family. There will be plenty of time later for your friends to meet your baby.

You'll need to rest whenever you can, because it's an almost sure bet your night sleep will be frequently interrupted for a while. As difficult as it might be to rest when your baby rests—especially if you have other children—you must try. Get help with laundry, cooking and cleaning, if possible, during the first couple of weeks. Don't try to do everything yourself.

Postpartum

The first week after giving birth may not be a particularly comfortable time. You can expect

- Vaginal discharge.
- Cramps as your uterus contracts.

- Pain in the perineal area, or, in C-sections, around your incision.
- Urinary problems for a day or two.
- Constipation.
- Breast discomfort.
- Discomfort from stitches.
- General stiffness and soreness.
- Exhaustion.

Although some women bounce right back after childbirth and seem to hit the ground running, most new mothers will have considerable discomfort, at least in the beginning. Take it easy and rest whenever possible, and it won't be long until you're back up and able to care of everyone and everything you did before your baby was born.

You'll start to get a bit of confidence once you've had your baby at home for a week or so, and you may be establishing some sort of routine or means of coping with chores and caring for your baby. You'll probably still be tired, but your fatigue may seem easier to deal with. As time goes on, you'll have less discomfort. You'll gradually begin to lose weight, and your abdomen will begin to flatten somewhat.

This doesn't mean, however, that everything will be rosy. Having a baby has major implications on your life, and, if you're not ready or willing to deal with them, you may find yourself feeling impatient, resentful, and disappointed. You might be unhappy with the way you look, and feel trapped and confined. Some things you might try to help relieve those feelings include

- Eating healthy: Avoid (especially if you're nursing) caffeine, too much sugar, and alcohol.

Bright Idea
New mothers who resume exercising after they deliver their babies lose more weight and have more positive outlooks, compared to those who do not exercise, according to University of Michigan researchers.

- Exercising: Take your baby for a walk, if feasible; if not, enlist a relative or your partner to baby-sit while you take a stroll. Some mild, postpartum exercises will help you start getting your body back in shape.

- Pampering yourself: Consider getting a new haircut (preferably one that requires minimum effort) or a massage, if you can find someone to watch your baby for an hour or two. Walking around in a milk-stained bathrobe with uncombed hair until four o'clock in the afternoon is bound to make anyone feel depressed! Shower and dress in the morning so you feel ready for the day.

- Staying close to your partner: Remember, you're in this together.

- Laughing: Things will seem more normal soon.

- Above all, don't isolate yourself—stay in touch with friends and co-workers. Telephone them when you get a minute, just to say hello and keep in touch. This will help you feel less isolated, and that you're still involved with the world outside.

If you feel depressed...

Mild depression following childbirth is common and will soon pass. However, if you feel you're more than a little depressed, or if your depression is causing you to feel angry and aggressive toward your baby or other children, talk to your practitioner immediately. You may need professional help.

Make sure you make some time for yourself every day, even if it's only a half hour. Let dad, grandmom, or a neighbor take the baby and spend some time doing what you want to do. This can help prevent serious postpartum depression.

What your baby might do

While you're dealing with postpartum changes, your baby is dealing with the first few days and weeks of its life. It's sometimes difficult to balance your needs with those of your baby. Knowing what you might expect can help.

Babies have very different habits and personalities; some sleep most of the time and rarely fuss, while others are demanding and noisy. An average newborn sleeps about 15 out of every 24 hours, and fusses for two or three hours at different times during the day (and night!). There are, however, many variations when it comes to babies:

- Personality: Some are calm and tranquil, while others squirm, arch their backs, and scream. Again, this variation is normal.

- Attitude: Some babies like to be held often and close, while others prefer to keep some distance. Both are normal.

- Sleep habits: Some babies settle down to sleep quickly and easily, while others don't.

You'll very soon get to know your baby and his or her likes and dislikes. Contact your pediatrician with any questions or concerns, and give your baby a lot of love and attention. There are many good books and guides concerning baby care—see the resource guide in Appendix B for some suggestions.

Wrapping it up

While you're pregnant, you think it will never end—but before you know it, nine months have passed, and you're a mother. It's a gift to be able to enjoy your pregnancy, despite the discomforts, anxieties, and challenges it may present.

Pregnancy isn't something you need to do alone. There is plenty of help available if you need it, and your partner should play an active role. Feel each of your unborn baby's movements with pleasure and wonder, remember the first time you heard your baby's tiny heart beating inside your abdomen, and anticipate the sound of his or her first cry. Treasure and remember as much as you can about your pregnancy and childbirth experience.

Just the facts

- Discuss with your practitioner your feelings about forceps and episiotomies, and breastfeeding and bottlefeeding.
- If you're not sure if your contractions are the real thing, err on the side of caution—get to the hospital or birthing center.
- Many potential birth defects can be avoided or corrected with proper treatment.
- Most women who have had a miscarriage or stillbirth go on to have a subsequent healthy baby.
- A certain amount of anxiety and depression are normal following childbirth, especially if your labor and delivery were particularly long and painful.

PART III

Not All in Your Head: Mental Health Issues

GET THE SCOOP ON...
How to tell if you're depressed ▪ Why women have higher rates of depression ▪ How to decide if you're at risk ▪ What the experts say about counseling ▪ The pros and cons of the newest antidepressants ▪ Whether natural depression remedies work

Depression

It's normal to feel sad from time to time—everyone does. But for almost one in four women, this sadness will deepen into a clinical depression. Unfortunately, far too many women (as many as 100,000 in the United States) haven't been correctly diagnosed and aren't receiving treatment that could help them return to a normal life.

Your dog dies . . . you lose out on a promotion . . . you break up with your partner . . . the next thing you know, you're home alone at midnight, digging into a quart of rocky road ice cream and wondering if life's worth living.

Sometimes you have a real reason to feel blue. But temporary sadness should be just that—temporary. After a few days, the fog should lift and life should start looking good again. If you're clinically depressed, the sad or hopeless feeling doesn't go away—or if it does, it comes right back. Symptoms can range from uncomfortable to debilitating. In serious cases of depression, suicide is a real risk.

Depression quiz

To find out if your symptoms are transitory sadness or true depression, take this quiz. If you can answer yes to several of these questions (and you've had the symptoms for more than two weeks), you may be depressed:

- Do you feel terribly sad and cry a great deal?
- Do you have trouble sleeping, or you sleep too much?
- Are you tired all the time, no matter how much sleep you get?
- Do you experience outbursts of complaints and shouting?
- Do you feel worthless, unattractive, or guilty all the time?
- Have you lost interest in eating—or do you overeat all the time?
- Have you lost interest in hobbies and activities you once loved?
- Do you have trouble concentrating?
- Are your thoughts muddy or foggy?
- Do you feel restless?
- Do you have phobias, delusions, or extreme fears?
- Have you lost interest in having sex?
- Have you had suicidal thoughts?

Why are women so depressed?

Most of us have watched a relative or friend struggle with depression—and many of us have experienced it ourselves. In fact, as compared with American men, twice as many American women have at least one depressive episode in their lives. The typical

> " I ask people if there are cobwebs in their house. If patients aren't bathing, if their house isn't clean, if they can't get out of bed—that's a good indication that they're depressed.
> —North Carolina psychiatrist "

depressed woman is between 25 and 40, married, and has children. She could be on either end of the economic continuum: very successful or fairly poor. She may have too little personal support, or a problem with drugs or alcohol.

Careful epidemiological studies have shown that the higher depressive rate in women is not due to a woman's greater willingness to report depression. Instead, scientists have discovered that women really do get depressed at a higher rate than men.

There isn't one single cause of depression, and there probably isn't one reason why women experience the problem more often then men. Data from a variety of studies show that depression clearly has psychological, environmental, genetic, and biological roots, and a woman's higher risk of depression might be caused by some combination of all three.

Serotonin story

The language of emotion is written with chemicals found in your brain; when the level of these chemicals drops, scientists believe, depression occurs. While there are as many as 100 different kinds of these neurotransmitter chemicals, three are the most important in the onset of depression:

- Serotonin
- Norepinephrine
- Dopamine

Of these, serotonin is perhaps the most critical chemical in the development of depression. It appears as if environmental and psychological experiences can alter a woman's brain chemistry, lowering levels of neurotransmitters.

There seem to be significant gender differences in the serotonin system. Recent studies have

Unofficially...
A woman's body seems to be particularly sensitive to environmental changes, including stress and daylight, both of which affect the level of serotonin.

suggested that women produce lower levels of serotonin than men. In fact, studies at McGill University found that the average synthesis rate of serotonin was 52 percent lower in women than in men—one of the largest gender differences in the brain ever reported.

This lower rate of serotonin synthesis might increase a woman's overall risk for depression—especially if serotonin stores are also depleted during stress and winter darkness.

If serotonin is the link between you and your environment, and if this neurotransmitter is regulated differently in men and women, it might explain gender patterns not only in depression but also in a range of psychiatric illnesses.

For example, depression and anxiety are more common among women, but alcoholism and aggression are more common among men. At the same time, low serotonin levels have been found in depression and anxiety disorders in women—and low levels are also found in the brains of men with severe forms of alcoholism and aggression.

Wintertime blues: The inside scoop

If you've ever noticed that you start feeling depressed and sluggish as winter approaches, you're not alone. As many as 12 million Americans may suffer from seasonal affective disorder (SAD), also known as winter depression. Up to 35 million more may experience it in its milder forms. It's a type of depression that's three times as common in women as in men, and until recently no one knew why.

Women with the problem usually begin to notice seasonal depression in their 20s and 30s; some experts believe as many as half of all women in northern states experience pronounced winter depression. Unfortunately, very few get the proper treatment because doctors often can't tell the difference between typical depression and SAD.

This gender difference, according to scientists at the National Institute of Health, may occur because women might be more sensitive than men to changes in exposure to light and dark.

For some time, we've known that the hormone melatonin seemed to play a role in SAD. (Melatonin is a hormone that helps us sleep deeply; in animals, it's also related to reproduction control.) Humans secrete melatonin only in the dark, and only when the body's internal clock (located in the hypothalamus) thinks it's night. Melatonin levels drop again in the morning, as light hits the retina of the eye. (Also at night, the level of serotonin drops as melatonin increases.)

Interestingly, scientists have found that under normal conditions, women had longer episodes of melatonin secretion in winter than in summer, but men had no seasonal difference. This suggests that women are more sensitive to natural light than men, and that even when surrounded by artificial light, women somehow still detect seasonal changes in natural day length.

The best treatment for SAD is light therapy—exposure to special types of light during the winter will reverse this type of depression in most people. However, you must get an accurate diagnosis and the right kind of light box to get enough high-intensity light. Typically, you should sit about three feet from a bank of special lights (between six and eight fluorescent bulbs) for about three hours a day. Ordinary room light is not bright enough to affect SAD. After a few days of sitting for several hours under these

Moneysaver
A full-spectrum 10,000 lux lightbox is most commonly prescribed for SAD; a good one should cost between $400 and $500. This may be tax deductible or covered by insurance, and payment plans are usually available.

high-intensity fluorescent lights, symptoms should begin to subside. Treatment should always be under the supervision of an expert.

Since light therapy may be only partly successful in easing symptoms, your doctor may want you to take an antidepressant as well. While antidepressants may be used without light therapy for people with SAD, your doctor can usually use lower dosages of drugs if combined with phototherapy. Often, your doctor will need to adjust the dose of antidepressants with the changing seasons, increasing the dose as the days get shorter. Many doctors consider Prozac and other serotonin reuptake inhibitors (SSRIs) to be the best choice for treating SAD, since these drugs affect the serotonin system, which is thought to be linked to the cause.

A few depressed people seem to be at least temporarily helped by staying up all night, and then resuming their regular sleep-wake cycle, but others don't respond to this at all.

Hormones: The female difference

As much as some women may hate to admit it, it appears that a woman's different hormonal makeup may indeed be linked to an increased tendency toward depression. In fact, depression and problems with hormone regulation seem to go hand in hand. It shouldn't be surprising; hormones affect neurotransmitter activity, and neurotransmitters affect the timing and release of hormones.

Since women have higher levels of circulating hormones, this may be another reason why women are at higher risk for depression. This also may be why girls become more susceptible to depression than boys only after puberty, when their hormones begin to rise. Indeed, women appear to be especially vulnerable to depression during events related to reproduction (menstruation, ovulation, pregnancy, and menopause). Altered levels of hormones during these times can affect mood-regulating neurotransmitters, but just how they do this isn't clear.

Estrogen also may lead to depression by triggering the body's stress response. During stressful times, the adrenal glands secrete higher levels of the hormone cortisol, which increases the activity of the body's metabolic and immune systems. It's possible that high levels of estrogen might both increase cortisol secretion and decrease cortisol's ability to return to normal levels. The result would be a more pronounced, long-lasting type of stress response. It's not clear whether depression is a cause or the result of high cortisol levels, but the two are undoubtedly related. Over the past few decades, a number of studies have shown that cortisol levels are elevated in about half of all severely depressed people. And if estrogen raises cortisol levels after stress, then estrogen might render women more prone to depression—particularly after a stressful event.

Some women appear to have inherited a greater tendency than other women to get depressed after stressful events. In research with female twins at the Medical College of Virginia, experts found that women with a family history of depression had a higher risk of becoming depressed themselves after stress than did women without such a family history. In other words, these women seem to have inherited a vulnerability to become depressed after a crisis.

Depression after delivery
Nowhere is the link between hormones and depression more evident than in postpartum depression. Most women experience a wide range of emotions

during pregnancy and after the birth. Regardless of how prepared you were or how much you looked forward to your pregnancy and your baby's birth, you may hit some dizzying highs and frightening lows.

On the third or fourth day after the birth, many women experience the "baby blues"—an extremely common reaction that happens to almost three quarters of all new mothers. It's sort of a letdown feeling after the incredible experience of birth. You may cry for no apparent reason, or feel impatient, irritable, restless, or anxious.

The blues usually disappear on their own—often as quickly as they came. However, in 1 in 10 new moms, that blue feeling deepens into true depression. What many women don't realize is that this more severe postpartum depression may not appear until up to a year or so later, often beginning gradually and getting worse.

Symptoms may include

- Overconcern or lack of interest in the baby.
- Fear of hurting the baby or yourself.
- Sluggishness, fatigue.
- Sadness, hopelessness.
- Appetite and sleep disturbances.
- Poor concentration, memory loss.
- Uncontrollable crying, irritability.
- Guilt feelings.
- Feelings of inadequacy or worthlessness.
- Mood swings.
- Lack of interest in former enjoyments (including sex).

If you have several of these symptoms (either mild or severe), you could be experiencing postpartum depression.

Many women don't realize that it's possible to start having these symptoms while they're pregnant, after a miscarriage or abortion, or even a year or more after delivery. The baby blues can happen almost any time, no matter how many previously uncomplicated pregnancies you've had. In fact, most women have never experienced anything like this at any other time in their lives.

Today, experts believe that postpartum depression occurs as a result of fluctuating hormone levels. During pregnancy, rapid changes in levels of estrogen, progesterone, and thyroid hormones appear to strongly affect a woman's moods. Fortunately, all of your symptoms, no matter how severe, are temporary and treatable with skilled professional help and support. Exactly what treatment you get depends on which symptoms you have and how severe they are.

Bright Idea
If you've got several of the postpartum symptoms (or they are severe), contact your doctor for a complete medical evaluation (including a thyroid screening), a mental health evaluation, and psychotherapy. Many women find that support groups can give extra emotional support.

Drugs and depression

Many women don't realize that depression can be caused by taking certain medications. Some drugs used to treat arthritis, heart problems, high blood pressure, and cancer can produce depression, but the effects of these drugs may not always be clear right away. If you're taking any medications and are feeling depressed, ask your doctor if the drugs could be triggering your sadness. Scientists also think that some illnesses themselves can bring about depression, including Parkinson's disease, stroke, and hormonal disorders such as thyroid disease.

Are you at risk?

Your doctor may not tell you this, but there are some women who have a higher chance of developing depression than others. Knowing what you're up against can help you recognize the problem if and when it occurs. First of all, if you've had one episode of depression, you've got a 50 percent chance of having another—sometimes as many as four or five episodes in one lifetime.

Second, if depression seems to run in your family, you may be at higher risk, since many cases appear to be genetic. While there doesn't seem to be just one "depression gene," it's certainly true that you can inherit a vulnerability to depression. In a 1992 study of identical female twins (who share all genes), researchers found that if one twin has a major depression, the other is 66 percent more likely to suffer from the same problem than are unrelated children. But among fraternal twins (who share no more genes than other siblings), one twin had only a 27 percent higher chance of sharing her sister's depression.

Of course, your chance of inheriting depression varies depending on which relatives are affected:

- Close relatives of depressed people have a 15 percent chance of having major depression.
- Close female relatives of depressed women have a one in four chance of developing major depression, and a 90 percent chance of being mildly depressed.
- If your identical twin is depressed, you're 67 percent more likely to be depressed.
- If your depressed relatives abuse drugs or alcohol, you're 8 to 10 times more likely to do the same if you become depressed.
- If a depressed close relative has committed suicide, you're much more vulnerable to suicide yourself if you become depressed.

Counseling: What the experts say

Figuring out that you're depressed is half the battle—the other half is getting effective treatment. The good news is that if you're depressed, counseling can help you improve your mood and learn better ways to deal with stress. In fact, studies have shown that counseling (or "talk therapy") works just about as well as taking antidepressants.

However, if you want to cure your depression as fast and effectively as possible, recent studies have shown clearly that the best way is to combine counseling with antidepressants in a sort of one-two punch. The drugs can help normalize the chemicals in your brain, and counseling can help you address the issues that may contribute to your sad feelings.

Studies have shown that it's possible to affect the chemical levels in your brain by talking about problems and reducing stress, which could be one reason why talk therapy helps.

Counseling is also helpful because being depressed for a long period of time can actually affect the way you learn to cope with life. Counseling can help women learn what "normal" feels like.

Finding a therapist

Selecting a therapist is highly personal. A professional who works very well with one woman may not be a good choice for another. There are several ways to get referrals to qualified therapists such as licensed psychologists, psychiatrists, social workers, and other types of counselors, including the following:

- Talk to close family members and friends for their recommendations, especially if they have had a good experience with psychotherapy.

Timesaver
Short-term talk therapies (12 to 20 weeks) have proven useful in treating depression. One method helps patients recognize and change negative thinking patterns that have led to the depression. Another approach focuses on improving a patient's relationships with people.

- Many state professional associations operate referral services which put individuals in touch with licensed and competent mental health providers.

- Ask your primary care physician (or other health professional) for a referral. Tell the doctor what's important to you in choosing a therapist so he or she can make appropriate suggestions.

- Inquire at your church or synagogue.

- Look in the phone book for the listing of a local mental health association or community mental health center and check these sources for possible referrals.

Therapists: Heroes or healers?

Therapists are specially trained to deal with people, but this doesn't make your counselor a magician. He or she is a human being, with normal strengths and weaknesses. Therefore, if you really want to feel better, don't play mind games or try to trick your therapist. Be as honest, direct, and open as you can.

On the other hand, it's important that you understand your rights in a therapy situation. You have the right to

- Understand the therapist's therapeutic orientation and specialization.

- Ask questions about your therapist's background, attitudes, and values that may be relevant to your treatment.

- Understand the limits of confidentiality, and with whom (and under what circumstances) the therapist may discuss your case.

- Be fully informed about written or taped records and who else may see them.

- Understand the approximate length of treatment.
- Negotiate treatment goals.
- Be fully informed of a diagnosis.
- Be fully informed of treatment strategies.
- Refuse any treatment or intervention.
- Ask the therapist to evaluate your progress.
- Consult with another therapist about your therapy.
- See your written files.
- Ask the therapist to send a written report about treatment to anyone you wish.
- Refuse to allow your therapist permission to use aspects of your case for publication or a speech.
- Refuse to answer any question.
- End therapy any time.

Analysis or talk therapy?

Different therapists have different ideas about how to treat depression based on their orientation. Depending on the therapist, you may engage in role playing, psychoanalysis, discussion, dream analysis, or body-awareness activities. Some therapists may want your family members to come to sessions, others may ask you to attend group therapy sessions.

The therapist's orientation also will affect the way he or she treats your depression and its cause. Some therapists focus more on the biochemical origin of depression, others may also want to talk about your childhood or the present. Many therapists borrow from a variety of orientations.

These different schools of thought may include

Bright Idea
Be sure to ask your therapist to explain his or her basic orientation. If you're not comfortable with this information, consult a different therapist.

- Behaviorism: You may be given specific tasks to accomplish between sessions; not much time will be spent on your early life. You may be asked to try relaxation, assertiveness training, or behavior modification.

- Humanism: Who you are as a person is important; you may be asked to think about your behavior in certain ways.

- Psychoanalysis: Your early life and how you resolved major issues are believed to be important in how you now feel. You may be asked to do free association and dream analysis. Treatment can continue for many years.

Treatment can last anywhere from one or two sessions (short-term therapy) to a number of years (psychoanalysis). These days, the trend is definitely toward brief therapy. It's a good idea to ask your therapist how long he or she expects you to need care. If you don't relish the thought of spending the next five years in therapy, then you may need to find a different specialist.

Paying for treatment

One of the problems in getting help for depression is not just the high cost of mental health care, but the reluctance of most health insurance companies to pay for counseling. And despite the fact that depression strikes far more women then men, the nation's largest managed care groups don't have any gender-specific guidelines for treating the problem.

Don't avoid seeking help because you're afraid how much treatment might cost. Often depression can respond to treatment within weeks—not months or years—of beginning therapy and medication.

Fees for therapy vary and depend in part on what kind of expert you consult. Private practitioners may charge $50 an hour on up; mental health clinics will be less expensive. Community mental health centers offer treatment based on a patient's ability to pay.

Is your therapist really helping?

Sometimes women feel as if they have spent a long time in therapy without much benefit. Anyone receiving counseling who isn't sure if the treatment is helping can request a consultation with another therapist to help evaluate the situation. You should feel free to bring this up with your therapist. Remember, you aren't helpless in this situation. Here's what to do:

1. Discuss the situation with your therapist, explaining what you're uncomfortable with.
2. If you're still not satisfied, get a second opinion from another therapist.
3. If you're in a clinic or mental health agency, ask to meet with the therapist's supervisor or administrative superior.
4. You may complain to a community advocate.
5. End therapy or transfer to another counselor.

Therapists certainly use a variety of techniques during treatment. However, if any technique makes you uncomfortable or seems ineffective, you should talk about your feelings. You can also ask a different therapist whether the technique seems reasonable, or you can contact an ethics committee of a professional association (such as the American Psychological Association and the American Psychiatric Association). (See Appendix A for contact information.)

Moneysaver
Costs vary due to location and the type of training a person has, and some therapists and many mental health clinics have sliding fee scales based on income. Clinics charge less than private practitioners; masters-level social workers charge less than Ph.D.-level psychologists, who, in turn, charge less than psychiatrists (M.D.s).

Watch Out!
You also have the right to ask your therapist about his or her opinions about sexism and its effects. If your question isn't treated with respect, that could be the first clue that this therapist may not be the right one for you.

If you can't imagine yourself bringing this up, or your therapist gets upset when you mention your concern, you need to question whether you should continue in therapy with this person. If you don't feel free to bring up doubts, you may want to seek a consultation with someone else.

Squeezing out sexism

Many women wonder privately what to do if they discover their therapist seems to have an uncomfortably traditional outlook toward women. While most psychologists would insist that sexism doesn't play a part in their treatment, in fact it's almost impossible for anyone in our society—man or woman—to be raised entirely without any sexist influence, according to the American Psychological Association.

You may notice what you feel are sexist ideas creeping into your therapist's conversation. Perhaps your therapist believes that women possess certain "feminine" personality traits, that it's a "woman's nature" to want to be dominated by a man, or that women who complain a lot are "hysterical." If this troubles you, remember: You're the consumer. You have the right to choose a particular therapist or counselor.

During treatment, if you feel your therapist is behaving in a sexist way, talk about your feelings. Express your concerns right away—don't just quit therapy the first time it happens without discussing the problem. You don't want to leave someone who is helping you, but you don't need to stay with someone whose attitudes are destructive to you, either.

If your therapist acts inappropriately...

It's normal for you and your therapist to have lots of different kinds of feelings for each other, from strong dislike to intensely caring feelings. You may even find yourself sexually attracted to your therapist—or find that your therapist is attracted to you. Maybe you're attracted to each other. If this is the case, it's helpful to talk about these feelings with each other.

However, it is unethical for your therapist to ever engage in any kind of sexual relationship or erotic contact with you, either as part of your treatment or outside regularly scheduled appointments. Even if you and the therapist want to have this relationship, it's unethical. Any well-trained therapist knows that a woman can be deeply damaged in therapy by developing a sexual contact with a therapist, no matter how much she might want to do so.

Inappropriate contact is not common, but if your therapist ever uses inappropriate or uncomfortable body language, or tries to kiss, caress, or fondle you, quit treatment right away. Therapists should never, under any circumstances, make sexual overtures toward a client.

If the therapist is a member of a professional group or organization, you can report an ethics violation to the ethics committee of that professional group. (You can find a list of names and address of all the major professional organizations in Appendix A.)

If your therapist is licensed or certified by your state, you can also file a complaint with the state licensing board. The board will investigate the matter; if the board finds that the therapist violated ethical standards, it may revoke the therapist's license.

Remember: If you choose to report your therapist, you may be required to participate in long and sometimes painful proceedings. You may lose the

> **Watch Out!** You should contact your doctor if you're taking antidepressants and you're thinking of taking any over-the-counter or prescription drugs, you get pregnant or plan to, you plan to breastfeed, or you have a serious side effect.

right to confidentiality during the process. Be sure to weigh the costs and benefits of your actions carefully. You might find it helpful to talk to someone you trust before making a decision.

Do antidepressants work?

Depression responds well to counseling, but antidepressants are essential in treating the condition.

Only a physician can prescribe drugs, however, so if you are seeing a psychotherapist you will need a referral to a psychiatrist, who is a medical doctor with a specialty in mental health. While any physician is legally permitted to prescribe antidepressants, a psychiatrist has the most training in the enormously complex art of correctly prescribing and managing antidepressant medication.

Antidepressants can improve mood, sleep, appetite, and concentration, but they often take at least 4 to 12 weeks before there are real signs of progress. Most need to be continued for six months or longer after symptoms disappear. They work by correcting a chemical imbalance in the brains of depressed people, boosting the level of neurotransmitters important in fighting depression.

Each antidepressant on the market today helps between 60 and 80 percent of all depressed people. The hard part is that no one knows which drug will work best for which person—or why.

Each of the major classes of antidepressants—monoamine oxidase inhibitors (MAOIs), tri- and tetracyclics, and SSRIs—affect different neurotransmitter systems in different ways. The more neurotransmitters the drugs affect, the more side effects you're likely to have.

So how does your doctor know which one to try? It's a case of educated guesswork. Most doctors today will start with one of the very newest types of antidepressants, the SSRIs (Prozac is in this class), mostly because they work well with the fewest side effects.

But if the first drug doesn't work (and it may not), your doctor should keep on trying different drugs in different combinations. Many times, you may need to switch four or five times before you find the antidepressant that works best for you.

Most doctors have a favorite antidepressant that they'll start their patients out on, generally because they've found it seems to work best for the majority of their patients. Sometimes, your doctor will combine drugs with different side effect profiles so that each offsets the other's negative effects. (For example, one drug that causes drowsiness will be combined with another antidepressant that causes wakefulness.)

The most important consideration is to find the medication that deals best with your individual symptoms. Beyond that, the various drugs may cause side effects that differ significantly. Different women respond to different medications, but fortunately there are many different drugs to try.

What to ask your doctor

Before you begin taking any antidepressant, you should fully understand what to expect from the drug. It's important to be able to ask your doctor all the questions you have. Don't worry about how busy the doctor is or that there's a roomful of clients waiting to see him or her. Get all your questions answered right away.

Because different drugs have different side effects, make sure you discuss the side effects fully with your physician before opting for any particular medication. Some doctors don't like to discuss side effects, fearing that this may unduly frighten you or make you more likely to experience that side effect. If your doctor is reluctant to discuss side effects with you, then find another doctor who will. The more you know about possible side effects, the better prepared you will be to deal with them.

When you go for your first appointment for an antidepressant, take along a sheet of paper with these questions:

- How dangerous is this drug if taken in slightly higher than normal doses?
- How will it affect my sleep?
- Will it affect my level of anxiety?
- Will it affect my sex life? If so, how?
- Will I gain or lose weight?
- How will it interact with the other drugs I take?
- How will it affect the other medical conditions I have?
- How soon can I expect to notice an improvement?
- How long do I need to wait before you decide it is or is not working?

Hot off the lab table: The newest drugs

Mention "antidepressant" and most people think of Prozac—it's certainly the best known drug of its kind in recent memory. But science has been coming up with even newer antidepressants that work just as well (with fewer side effects) that you may not have heard about.

In fact, Prozac is only one of a large group of new antidepressants known as the SSRIs, which work by interfering with the reabsorption of serotonin. This boosts the brain levels of serotonin, easing depression. The SSRIs are the newest and most powerful drugs, and the ones with the fewest side effects. Unfortunately, they are also the most expensive. The truth is, however, that it's often impossible to tell which drug you will respond to best.

Drugs in the SSRI class include

- Celexa (citalopram).
- Prozac (fluoxetine).
- Zoloft (sertraline).
- Paxil (paroxetine).
- Luvox (fluvoxamine).
- Serzone (nefazodone).

Citalopram, or Celaxa, is the very newest antidepressant granted approval by the U.S. Food and Drug Administration. Celexa is chemically similar to Prozac, Paxil, Zoloft, and other SSRIs, but while all these drugs are chemically similar, they aren't identical. Some provide more relief with fewer side effects than others, but it's impossible to tell ahead of time which drug will work best for whom.

Celexa has been marketed since 1989 in Europe, where it has already surpassed Prozac as the most popular type of SSRI; it's used by about eight million people worldwide. While Celexa should be used cautiously with certain other drugs such as ketoconazole, some data show that among the SSRIs, Celexa may be the least likely to cause potential drug interactions.

Celexa works as well as the tricyclic antidepressants imipramine and maprotiline, but not as well as the tricyclic clomipramine. (Tricyclics are discussed below.) It worked as well as Prozac with about the

Watch Out!
While all drug overdoses are potentially dangerous, some drugs are more dangerous than others in excessive levels; Celexa is especially dangerous (there have been 12 overdose deaths associated with this drug in Europe).

> We don't have good guidelines about which person will do well on which drug. If the first drug doesn't work, don't give up. If your doctor won't help you, go to someone else.
> —North Carolina psychiatrist Andy Myerson

same side effects, but Celexa had a higher rate of complete recovery after two weeks.

The side effects are linked with how much of the drug you take, but the most common are similar to other SSRIs: nausea, dry mouth, increased sweating, sleepiness, and insomnia. Six percent of men experienced difficulty with ejaculation, and 3 percent reported impotence. (In fact, various problems with reduced libido and sexual performance are common among almost all SSRIs.) Some patients may experience a slight weight loss during therapy. You may notice an improvement as soon as a week up to a month, but you should continue taking the Celexa until your doctor says it's okay to quit.

Cyclics: Do they still work?

Before Prozac, tricyclics were the antidepressants of choice—and had been ever since they were first introduced in 1958. Today they're less popular than the SSRIs, but they are still used for women who don't respond to anything else.

Common cyclic antidepressants include

- Amitriptyline (Elavil, Endep, Emitrip, Enovil).
- Amoxapine (Ascendin).
- Clomipramine (Anafranil).
- Desipramine (Norpramin, Pertofrane).
- Doxepin (Adapin, Sinequan).
- Imipramine (Tofranil, Tipramine, Janimine).
- Maprotiline (Ludiomil).
- Nortriptyline (Pamelor, Aventyl).
- Protriptyline (Vivactil).
- Mirtazapine (Remeron).

The cyclics (tetracyclic and tricyclic) work by beefing up the brain's supply of norepinephrine and serotonin levels (chemicals that are low in depressed women). But they also interfere with many other neurotransmitters and systems in the brain, which causes more side effects.

Common side effects include tremor, headache, sensitivity to light, dry mouth, nausea, fatigue, weakness, anxiety, diarrhea or constipation, indigestion, insomnia or sedation, nervousness, and excessive sweating. More infrequent side effects include shakiness; dizziness; vomiting; abnormal dreams; pain in eyes, joints, abdomen, muscles, or back; diminished sex drive; slow pulse; hair loss; rash; palpitations; irregular heartbeat; fever; chills; and more. If you're taking these drugs, you should stay out of the sun to avoid skin sensitivity.

Because these drugs have a pronounced sedative effect, be extra cautious about driving, using machinery, or engaging in any activities that require alertness, judgment, or physical coordination until you feel confident that the drug does not impair your abilities. Don't drink alcohol while taking these drugs.

Contact your physician immediately if, while taking these drugs, you develop a fever, chills, or any flulike symptoms.

MAO inhibitors: Are they safe?

Soon after researchers developed tricyclics, they came up with another very different set of antidepressants—monoamine oxidase inhibitors (MAOIs). These drugs affect the same two neurotransmitters as tricyclics (serotonin and norepinephrine), in addition to a third—dopamine.

Common MAOIs include

- Isocarboxazid (Marplan).
- Phenelzine (Nardil).
- Tranlcypromine (Parnate).

A protein in the brain called monoamine oxidase burns up these neurotransmitters. Since depression is linked to a low level of neurotransmitters, blocking the monoamine oxidase with MAO inhibitors boosts the level of the neurotransmitters, easing depression.

Unfortunately, monoamine oxidase also burns up tyramine, a molecule that affects blood pressure. So when monoamine oxidase gets blocked by the MAOI, the level of tyramine begins to rise, which can cause a sudden blood pressure spike so severe it can burst blood vessels in the brain.

A wide range of foods boosts tyramine in the brain, which isn't harmful unless you're taking an MAO inhibitor. To avoid a fatal reaction, anyone who takes MAOIs must follow a rigid diet, avoiding:

- Alcoholic beverages, especially sherry, liqueurs, and beer (many cough syrups are 25 to 30 percent alcohol).
- Anchovies.
- Bologna, pepperoni, salami, and any fermented sausage.
- Cheese (especially strong or aged).
- Chicken liver.
- Fermented food (such as beer and some sausages).
- Fruit (especially overripe fruit).
- Meat prepared with tenderizers.
- Smoked or pickled meat.
- Soy sauce.

You shouldn't take MAOIs if you've got serious heart problems, epilepsy, bronchitis, asthma, or high blood pressure, or if you have trouble following a rigid diet.

MAOIs have many side effects, including making you feel drugged or sluggish. In addition, the drugs can be toxic at fairly low doses, which means they're not a good choice if you're suicidal.

On the other hand, a few people don't respond to any other drug. If you're willing to deal with the diet and the other side effects in order to ease your depression, MAOIs may work for you.

Lithium: What you need to know

Lithium is an extremely effective drug used to treat manic depression, a type of mental illness that includes mood swings from deep depression to mania. Lithium can quickly reverse mania in 80 percent, and stabilize mood in 60 to 70 percent, of women.

Scientists aren't exactly sure how lithium works, but they believe it may correct chemical imbalances in certain neurotransmitters (serotonin and norepinephrine) that influence emotion and behavior. It works best by controlling a person's mania. Sometimes your doctor may add Prozac or another antidepressant to control depression in addition to the lithium.

Unfortunately, lithium doesn't work for everybody (it's most effective if you haven't had more than three episodes of mania).

There are a number of side effects with lithium, the most serious of which is the very narrow range between a dose that works (and is safe) and one that is toxic. It's easy for lithium to build up in your body (especially if you have kidney problems). Signs that you're getting too much include

- Diarrhea and vomiting.
- Drowsiness.

> **❝** When I went off lithium, the manic depression came back. It was terrible. I would stand there at work and pretend I was alive.
> —Jack, 48 **❞**

Watch Out!
Don't lose too much salt if you're taking lithium because to do so will alter the blood-lithium concentration, leading to lithium toxicity. Don't overexert yourself and sweat too much, either, and avoid extremely hot weather and saunas.

- Muscular weakness.
- Lack of coordination.
- Giddiness, confusion.
- Blurry vision.
- Ringing in the ears.
- Seizures.
- Staggering.

Other side effects include thirst, frequent urination, weight gain, and drowsiness. People with psoriasis or diabetes may notice that their symptoms get worse with lithium.

Electroconvulsive treatment

Many people have a profound, negative knee-jerk reaction to the idea of electroshock, now known as electroconvulsive treatment (ECT). However, ECT is still used today because it appears to work for people with very serious depression who don't respond to any other treatment.

In modern ECT, the patient is given an anesthetic and muscle relaxant before padded electrodes are applied to one or both temples. A controlled electric pulse is delivered until a brain seizure occurs. Patients usually have 6 to 12 treatments.

Pros and cons

Doctors still use ECT because it works for some people who don't respond to anything else. On the other hand, treatments do cause temporary memory loss. More ominously, some patients say that after several treatments they experience a more serious memory loss—but this, too, disappears a few weeks after treatment ends. It's not clear whether ECT causes permanent memory loss, although all patients show some amount of amnesia for events right before treatment.

If your doctor is considering ECT, remember that it doesn't combine very well with most antidepressants (including Prozac), and a few people on Prozac have had prolonged seizures after ECT.

ECT and your pregnancy

If you're depressed and pregnant, you may not want to take antidepressant drugs, which carry certain risks to your unborn child. In this case, ECT is an option, because it has been found safe during all trimesters of pregnancy by the American Psychiatric Association. Your doctor can minimize the risk of the procedure by modifying the technique, and medications used during ECT are safe to use during pregnancy.

Nevertheless, all pregnant women should have ECT in a hospital where a fetal emergency could be managed if necessary. If you are considering ECT and you're pregnant, you should contact an obstetrician about the possible complications related to ECT in pregnancy.

Alternatives

Certainly anyone who is more than mildly depressed should consider having psychotherapy and taking antidepressants. However, mildly depressed women may want to first try treating their depression with alternative methods before resorting to antidepressant medication and/or therapy.

A word of caution: If you have suicidal thoughts, you should not risk treating your depression with alternative methods. Serious depression must be treated aggressively with a combination of

Unofficially...
Some people associate ECT with the ancient Roman tradition of applying electric eels to the head to cure madness, but it was actually invented in the late 1700s when Ben Franklin was shocked into unconsciousness during one of his electricity experiments.

antidepressants and therapy, which have been shown to work best for severe depression.

St. John's wort: Does it work?

St. John's wort is an ancient herb associated with magic, mysticism, and mysterious rituals. Today it's made a comeback as "nature's Prozac" because of its apparent ability to combat depression. One reason why St. John's wort is so popular is that the herb costs only about $10 a month—considerably less than pharmaceutical antidepressants—without many of the side effects of other antidepressants. St. John's wort burst onto the medical scene in 1996 after the British Medical Journal published an overview of 23 clinical studies of 1,757 patients comparing an extract of St. John's wort with placebos and certain older antidepressants. The journal concluded that the extract worked better than the placebo in mild to moderate depression, with only a few mild side effects.

Since then, other studies have found that the herb works as well as certain older antidepressants (the tricyclics, including imipramine), with fewer side effects. In fact, in the last 2,000 years that herbalists have used St. John's wort, there has never been a reported human death attributed to it.

However, there is still much that we do not know about St. John's wort. For example, it's not known which components of the herb are active. The extract from St. John's wort contains polycyclic phenols, hypericin, and pseudo hypericin (the presumed active components), in addition to flavinoids (hyperoside, quercitin, isoquercitrin, rutin), kaempferol, luteolin, biapigenin, and hyperforin. Recent data suggest that hyperforin may play a significant role in explaining the effects of hypericum extracts on mood.

Because there have been no long-term studies comparing Prozac and other SSRIs with St. John's wort, the United States government launched a three-year study in October 1997 to test the herb head-to-head against the newest antidepressants, including Prozac and Paxil. These drugs are believed to act in the brain very much like St. John's wort.

Using standardized doses of research-grade hypericin in well-controlled populations, scientists at the National Institute of Mental Health and the National Center for Complementary and Alternative Medicine (formerly, the National Office of Alternative Medicine) will find out whether a longer course of treatment with the plant causes more serious side effects, and which works better: St. John's wort or SSRIs.

It's best to take 900 mg of St. John's wort a day, divided into three equal doses of 300 mg. each. Take the herb during meals to avoid stomach upset, which is the most common side effect. Other side effects—which are very rare—include a slight skin sensitivity to the sun in very delicate-skinned women.

While it's possible to use St. John's wort that you grow yourself, it's hard to make sure you're getting the right amount of hypericin (the herb's active ingredient). If you do choose to grow your own, make sure you're buying the right variety of the herb used to cure depression; be sure to purchase Hypericum perforatum, which can reach 32 inches tall. This variety is often not the one you'll see in nurseries, because it looks so unattractive. (There are more than 200 varieties of Hypericum.)

You should never take St. John's wort with any other antidepressant (and you should wait two weeks when switching from an MAOI to St. John's

Moneysaver
When buying St. John's wort, compare brands for the best value. Make sure you purchase 300 mg. tablets, standardized to 0.3 percent hypericin (the active ingredient in St. John's wort).

wort, or vice versa). You may notice an increase in nervousness if you take this herb together with large doses of caffeine. Women who are very sensitive to caffeine or to the anxiety-producing effects of Prozac may feel nervousness or insomnia with St. John's wort. Don't take St. John's wort if you're pregnant without consulting your doctor.

Ins and outs of acupuncture

Many women think of acupuncture as primarily as a treatment for pain. However, some studies from the former Soviet Union and China have found that acupuncture seems to be an effective method for treating mood disorders.

Since cognitive and behavioral therapies can affect brain function and level of neurochemicals, it's certainly possible that acupuncture may do the same. In at least one Chinese study, more than half of depressed acupuncture patients stopped feeling depressed after eight acupuncture treatments. However, acupuncture as a treatment for depression is still in the research stages; experts don't recommend relying solely on acupuncture. Larger studies are planned to compare acupuncture with established treatments, and to test whether it can prevent relapses.

Seeking support

Social support has profound psychological benefits which can help anyone who feels depressed. Antidepressants and counseling are very effective, but you might find that joining a support group can really turn your life around.

Many women don't feel comfortable talking about depression with others. However, talking about your depression with women who've been there can be far more comforting than sitting on a therapist's couch.

Over the past 25 years, many studies have shown that social isolation raises the level of stress hormones in the blood, triggering feelings of depression and anxiety, increased heart rate, higher blood pressure, and impaired immune function. When social isolation becomes chronic, stress hormones circulate constantly in your body, interfering with your ability to cope with depression. On the other hand, well-developed social networks of all types lower the flood of stress hormones, allowing the body to better cope with stress.

Can you relax depression away?

Since stress hormones can lead to depression, it's not surprising that women who meditate (or who practice some type of relaxation method) often report feeling happier and more positive. In fact, many studies have shown that mood improves in depressed people who regularly relax through meditation or by doing yoga or other exercises.

Watching funny videos or listening to humorous records can also have a measurable effect on brain chemical levels and health.

Vitamins

Because some vitamin deficiencies can cause depression, you may consider taking vitamin supplements if you're mildly depressed. Even a minor B6 deficiency can lower serotonin levels. As little as 10 mg of vitamin B6 a day can relieve depression.

Folic acid (another B vitamin) also can help ease depression. Several studies have shown that depressed people tend to have low blood levels of

Watch Out!
If you use gingko, you should not take more than 240 mg per day or you might develop diarrhea, restlessness, and irritability.

folic acid, and other studies have shown that supplementation helps relieve depression.

Getting better with gingko

Herbalists believe that the herb ginkgo biloba improves blood flow through the brain, but research suggests it also appears to normalize neurotransmitter levels linked to depression.

Banish depression with a cuppa Joe

Coffee is the nation's most popular pick-me-up, providing a mild but noticeable antidepressant effect. The addition of caffeine to aspirin has been shown to produce better pain relief than aspirin by itself, and since caffeine isn't known to relieve pain, researchers believe its mood-elevating action accounts for its pain-relieving benefit.

Caffeine has also been used in some physician-supervised weight-loss programs with modest but statistically significant success. Again, because the drug has no known appetite-suppressing response, scientists attribute its action to its mood-elevating effect.

Of course, some people are more sensitive to caffeine; anyone who uses too much may experience insomnia, agitation, restlessness, and irritability. In addition, women with cystic breasts should not use too much caffeine.

Exercise—is it enough?

It's possible to ease some cases of mild depression by exercising regularly (running, biking, and swimming are good choices). Aerobic exercise boosts the level of brain chemicals related to mood—some of the same chemicals that are affected by antidepressants.

No time for an exercise program? Even a brisk 10- or 20-minute walk can help, although to be most effective you should exercise at least three times a week for at least half an hour each time. (Five or more times a week is better.) Sadly, exercise alone isn't going to help a severe depression, however.

Down the road: What you can expect

About two-thirds of women who experience serious depression recover with antidepressants and psychotherapy. While it is quite possible that depression will recur, most women will find that their depression will respond again to retreatment with antidepressants and therapy. The important thing to remember is that almost everyone who is depressed can be helped by medication—and the sooner treatment is started, the sooner you'll be feeling better.

Just the facts

- Women are twice as likely as men to be depressed.
- Depression is caused by a combination of genetic, biological, psychological, and environmental factors.
- The best treatment for depression is often a combination of therapy and antidepressants.
- Seasonal affective depression is caused by high melatonin levels during winter and responds well to a combination of light therapy and antidepressants.
- The herb St. John's wort appears to work as well for mild to moderate depression as placebo, with fewer side effects.

GET THE SCOOP ON...
The best treatments for anxiety ▪ Breathing tips to ease stress ▪ Spotting domestic abuse ▪ Getting help for domestic abuse

Stress, Anxiety, and Violence

Stress is healthy—as long as you can keep it under control. But when stress builds up to the point where you feel like you're going to explode, it can have a negative affect on your mental and physical well-being. Our stress response has been around since the dawn of time, when the cave-dwellers who responded best to stress lived longest. In prehistoric time, there was a real need for our body's quick response to danger; stress today exists as an ancient holdover from our ancestors as one of the ways our bodies protect themselves. When danger threatens, "stress hormones" are released into the bloodstream to prepare you for action and to evade danger. These hormones (including adrenaline) are pumped throughout the entire body to

- Speed up breathing.
- Increase heartbeat and blood pressure.
- Tense muscles (so you can run away from danger).

> Stress as a scientific concept suffers the misfortune of being too widely known and too poorly understood.
> —Scientist and stress expert Hans Selye

- Slow down digestion in order to shunt blood to vital muscles and your brain (you may experience this as butterflies in your stomach).
- Energize the brain (so you can plan and think your way out of trouble).
- Clot blood more quickly.
- Pour sugar and fat into the blood (to give your body fuel to defend itself).

How stress affects you

These physical and psychological changes help you if you're actually threatened by danger, but today we've got those same unconscious body responses to normal, everyday stress, but no way to get rid of all that tension. Many women don't even realize how many inconsequential, annoying stresses they deal with, and just move on. But each one can take its toll on your body. Most situations that cause stress don't provide you with an outlet for all that extra energy your body is producing. This kind of unresolved stress can

- Kill your appetite.
- Cripple your immune system.
- Shut down the processes that repair your tissues.
- Interfere with your sleep.
- Break down your bones.

When your stress is over, the stress hormones should drop down to normal levels. Sometimes, however, they stay at high levels in the blood, and when stress builds up, the stress hormones never drop below "crisis" level. Continued exposure to these stress levels can lead to mental and physical symptoms, including

- Anxiety.
- Depression.
- Heart palpitations.
- Muscular aches and pains.

Stress doesn't usually directly cause illness, but it can certainly contribute to some diseases and worsen conditions that you already have. Stress has been directly linked to triggering or worsening

- Allergies.
- Asthma.
- Migraines.
- Irritable bowel syndrome.
- Eczema.
- Psoriasis.
- Hives.
- Herpes simplex types I and II.
- High blood pressure.
- Heart disease.

How stressed are you?

Most women underestimate the amount of stress they encounter in their daily lives. You'd be surprised how much stress you can experience without even realizing it—so the first step in handling stress is to identify it so that you can take responsibility for your own thoughts, feelings, and behavior. The first way to do this is to take a "stress test" to see what sorts of life stresses you've been dealing with. Then, you need to take a look at your daily life to identify the fairly minor everyday stresses you experience that can be destructive as they build up.

Unofficially...
One out of five people responds to stress in a destructive way.

Stress test

Mental health experts have devised a test that looks at life changes to show you how stressful many seemingly everyday life events can be. Keeping in mind the idea that any change usually brings about stress (even if it seems like fun, such as taking a vacation), complete the following test. Check all the events that have occurred in your life in the past year and then total the points:

Death of a spouse	100
Divorce	73
Martial separation	65
Jail term	63
Death of a close family member	63
Personal injury or illness	53
Marriage	50
Fired from job	47
Marital reconciliation	45
Retirement	45
Change in family member's health	44
Pregnancy	40
Sex problems	39
New family member	39
New business	39
Change in financial status	38
Death of a close friend	37
Different line of work	36
More arguments with spouse	35
Mortgage or loan for major purpose	31
Foreclosure	30
Change in job responsibility	29
Son or daughter leaves home	29
In-law trouble	29
Outstanding personal achievement	28
Spouse starts or stops work	26
Begin or end school	26

Change in living conditions	25
Trouble with boss	23
Change in work hours or conditions	20
Change in residence	20
Change in school	20
Change in recreation	19
Change in church activities	19
Mortgage or loan for smaller purchase	17
Change in sleeping habits	16
Change in number of family get-togethers	15
Change in eating habits	15
Vacation	13
Holidays	12
Minor violations of law	11

Points total more than 300: Your stress level is high. You need some stress intervention techniques now!

150–300: Borderline high stress. You need to reduce the number of high-impact changes, if possible, and learn stress reduction techniques.

0–150: Your stress level based on life changes at the moment is low.

Keep a stress log

You may have been surprised at how many major life stresses you're juggling. Now it's time to identify actual day-to-day stressful situations you handle by keeping a "stress log." This is one strategy often recommended by psychologists as a starting point to understand exactly where your stress is coming from. Before you can hope to deal with your stress, you need to know exactly what areas of your life you find challenging.

In your diary, note the stress you experience and how it makes you feel throughout the day. If you keep this diary faithfully for two weeks, you should

Bright Idea
Put a piece of colored tape on your watch and on your clock at work as a reminder to relax. Now each time you glance up to see what time it is (a guaranteed stress builder), you'll see the reminder. Say the word "relax" to yourself and feel your tension fade...

begin to see patterns emerging. Whenever a stressful event occurs at any time during the day, write down

- What happened.
- Where it happened.
- How stressed you are on a 1 to 10 scale.
- How you handled it.

Then, every hour (regardless of whether or not you think you're feeling stress), record the following:

- The time
- How happy you are right now (on a 1 to 10 scale)
- How stressed you are right now (on a 1 to 10 scale)
- Whether you are enjoying what you're doing
- How efficient you are right now

Dealing with stress

Now that you've got a good idea of the major areas of stress in your life and the precise areas of stress you encounter on a daily basis, you're ready to work on dealing with it. Of course, you can't get rid of stress—but you can learn how to manage it.

Although other people and situations do contribute to stress, the events that affect you from the outside are beyond your control. It's all too easy to blame stress on others or situations that you can't control. It's more productive to take personal responsibility for your stress and to look for things that you can change—and it's more effective to learn to manage stress than to simply lessen it. You might be able to lessen stress briefly by taking a vacation, for example, but your vacation won't last forever, and eventually you need to face all the things you wanted to escape in the first place. Your success and happiness will depend not on making stress disappear, but on learning how to manage that stress.

Once you've identified the stress in your life, you need to commit yourself to creating change. For many women, the hardest part of learning to manage stress is finding the time to tackle the problem. In fact, this sort of time pressure is often a main source of stress. When you feel overwhelmed, it can be hard to take the first step in any healthy direction.

It's a fact that many women spend far more time, energy, and money on their home than they do on themselves. They are more likely to take the time to wash the windows or scrub the woodwork than to take a few minutes and give themselves a break. For many women, spending time on themselves when there is work to be done seems selfish. It's not. It's just as important to take care of yourself as it is to take care of your home and your job—or everything will eventually break down. Taking the time to manage stress is just good preventative maintenance for life. Eventually, unmanaged stress will affect your health, and if you're in the hospital you're not going to be able to be effective at home or on the job.

Many techniques can help to manage stress, and there's no one magic technique that's right for everybody. Remember, all stress management techniques are simply tools to help you learn to handle stress more skillfully and to have new and more effective ways to deal with difficult situations. But any technique will only work if you use it consistently.

Breathing can help

Without thinking about it, you automatically breathe in and out—but if you want to, you can control your breathing. This in turn can control your

Unofficially...
Yawning doesn't mean you're bored; it's also a sign that you're not breathing correctly. It means your body is trying to take in more oxygen because you're not providing enough from normal breathing.

heart rate, which can affect how stressed you feel. Deep breathing is essential for your health and for stress management. In fact, of all the things you can do to alleviate anxiety, forming healthy breathing habits will likely produce the most dramatic results. There is probably no single step that will so profoundly affect your body.

When stress builds and you begin to get anxious, most of us take shallow "chest" breaths. This means you're using your chest muscles to inhale instead of breathing from your diaphragm, so that only the top part of your lungs fill with air. As anxiety builds and you begin to breathe more and more shallowly, oxygen levels fall and stress chemicals pour into your blood. This sets up a vicious cycle: The more pronounced your shallow breathing, the more your brain pumps out stress hormones—and the more anxious you become. You feel more tense, you have trouble concentrating. Your brain gets less oxygen than ever, and sends out even more stress hormones.

When you're tense, do you ever feel constricted, lightheaded, or anxious? If you do, you know you've been shallow breathing. As you forget to contract your abdominal muscles and completely exhale, this leaves old, stale air in your lower lungs. You need to learn to inhale and exhale correctly in order to take in more oxygen and remove all of the carbon dioxide.

When you don't breathe deeply enough and your diaphragm doesn't move correctly, it affects more than your state of relaxation. The downward movement of your diaphragm massages and stimulates the liver, stomach, spleen, kidneys, adrenal glands, pancreas, and colon—this pressure is crucial for proper functioning. When you interfere with the movement of the diaphragm because you have poor posture, tense abdominal muscles, and poor breathing habits, you interfere with the normal functioning of all these organs.

Deep breathing is a very effective method of relaxation that can include everything from simply taking a few deep breaths to yoga and Zen meditation. Deep breathing

- Boosts your oxygen exchange.
- Lowers your heart rate.
- Lowers your blood pressure.
- Distracts you from stressful situations.
- Boosts your sense of self-control.

When you know you can count on deep breathing to calm down, you regain a sense of control over your emotions, and the cycle of anxiety and stress is broken. There are a variety of ways you can practice deep breathing (also called diaphragmatic breathing). You can practice the following exercises in any position, but it's easiest to lie down while you're learning them.

To increase the amount of oxygen you receive, do this exercise at least once a day for three weeks. The more often you do it, the better the results:

1. Sit in a chair with back straight, hands in your lap, feet flat, and thighs parallel to the floor.

2. Inhale deeply and slowly through your nose, without forcing. Let your abdomen expand—push it out! Imagine air filling your abdomen. Don't worry about looking fat.

3. In one continuous breath, imagine filling your chest and lungs with air. Feel your chest expand fully and your shoulders rise.

Unofficially...
Our legal system now recognizes stress as a consequence of crime. Courts have ruled that a victim really can be "scared to death."

4. Exhale slowly through your nose. Breathing out should take longer than breathing in.

5. Do this for at least one minute. Keep a comfortable rhythm; don't strain. Focus on keeping your breathing deep and full and your body relaxed.

It's hard for most of us to breathe this way all the time, but it can come in handy whenever you're feeling mildly tense, anxious, or upset. You can even prevent some stress symptoms such as stomach butterflies, dry mouth, or pounding heart by practicing deep breathing before a stressful situation.

You can also use deep breathing in the face of severe stress; it's one of the techniques that experts teach women who are trying to control phobias, the most severe type of stress situation there is.

Deep breathing isn't magic or hypnosis. You won't be unconscious or in another state of consciousness. What the technique will do is to restore your natural, healthy style of breathing, distract you from pain or anxiety, give you an energy boost, and sharpen your awareness. It's one of the best stress managers around.

You can practice anytime, not just in the middle of a stressful crisis. Try deep breathing

- While commuting. Sitting in traffic is a perfect time to practice your deep breathing (especially if you're in the middle of a stressful traffic jam!).

- Before eating. Taking some deep breaths before eating not only reduces any stress you may be feeling, but can help you savor what you're about to eat and not gulp your meal.

- During sports. If you're playing sports and you have a few seconds before hitting a golf ball or serving a tennis shot, do some deep breathing.

- Before performing. Most of us get nervous before a performance of any kind. Taking some calming, deep breaths can help control those stress-related fears.

Just relax...

Relaxation training is a very important part of stress management. There are different approaches to relaxation, ranging from simple relaxation strategies to self-hypnosis.

When you relax, you focus your thoughts on something besides stressful thoughts. As you practice relaxation, breathing slows, blood pressure drops, muscles relax, anxiety lessens, stressful thoughts disappear, irritability eases, stress headaches fade, and you begin to think more clearly.

Most women find it helpful to schedule a relaxation time because, otherwise, it just doesn't seem to fit into the day. Some women like to start off the day with a relaxation period of about 20 minutes, while others use prefer to use it to unwind after a tough day. Some find it best to use their lunch hour in the middle of the day to de-stress.

The first step is to learn how to relax your body. You'll probably be surprised at how much tension there is in your muscles. Until you relax them, you may not realize how taut they are. Here's how to begin:

1. Find a position that feels comfortable (either sitting or lying down).
2. Close your eyes.
3. Relax your arms with hands lightly folded on your lap.
4. Begin taking slow, deep breaths.

Unofficially...
Americans make 187 million visits to their health care providers each year for stress-related complaints.

5. Breathe rhythmically from the abdomen (not the chest).

6. As you say the word "relax" silently to yourself, focus on the muscles which control the forehead, neck, and scalp.

7. When you feel the top of your head relax, move down to the eyes. Keep repeating "relax" as you consciously focus on each muscle group. Don't move on until you feel the area relax.

8. Move on to the sinus area of your face.

9. Move to the muscles of your ears and the back of your neck. This is the seat of quite a lot of tension; spend some time here. Don't move until you can actually feel those muscles loosen.

10. Move down the shoulders, arms, and hands, all the way to toes, relaxing each section.

Some women say they have trouble simply focusing on a muscle and willing it to relax. In this case, you could try the alternative practice of progressive muscle relaxation—basically, this is simply the rhythmic tightening of one set of muscles in your body while relaxing the others. Start with your fist to get into the swing of it; tighten one fist while relaxing the rest of your body. As you relax your muscles, imagine white light or warm energy filling the area. (If you can't imagine white light, try thinking of a mist or fog.)

Bright Idea
Try making your own meditation tape. With soothing background music, give yourself a few relaxation suggestions, and then record your voice counting backward from 10 to 0. Then give yourself a few affirmations.

Meditate

It may sound exotic, but actually meditation is a very effective stress management technique. It's really just a way to learn to relax and ease your mind so that you'll feel less anxious and better able to cope with stress:

1. Follow the above steps in relaxing your body.
2. After you've relaxed your muscles, start counting backward slowly from 10 to 0.
3. As you count, visualize yourself descending (such as riding on an escalator or floating downward).
4. As you descend, visualize each number as you say it.
5. Every few numbers, tell yourself, "I'm becoming more relaxed. When I get to zero, I'll be totally relaxed."
6. When you get to the bottom of your descent and reach zero, imagine a peaceful scene.
7. Now, focus on your breathing. As you breathe out, silently repeat a word or a phrase.
8. When thoughts pop into your head, calmly let them go. Return to your word.
9. Continue for 10 to 15 minutes. At the end of this period, suggest to yourself that you will open your eyes and feel completely refreshed. Now open your eyes.

After several weeks of practice, most women say they feel not only more relaxed after meditating, but more likely to stay calm when stressed out. However, meditation doesn't work for everybody. Some women get so relaxed they simply drift off to sleep. Others tie themselves into knots because they can't master the art of thinking about nothing. If this is your problem, you can try visualization instead.

Visualization

This technique is a more active procedure than meditation, so many women find it easier than meditating.

Unofficially...
A recent report from the National Institutes of Health concluded that meditation and similar forms of relaxation can lead to better health, higher quality of life, and lowered health care costs.

Basically, visualization involves relaxing yourself and then imagining a calming scene. The principle behind visualization and imagery is that you can use your mind to recreate a relaxing place. The more intensely you call up the scene in your mind, the stronger and more realistic the experience will be. In active visualization, you can give yourself suggestions (called affirmations) while you're in the scene:

1. Relax your body as described above.

2. When you are fully relaxed with your eyes still closed, imagine a calm, beautiful scene in full detail. Pick out a place you have visited or make one up—it doesn't matter. This may take practice; some people seem to be natural visualizers and others aren't.

3. Make it as real as possible. Don't just imagine a picture. Listen to the wind blow, smell the scent of freshly mown hay or the surf, feel the spray of the waves.

4. If you wish, still in the scene with your eyes closed, give yourself a positive suggestion: "I feel peaceful" or "I feel completely relaxed." It doesn't matter what the suggestion is, as long as you frame it in a positive way. Don't say "I won't be nervous," but say "I'm completely calm."

5. At the end of the visualization, tell yourself: "When I open my eyes, I will feel calm, peaceful, and completely refreshed." Then open your eyes.

While visualizations work well to de-stress, you also can use them to prepare yourself for stress. In this case, instead of visualizing an imaginary scene, you'd preview the upcoming stressful situation, watching yourself be confident and calm. The more chances you have to preview such a situation, the more likely you'll be able to get through it with a minimum of stress—just the way you imagined it.

Visualization works because your sense organs convert signals from your environment into nerve impulses that feed into the areas of the brain that, in turn, interpret the environment. When you visualize, you're creating a similar set of nerve impulses that feed into those same areas. Because your brain can't tell the difference between what is real and what is actively imagined, this type of active visualization can truly make a difference in the way you deal with everyday situations. It's a trick professional athletes and top business executives use regularly to boost their performance. You can do the same thing.

Exercise stress away

Exercise is one of the best ways to manage stress. Aerobic exercise (exercise that makes your heart and lungs work harder) actually helps your body use up excess stress hormones. Regular exercise helps your body react less dramatically to stress, while helping you feel better and decrease depression. Exercise is most helpful if it's practiced consistently over a long period of time.

If you start exercising regularly, you'll be better able to fight stress because exercise

- Improves lung capacity.
- Lowers blood pressure.
- Lowers fat in the blood.
- Increases capillary circulation and blood flow in the arteries.
- Conditions the heart.

Start slowly in the beginning, because you'll want to keep at it—not give up because the whole

Bright Idea
Give yourself a one-minute stress-buster when you feel tense: Think "happy" and pull your lips into a smile. Visualize yourself looking happy, with your eyes dancing. Say, "I'm just fine." When you think happier, it's harder to feel stressed.

business is just too stressful. While you should check with your doctor if you're in doubt, almost no one is too old or too flabby to start exercising. Twenty or 30 minutes of exercise four or five times a week is ideal, but even much less can help you relax and cope with stressful situations more effectively.

The specific type of exercise or the amount of time spent exercising isn't as important as doing it regularly. It may not seem like you're doing much, but brisk walking is the perfect exercise for many women. Jogging, swimming, and bicycling are other popular choices. Choose an exercise you enjoy so it's more likely that your program will succeed.

If you think you don't have the time to exercise, try these 10 stress-busting exercises:

1. Snap on your dog's leash and walk him one block farther than usual, faster than usual. Then add another block tomorrow. Or try walking your pet more often.

2. On your way to the basement in your favorite department store, take the stairs instead of the elevator.

3. Park in the garage two blocks from your office instead of the lot next door.

4. If you're thinking about ordering takeout, don't have it delivered—walk to the restaurant and pick up your order.

5. At the office, take a coffee break by walking outside for a brisk 15 minutes.

6. If you take the subway or bus to work, get off one stop earlier and walk the rest of the way.

7. Take the stairs to and from your office every day instead of the elevator. (But start gradually, especially if you work on an upper floor.) Add

Unofficially...
You burn almost the same number of calories whether you walk or jog a mile (and walking is much less stressful on your joints, especially the knees).

one more flight each week until you're walking the whole way.

8. Use the bathroom on the floor above or below yours.
9. Don't use a riding lawnmower when you can push one.
10. If you do use the elevator, get off one floor above or below where you want to go and walk the rest of the way.

While exercising is a good idea, if you're over 55 or in poor physical condition, don't start an exercise program before you see a doctor for a physical and a treadmill test. Once you start exercising, you need to be aware of potential problems, especially if you've just started moving around after years of inactivity. Watch out for any of the following signs:

- Excessive tiredness
- Unusual joint, muscle, or ligament pain
- Chest pain
- Pain in teeth, jaws, or ears
- Lightheadedness, dizziness, or fainting
- Nausea or vomiting
- Headache
- Shortness of breath
- Sustained increase in heart rate after slowing down or resting
- Irregular pulse

Diet and stress

Unfortunately, the foods you turn to when you're under stress are usually the ones you won't find on any government food group chart. The blunt truth is that to master stress, you have to change. You have

Bright Idea
Yoga is another popular stress-management tool that combines aspects of both exercise and meditation; it can help you slow down your mind and relax your body.

to figure out what you're doing that's not healthy, and make different lifestyle choices. A healthy diet is one way to do that, one that includes only moderate use of caffeine, nicotine, and alcohol.

Caffeine is a stimulant drug that triggers a stress response and draws the B vitamins out of your body. Studies talk about the amount of caffeine in a cup of coffee—but most people these days drink coffee in mugs, which hold almost twice the amount of coffee (and caffeine).

If you want to cut down on caffeine, do it slowly to avoid headaches and other withdrawal symptoms. Cut out chocolate while you're at it, since it has less caffeine than coffee and tea. Coffee and tea have varying amounts of caffeine depending on what type of coffee beans are used and how the beverages are prepared. Specialty coffees (as well as most coffees sold by restaurant franchises) are made from arabica beans instead of the robusta beans used in coffees sold in cans in grocery stores, and arabica beans contain less caffeine. In addition, the process of dark roasting to which specialty coffee is subjected burns off some of the caffeine. Instant coffee has between 65 and 100 mg of caffeine; percolated, 80 and 135 mg; filtered, 115 and 175 mg; drip brewed, 154 and 210 mg; and decaf, 1 and 5 mg. Instant tea has between 35 and 70 mg; brewed tea between 28 and 154 mg; and iced tea, 39 and 44 mg. Here's how to cut back:

1. Tomorrow morning, sip on juice instead of coffee. Then have your regular amount the rest of the day.

2. In a day or two, cut back by a second cup of coffee.

3. If you start to crave a cup of coffee in the morning, pour sparkling water in your mug and sip

on that all day. (You can never get enough water.)

4. If you miss the taste of cola drinks and coffee, try drinking caffeine-free colas, a soda that's naturally caffeine-free, or decaffeinated coffee. (There is some residual caffeine in decaf coffee, but not much.)

Bright Idea
If you can't go caffeine free the cold turkey route, try drinking half regular strength coffee, half decaf.

While in the short term, nicotine does have a relaxing effect on the body, in the long run, the toxins in smoke raise your heart rate and begin to stress your entire body, from your brain to your immune system. Anyone who doubts this effect should try this exercise:

1. Before smoking your first cigarette in the morning, take your pulse.
2. Now smoke a cigarette.
3. Take your pulse again.

Your heart on nicotine beats faster, and this increase happens every time you light up. Of course, giving up cigarettes is not easy and can be stressful in and of itself, but once you get through the acute nicotine withdrawal period, most people report feeling much more relaxed in general.

In small amounts, alcohol can help you relax, but some people can't stop there. Alcohol in large doses is a stimulant and too much liquor can boost stress by interfering with healthy, normal sleep.

Instead, here are the foods you should be eating to help you relax:

- Starch and sugar: Recent brain chemistry research has found that both sugar and starch can induce relaxation. You may think of sugar as an energy food, but it's really more of a tranquilizer. While sugar can boost your energy in the short run, your body then copes with the sugar rush by secreting insulin, which cuts the amount of sugar in the blood. This gives you a quick energy boost followed by a low-energy feeling.

- Calming foods: For a natural tranquilizer, eat a small amount of carbohydrates (just one small roll or two small cookies).
- Energy-boosting foods: For a natural boost, eat a small amount of protein (some peanut butter, tuna, or meat).

Anti-stress vitamins/herbs

Stress can affect how you process nutrients in your food. Many women under stress don't absorb or digest food as they should. This means the vitamin B in your body can become depleted. (Vitamins B1, B2, B3, B6 and B12 are all involved in digestion and metabolism; B1 helps carbohydrate digestion; B2 helps release energy to cells; B3 helps metabolize carbohydrates; B6 helps metabolize protein, fat, and carbohydrates.

To make sure you're eating a good diet to combat stress, choose

- B-complex vitamin supplements (the "anti-stress vitamin").
- Vitamins A, C, and E.
- Calcium.
- Trace elements.

B-complex vitamins are very important, and you can get them in a healthy diet that includes

- Beans.
- Lean meat.
- Whole grain and enriched cereals.

- Poultry.
- Fish.
- Dairy products.

Social support—Does it work?

When stress builds up, having someone to turn to can have profound effects on your health. A live-in partner, friends, and family are all good support sources, provided the relationships are fairly positive. Pets are also helpful, and so are religious organizations and other groups.

If you don't have a solid support system, you could turn to a professional—a therapist such as a social worker or a psychologist. These experts can help you learn stress management strategies and coping techniques. Support groups of various types are also available.

The value of social support is enormously important in combating stress; studies have found that counseling alone—without modifying diet or exercise at all—can reduce the risk of heart attacks.

Stress can be good

Some stress is inevitable and actually beneficial when it helps you grow, attain difficult goals, and perform your best. Stress or nervousness before a big presentation may help you perform better or think with more clarity and precision. Eliminating all stress from your life would leave you sluggish and bored. Stress can boost your performance—but only up to a point. If, for example, you're getting ready to give a speech and you get too stressed and anxious, you may have trouble remembering what you planned to say.

Ideally, you should be able to adjust the amount of stress you face. If you learn to recognize the

Bright Idea
Nutritional yeast is an excellent source of B vitamins, and can be sprinkled in soups or salads or added to casseroles.

warning signs of increasing stress, you'll be able to cope intelligently with your stress before it wears you out.

Anxiety: What's normal?

If you've ever stood up in front of a lecture hall, you probably are intimately acquainted with the symptoms of anxiety: sweaty palms, twisted stomach, and dry mouth. It's your body's way of preparing you to confront perceived danger.

But sometimes, normal anxiety builds up to the point where it can seriously interfere with your life. This is the case with about 30 percent of women who develop an anxiety disorder sometime in their lives. In fact, anxiety disorders are the most common of all mental illnesses, according to the National Institute of Mental Health.

In its general form (called generalized anxiety disorder), you experience chronic worry and tension, often without provocation, lasting for six months or more. Physical symptoms can include everything from headaches, nausea, and frequent urination. The panic attack, another form of anxiety disorder, affects between three million and six million Americans each year—and two-thirds of them are women. Without warning, the sufferer suddenly and repeatedly experiences an overwhelming sense of terror.

Anxiety disorders: Are you at risk?

Some scientists believe that anxiety disorders can be traced back to a stressful or traumatic experience in your childhood that you have pushed out of your conscious mind—only to have it pop back years later as anxiety. In other cases, a more recent emotional shock, such as death or divorce, may trigger an anxiety disorder. In addition, your genes and biochemical makeup most likely play an important part in whether or not you develop a problem with anxiety. This is especially true if you develop panic attacks.

Panic disorder

Panic disorder, a condition in which a person experiences repeated episodes of intense terror, affects twice as many women as men. Panic disorder usually begins in early adulthood and often runs in families. If you experienced panic disorder before or during your pregnancy, you may well have much more severe attacks after the birth of your baby. The panic attacks are triggered without warning and are accompanied by a range of physical symptoms that may include

- Shortness of breath.
- Racing and/or irregular heartbeat.
- Chest pain.
- Sweating.
- Chills.
- Hot flashes.
- Dizziness.
- Nausea.
- Feeling of impending doom.
- Fears of going crazy or dying.

The attacks may come as often as once a week, or as seldom as every six months or more. No matter what the pattern, usually the woman begins to live in fear of the next attack to such a degree that the fear of the incident becomes worse than the attack itself.

Watch Out!
Up to 65 percent of all people with panic disorder also have a substance abuse problem or depression.

Sometimes a person who has many panic attacks begins to develop phobias related to the place where the attacks have occurred. A woman who's shopping when she has a panic attack may associate the mall with her fear and develop a phobia about going near it again. As she becomes increasingly fearful, she may then become afraid about driving near the mall, and then afraid to drive at all. Eventually, the fears may become so all-pervasive that the woman is afraid to leave the house and begins to avoid going out in public. At this point, her fear has become agoraphobia (literally, the "fear of the marketplace").

New research suggests that panic sufferers seem to experience false alarms of smothering, deep in the part of the brain that controls breathing. When people hyperventilate with panic disorder, they reduce their blood flow to the brain. The brain interprets this reduced blood flow as a sign of suffocation. This is one reason why breathing exercises can be so helpful in the treatment of panic disorder.

Phobias

Phobias usually begin in early adulthood between the ages of 18 and 34; phobias of all types are more common in women. You can suffer either from a specific phobia (such as a fear of dogs or airplane travel) or from social phobia—the fear of being in certain types of social or performance situations. Phobias tend to develop after a panic attack.

A phobia is an irrational fear. For example, if you're terrified of flying but you don't mind at all riding in a bullet train, that's a phobia. Common phobias include fears of being in enclosed places, heights, and elevators. If a phobia interferes with your life (say, you refuse to take on a certain assignment at work because it would involve air travel), professional counseling can help you cope.

Social phobia is a slightly different type of anxiety. Most people may feel a bit nervous about getting up in front of others—the difference between social phobia and stage fright is the degree to which the fear interferes with your life. You might feel a little apprehensive about addressing a group of business associates composed of 20 out-of-town vice presidents, but the woman with social phobia would be so anxious at being looked at in a social situation that she would be unable to eat in a restaurant, use a public bathroom, or sign a check in front of someone else.

Generalized anxiety disorder

Fear is one thing, but if you're struggling with a sort of generalized, free-floating anxiety, you may have a condition known as generalized anxiety disorder. Generalized anxiety affects about twice as many women as men. Although a third of victims eventually recover, men have a better recovery rate. Typically, a woman may have day-to-day feelings of generalized anxiety that continue constantly, interspersed with more acute panic attacks. The fear in this condition is not related to a specific object or situation (as in phobia).

Do you have an anxiety disorder?

If you think you have an anxiety disorder, you should make an appointment with a psychologist or psychiatrist for an evaluation. You'll also need to make sure your symptoms aren't caused by a physical disease, such as hyperthyroidism or heart problems. If you discover that you're physically healthy, your therapist will then need to rule out other psychiatric conditions that may share many of the same symptoms. Only after all other possible conditions are ruled out will your therapist reach a diagnosis of an anxiety disorder.

Treatment

Fortunately, anxiety disorders of all types can be treated with a form of counseling that can help you understand the anxiety reaction and what causes it. If the anxiety is more severe, medication can help control it and allow you to understand it.

Combining counseling and drugs

Most of the time, a woman with an anxiety disorder needs counseling to learn how to overcome her fear and anxiety. How quickly this works depends in part on the type of anxiety, how much it interferes with her daily life, and what contributes to the problem.

If the problem is so severe that therapy alone isn't enough to cope with the anxiety, anti-anxiety medication may be prescribed to control the anxious feelings (sometimes antidepressants are also used successfully to treat anxiety disorders). The problem with anti-anxiety drugs is that while they do work very well, they can pose a real risk of physical dependence or psychological addiction. Physical dependence can be treated by gradually tapering the dose of the drug, but psychological dependence is more difficult to handle.

The most likely of the anti-anxiety drugs to cause dependence are the benzodiazepines, such as Xanax and Valium. Long-term use of these drugs should be carefully monitored by your doctor, who will prescribe scheduled doses to be taken two or three times a day.

When it's time to stop using your anti-anxiety medication, never stop abruptly—it could lead to

Watch Out!
If you're taking anti-anxiety medication, don't drink alcohol or caffeinated beverages and never use over-the-counter drugs without checking with your health care provider first.

severe nightmares, insomnia, and seizures. Instead, taper off gradually under the advice of your health care provider.

Studies have shown that the best way to treat an anxiety disorder is by combining therapy with medication. With the drug helping to control symptoms, the patient then learns how to control symptoms using a variety of natural methods, such as relaxation and self-talk.

Phobias in particular are often treated successfully with a type of counseling known as desensitization. With this technique, the mental health expert helps a patient create a mental image of the thing that causes fear; as she concentrates on this image, her anxiety goes away and, eventually, she feels more relaxed. As she gradually retrains herself to handle the image, she can apply this method to real objects or situations, increasing her exposure until she can face the dreaded object or situation and handle her anxiety.

Kava

Kava is a popular herb that works well as a slight mood enhancer, without being hallucinogenic or addictive. Considered to be the perfect anti-anxiety treatment in Europe, the herb is now used to treat several ailments, including insomnia—but it's best known for easing anxiety.

Dealing with violent relationships

Every nine seconds in this country, a woman is physically abused. That adds up to almost four million American women who were physically abused by their husbands or boyfriends in the past year alone. Sadly, accurate information on the extent of domestic violence is difficult to obtain because women

Unofficially... European explorers of Polynesia in the 1600s were offered a ceremonial drink prepared by young virgins who chewed up the root of the kava pepper plant, spit it into a communal bowl, and mixed it with water and coconut milk.

Unofficially...
One recent survey found that 92 percent of women who were physically abused by their partners did not tell their health care providers.

tend not to report violent episodes, but we do know that about one-fourth of all hospital emergency room visits by women are caused by domestic assaults.

Contrary to popular opinion, domestic violence isn't confined to any one socioeconomic, ethnic, religious, racial, or age group. It is the leading cause of injury to women in the United States; women are more likely to be assaulted, injured, raped, or killed by a husband or boyfriend than by any other type of assailant.

Unfortunately, physical abuse isn't usually a one-time incident, but an ongoing pattern of behavior that escalates over time in both frequency and severity. Although most assaults on women don't end in death, they do cause injury and severe emotional distress. Physical injuries often aren't reported by women and go unrecognized by health care providers.

While most people think of domestic abuse as violent attacks, it can also include psychological abuse—a type of behavior that is underestimated, trivialized, and, at times, hard to define. In fact, psychological abuse has been reported by women to be as damaging as physical battering because of its impact on a woman's self-image. It often precedes or accompanies physical abuse, but it may occur by itself.

Is your partner an abuser?

There are some risk factors that make a man more likely to abuse a woman:

- A history of abusing women
- Being abused as a child
- Witnessing the abuse of his mother
- Being unemployed

Alcohol and drug use may also play a role—over one-half of the men accused of murdering their wives were drinking alcohol at the time of the offense.

Are you at risk?
Women who are abused don't share any particular characteristics or behavior that make them more susceptible to abuse. However, if you were abused or you witnessed domestic abuse as a child, you're much more likely to be abused as an adult—and to abuse your own children. You also may be more likely to have a problem with substance abuse or to have a relationship with someone who is a drug or alcohol abuser.

Although abuse can occur at any age, women between the ages of 18 and 24 are most at risk of being abused by their partners. Pregnant women are especially likely to be abused by a partner (or to have the abuse directed at the unborn child). Abuse during pregnancy carries the risk of not only of injuring the pregnant woman, but also of miscarriage or delivery of a low birth weight baby.

What's normal and what isn't
If your husband occasionally loses his temper and yells at you, is that abuse? If your boyfriend puts you down or treats you rudely, is that abuse? While it may be hard to tell in the beginning, there are some warning signs to tell if your relationship may becoming abusive.

No matter what the batterer says, women do not cause the violence against them. Instead, for the abuser it's about power and control, growing up in a cycle of violence and abuse, and having a distorted concept of what it means to be a man. An abusive relationship usually includes a pattern of behavior based on control—abusive people are usually trying to control the lives of others.

If you suspect that you or someone you know is in an abusive relationship, read the following list of abusive behaviors. The more questions there are that you answer yes to, the more dangerous the situation could be:

- Verbal abuse: Destructive criticism including mocking, name-calling, blaming, swearing, screaming, and humiliation
- Disrespect: Twisting your words and putting you down in public; insulting your friends and family; interrupting or changing the topic; not listening or responding; not recognizing feelings or opinions
- Emotional withdrawal: Not supporting or giving attention; not expressing feelings
- Minimizing or blaming: Denying the abuse; joking about poor behavior; shifting responsibility for abuse to someone else
- Abusing trust: Withholding information; seeing other women; being jealous
- Pressure: Intimidating you through guilt, sulking, or threats
- Economic abuse: Not letting you work; refusing to give you money or taking your money away; interfering with your work
- Isolating: Making it hard for you to see friends or relatives; monitoring your phone calls; telling you where you can go
- Harassment: Following you and checking up on you; embarrassing you in public
- Self-destructiveness: Substance abuse; threatening suicide

- Threats: Making or carrying out threats to hurt you or someone you know
- Intimidation: Making threatening gestures; driving recklessly; using superior size to intimidate you
- Destructiveness: Punching walls; destroying your possessions; breaking things
- Sexual abuse: Using force or coercion to obtain sex
- Weapons: Using weapons to threaten you

Symptoms of abuse

Bruised skin, broken bones, and black eyes are obvious signs of domestic abuse, but there are also a wide range of physiological complaints that often accompany such abuse. In one study, women with a history of abuse were four times more likely to have pelvic pain, backaches, and shortness of breath. Other studies have found abused women more likely to have had surgery and more likely to have been hospitalized for suicide attempts, gynecological problems, and undefined disorders. Other diseases or physical ailments more common among abused women include

- Abdominal pain.
- Irritable bowel syndrome.
- Bowel disease.
- Headaches.
- Sleeplessness.
- Tiredness.

Experts suspect this higher rate of physical disease and complaints may not be so much that abuse leads to physical symptoms, but that women who tend to complain about these symptoms also tend to

Unofficially... Women who had ended a relationship in the past year were seven times more likely to experience abuse from their estranged partner, according to a report published in the *Journal of the American Medical Association.*

Watch Out! Research has shown that using self-defense measures during rape reduces the chance of a completed rape, but increases the risk of other physical injuries.

speak up about abuse. Or, there may be some emotional factor that increases a woman's chances of developing these conditions and entering into an abusive relationship.

Not surprisingly, abused women also tend to have much higher rates of psychological problems, including depression, eating disorders, alcoholism, multiple personality disorder, post-traumatic stress disorder, and substance abuse. They are also more likely to abuse themselves through self-mutilation and self-starvation, or by returning to a partner for more abuse.

Moreover, women who have been battered appear to have a higher rate of personality disorders and a high number of psychosomatic disorders.

Getting help: Where to turn

One in four women in America will be assaulted by her partner in her lifetime. It doesn't have to happen. Domestic abuse can be very hard for health care professionals to spot, and many battered women are too afraid or unable to acknowledge the source of their trauma. They may not even admit it to themselves. Sometimes the abuser keeps a woman from getting medical help.

However, today it is easier for battered women to get support through shelters and support groups for battered women. Advocates from these programs can go with a battered woman to court to obtain a restraining order against the abuser. State and federal crime-victim programs can help women get back lost wages or uncovered medical or treatment costs.

If you or someone you know is experiencing or affected by domestic violence, call the confidential National Domestic Violence hot line at 800/799-SAFE (7233) (or TDD at 800/787-3224). In addition, you can contact the following organizations (see also Appendix A):

- National Coalition Against Domestic Violence: 303/839-1852
- The Battered Women's Justice Project: 800/903-0111
- The Resource Center on Child Custody and Protection: 800/527-3223
- The Health Resource Center on Domestic Violence: 800/792-2873

Just the facts

- You need to identify all the areas of stress in your life before you can learn how to manage it.
- Learning how to deep breathe can help you relax; deep breathing before a performance can help prevent stress.
- Relaxation, meditation, visualization, and exercise can lessen the effect stress has on your body.
- Eating a healthy diet and taking B-complex vitamins can help protect you from the effects of excess stress.
- A combination of medication and therapy can help you cope with anxiety disorders, including panic attacks and phobias.
- One out of four women will one day be abused by someone she knows.

GET THE SCOOP ON...
Why more women are dying from lung cancer ▪ Pros and cons of nicotine gum and patches ▪ Acupuncture and substance abuse ▪ Who to call when you have a drinking problem ▪ What are the best treatment plans for women

Substance Abuse

Substance abuse is an equal opportunity killer. Millions of women in the United States use substances to alter their mental state, their mood, or their behavior, and nearly half of all women have tried drugs at least once (including alcohol and cigarettes). Four million women have received treatment for drug abuse.

The problems from substance abuse are many: liver disease from alcohol; cancer and heart disease from cigarettes; hepatitis B virus and HIV from shared needles; heart attacks from illegal drugs; fatal overdoses from prescription drugs such as tranquilizers and painkillers.

What constitutes abuse?

If you have a beer or two at your outdoor barbecue with friends, do you have a problem? If you get so wound up from your job that once in a while you need a sleeping pill, is that substance abuse? Before you rush off to the nearest treatment center, here are four key factors to keep in mind:

- Loss of control: If you use more of the substance than you intend to or if your behavior changes when you're using it, this suggests you've lost control over your substance use.

- Craving: If you're addicted, you probably have an overwhelming desire for the substance, and spend lots of time thinking about how you'll obtain it and when you'll be able to use it next.

- Distorted thoughts: If you're addicted, you probably deny that you've got a problem or that you need help. If drinking has caused problems in your relationships or work life, you probably deny that they were caused by drinking; instead, you may say you drink because of these problems.

- Continued use: You'll continue to abuse the substance even if it means losing your job, losing custody of your children, having financial problems, or developing a serious illness.

Who's at risk?

There's no simple yardstick you can use to predict who is going to have a problem with drugs or alcohol and who isn't, but there are a number of factors that have been linked to substance abuse. Of course, these factors alone don't cause the problem, and just because you have one or more of these risk factors doesn't mean you're going to develop a problem. The odds, however, may be increased if any of the following situations apply to you:

Unofficially... Studies suggest that 70 percent of women who use hard drugs were sexually abused before age 16.

- Family history: If your parents or siblings have a substance abuse problem, you're more likely to have a problem yourself. Alcohol in particular is associated with genetic factors that can make you vulnerable to developing the addiction yourself.

- Stress: You're at higher risk of developing a substance abuse problem if you've been subjected to extreme stress, such as trauma, rape, physical abuse, or severe money problems.

- Poverty: Just because you're a blue color worker doesn't mean you're going to abuse drugs or alcohol, but statistics show that low income and lack of education are risk factors for substance abuse.

- Mental illness: Depression and anxiety in particular are more common in women than in men and increase your risk of substance abuse (perhaps as a way to ease the emotional pain). Still, the link between mental illness and substance abuse is complex and not yet completely understood.

The addictive personality

Certain personality traits seem to be linked to a tendency to become addicted, including

- Rebelliousness.
- Low tolerance for stress.
- Feelings of alienation.
- Impulsiveness.
- Problems in delaying gratification.
- Sensation-seeking.
- Indifference to social goals.
- Low self-esteem.
- Vulnerability to anxiety and depression.

Smoking

For many years, men were more likely to die of lung cancer than women, but recently the lung cancer rates for women have been rising—an ominous sign that more and more women are using tobacco.

In the short term, smoking can cause nicotine addiction, respiratory problems, coronary artery disease, dental problems, nervousness and depression, and a tendency toward health-damaging behavior. More obvious are the immediate changes in quality of life—bad breath, wrinkled skin, and stained fingernails. But the real damage from smoking is the long-term effects it can have on a woman's health:

- Lung cancer: Women who smoke heavily are 24 times more likely to develop lung cancer than nonsmoking women; lung cancer is now the leading cause of cancer deaths in women (surpassing breast cancer).

- Other cancers: Tobacco use is a major risk factor for other cancers such as cervical and esophageal/throat cancers.

- Hormone-related problems: The chances for infertility, an earlier onset of menopause, and the development of osteoporosis are all linked to smoking.

- Pregnancy problems: Smoking increases the risk of miscarriage, stillbirth, pre-term delivery, and low birth weight.

- High blood pressure: Women who smoke have a higher risk for high blood pressure and stroke.

- Heart problems: A woman who smokes is two to six times more likely to suffer a heart attack than a nonsmoking woman, and the risk increases with the number of cigarettes smoked each day. Women who smoke and use the Pill are 10 times more likely to have a heart attack.

Smoking can also mean big trouble for a woman's baby, both before and after birth. British researchers have found that potentially toxic tobacco compounds related to nicotine accumulate in the fluid surrounding a fetus as early as seven weeks, both in women who smoke and women exposed to smoke at home or in the workplace. Babies born to women who used tobacco during pregnancy are at a 2.5 times higher risk for sudden infant death syndrome and mental retardation. Children raised in a smoking household have twice the chance of getting asthma as those raised in a home with nonsmokers. They are also twice as likely to be hospitalized with pneumonia in the first year of life.

Watch Out!
Smoking during pregnancy is responsible for between $1.4 and $2 billion in health complications, according to the U.S. Centers for Disease Control.

How to quit

As hard as quitting may be, the results are well worth it—your smoking-related risks of disease quickly drop the longer you avoid tobacco. For example, in the first year after you stop smoking, the risk of coronary heart disease drops sharply. It then gradually returns to normal—that is, the same risk level as someone who never smoked.

If you decide that you're ready to stop smoking, there are a range of methods that work well. Some hardy souls quit cold turkey. Others use counseling, stop-smoking programs, hypnosis, or the newer nicotine replacement products described later. Once you've decided to take the plunge, here's how to start:

1. Make a commitment. If you want to quit, you've got to control your mind and your behavior. Don't focus on how hard it's going to be. (That makes it easy to give up!) Talk to yourself about the good things that come with quitting and

how much better you'll feel. Don't give yourself an "out" for failing.

2. Pick a stop-smoking date. Something like this is easy to put off, so choose a date to throw away your cigarettes. Slowly start tapering off before you reach the date, and when it arrives, get rid of all your smoking paraphernalia. Wash your clothes to get rid of the smell.

3. Build a support team. Odds are your friends and family have wanted you to quit for a long time, anyway; ask for their help. Look into counseling or hypnosis.

4. Persevere. If you find yourself in the bathroom sneaking a butt, don't beat yourself up—but don't allow this one indiscretion to throw you off your plan. If you start to light up, make yourself put it out. If you start to smoke, quit before you've smoked the whole cigarette.

Odds are, as you give up cigarettes you're going to have to deal with some unpleasant symptoms, including anxiety, hunger, irritability, restlessness, fatigue, and concentration problems. Once you smoke that last cigarette, your body starts repairing itself right away—it should be completely free of nicotine within two or three days. Withdrawal symptoms take longer to fade away, but they don't last forever—just about three weeks at the most. On the other hand, you'll notice some positive signs almost right away. You will

- Have more energy.
- Feel better physically.
- Begin to taste things more strongly.
- Smell better.

Patches and gum

Of course, knowing you should quit is one thing, but actually quitting is quite another. Modern science has come up with some new methods to help you—nicotine patches and nicotine gum. Both replace the nicotine that you would have gotten from cigarettes and can help you quit smoking by easing nicotine withdrawal symptoms while you deal with the psychological issues of smoking dependence.

Patches are considered to be a bit easier to use—you don't have to follow lots of rules as to how to use the product, as you do with gum. You simply apply the patch on your arm the first morning you plan to quit and leave it there for 24 hours. The patches have a fixed amount of nicotine, which is released in prescribed amounts and absorbed through the skin. Most patch systems are designed to be used for about two to three months, during which the dose contained in the patch can be gradually tapered off.

You may have to deal with some skin irritation, which you can treat with topical steroid creams, but the patch isn't appropriate for any woman with widespread skin irritations. A few women have found that the patch interfered with their sleep and made them nervous; one patch is designed to be removed at bedtime.

While the patches are easier to use than the gum, you've got to be very careful never to break down and sneak a cigarette while you're wearing one. Remember: The whole reason why you want to quit smoking is that nicotine is basically toxic. Several patients who wore a patch have died from heart attacks because they continued to smoke while wearing one, and the resulting overdose of nicotine was fatal. Nicotine acts on the central nervous system, first stimulating and then depressing it. It primarily acts on the autonomic nervous system, which controls involuntary body actions like heart rate.

Nicotine gum may be a bit harder to use the right way, but it's unlikely you'll be tempted to smoke a cigarette and chew nicotine gum at the same time. It's available in several strengths, but don't pop it in your mouth like a wad of Bazooka. Instead, here's the proper way to chew nicotine gum:

1. Chew the nicotine gum only briefly—long enough to release the nicotine (you can tell by the pepper flavor).
2. Once the pepper flavor is released, park the gum between your cheek and your gums for a few minutes until the pepper taste and tingle has faded.
3. Chew the gum a few more times until the nicotine is released again.
4. Park it in your cheek again.
5. Repeat the entire process for about a half hour, or until no more pepper taste is released.

You may need to chew between 9 and 12 pieces a day (try chewing one piece each hour) to prevent withdrawal—although some heavy smokers may need up to 30 pieces a day. After three months, you should start to gradually reduce the number of pieces you chew. About 5 to 10 percent of users develop a long-term dependence on the gum. Expect to deal with some side effects (some of which are related to withdrawal), including

- Nausea.
- Hiccups.
- Dizziness.

Watch Out! Don't drink any liquids while chewing nicotine gum; the liquid can interfere with the release of the nicotine from the chewing gum.

- Sore jaw (from all that chewing).
- Mouth ulcers.

Acupuncture and smoking

If you want to quit smoking and the thought of patches and gum makes your head swim, acupuncture may be a sensible choice. Through the trained use of specialized needles inserted into the skin, acupuncturists can treat disorders (including substance abuse) by stimulating certain areas in the body.

Research shows that acupuncture really can help you kick the smoking habit (not to mention alcohol and drug addictions, as well). In just 10 days of daily 30-minute treatments, some former smokers report they were able to throw away their cigarettes. The good thing about acupuncture is that, compared with various nicotine replacement methods, there are virtually no side effects or risks.

If you decide you'd like to try substituting pin pricks for cigarettes, be sure to choose an acupuncturist who has a state license and who has been certified by the National Commission for the Certification of Acupuncturists. This organization can give you referrals to more than 3,000 certified acupuncturists around the country (see Appendix A for contact information).

Alcohol abuse

Men make up 60 percent of the heavy drinkers in this country, but because it's so much more common—and more socially acceptable—men are more likely to seek therapy (or be forced to do so by the courts and bosses). Men who are alcoholics are more often viewed sympathetically, as people with a terrible disease. However, there is still a stigma

Watch Out!
A woman who abuses alcohol will die, on average, 15 years sooner than a woman who isn't an alcoholic.

against women alcoholics, who are generally viewed in U.S. society with scorn.

While alcohol is not a health beverage for men or women, the surprising fact is that it causes far more damage in a woman's body. Because a woman's body has more fat and less water, alcohol isn't diluted as much and more of it enters a woman's bloodstream. Moreover, her stomach produces less of an enzyme (called ADH) that breaks down alcohol before it reaches the blood. (In fact, studies show that women alcoholics have almost no ADH in their systems.)

Chronic alcohol abuse exacts a greater physical toll on women than on men. Even though a woman may drink less than a man, her liver and heart will be damaged much sooner from alcohol, and proportionately, women will die sooner from cirrhosis and other ailments of the liver and heart. Women alcoholics have death rates 50 to 100 percent higher than male alcoholics, and a higher percentage of female alcoholics die from alcohol-related accidents, circulatory disorders, and cirrhosis of the liver. Drinking to excess also carries a heavy emotional price. Women drinkers are proportionately more likely to commit suicide and more are apt to develop eating disorders and suffer from depression.

Alarmingly, even the most moderate drinking may increase a woman's risk of breast cancer (scientists suspect this is because of alcohol's interaction with estrogen). The risk of breast cancer increases when a woman drinks as little as one ounce of alcohol a day. Moreover, some studies suggest that the risk for breast cancer exists for even occasional drinkers of alcoholic beverages, although the results aren't clear.

Clearly, alcohol and hormones are interrelated, since alcohol abuse can also lead to fertility problems and early menopause. Of course, most women realize that drinking can cause serious harm to their unborn babies. The most serious risk is fetal alcohol syndrome, the most common cause of mental retardation in infants. Menstrual disorders, such as painful menstruation, heavy flow, premenstrual discomfort, and irregular or absent cycles, have been associated with chronic heavy drinking. These disorders can have adverse effects on fertility, as well.

With all this bad news, it may be surprising to hear that women today drink more than they used to. Those who do drink too much and seek help for their problem face stigma, so many women resist getting treatment. Western culture requires its women to step to the beat of a more saintly drummer. When they don't, society reacts with scathing condemnation. This makes admitting the problem and getting help much harder for women and their families.

As a result, some alcoholic women choose to seek help for more "acceptable" conditions, such as depression or anxiety, ending up with prescriptions for drugs which they then combine with alcohol. This only compounds their problem, so that now they struggle with a dual addiction where once there was just one.

What's your risk?

It's quite clear that alcoholism is related in some fashion to genetics, although the exact mechanism is not completely understood. Most studies have been done with male alcoholics and their sons, so the genetic pathway for women alcoholics is not clear.

In studies of drinking behavior among female twins, researchers found that being married seems to lessen the effect of an inherited tendency for drinking. Contrary to popular belief, women who have multiple roles (wife, mother, career woman, parent caretaker) may have lower rates of problems with alcohol than women who don't.

In fact, loss of a role as wife, mother, or worker may increase a woman's risk for abusing alcohol. Women who have never married or who are divorced or separated are more likely to drink heavily and experience alcohol-related problems than women who are married or widowed. But unmarried women living with a partner are more likely than any other women to engage in heavy drinking and to develop drinking problems.

Do you have a problem?

The following quiz was adapted from information obtained from the National Council on Alcoholism and Drug Dependence.

Bright Idea
You can call the Center for Substance Abuse Treatment at 800/662-HELP for information about treatment programs in your local community and to speak to someone about an alcohol problem.

QUIZ 10.1: IS YOUR DRINKING A PROBLEM?

- Have you ever decided to stop drinking for a week or so, but only lasted for a couple of days?
- Do you wish people would mind their own business about your drinking—and stop telling you what to do?
- Do you drink when you're depressed, hoping you'll feel better?
- Do you use alcohol as a medicine (such as to ease menstrual cramps)?

- Do you get someone else to buy alcohol for you because you're too ashamed to buy it yourself?
- Do you talk a lot about drinking?
- Do you feel sociable only when you drink?
- Have you ever switched from one kind of drink to another in the hope that this would keep you from getting drunk?
- Have you had to have an eye-opener upon awakening during the past year?
- Do you envy people who can drink without getting into trouble?
- Do you buy alcohol at different places so no one knows how much you drink?
- Do you plan ahead of time to reward yourself with several drinks after you've worked hard?
- Do you ever carry liquor in your purse?
- Do you drink to help yourself sleep or calm your nerves?
- Do you hide empty bottles or throw them away in secret?
- Do you drink when you're stressed out or under pressure?
- Do you ever wonder if anyone knows how much you drink?
- Do you worry about hurting your child when you've been drinking?
- If you drink occasionally, do you have a lot of drinks at one time?

- Have you had problems connected with drinking during the past year?
- Has your drinking caused trouble at home?
- Do you tell yourself you can stop drinking any time you want to, even though you keep getting drunk when you don't mean to?
- Have you missed days of work or school because of drinking?
- Do you drink more when you've been emotionally or physically abused?
- Do you feel panicky when you run out of money for alcohol?
- Do you get defensive when anyone mentions your drinking?
- Do you drive your car when you've been drinking?
- Do you use alcohol to have or avoid sexual activity?
- Have you fallen down or hurt yourself as a result of drinking?
- Are you absent or late for work more often after you drink?
- Do you take sleeping pills or tranquilizers with alcohol?
- Do you have blackouts?
- Have you ever felt that your life would be better if you didn't drink?

Did you answer yes to more than five of the questions? If so, you're probably in trouble with alcohol. Some experts believe that answering yes to even fewer than five questions may indicate there's a problem.

Bright Idea
Drug and alcohol treatment centers have reported that acupuncture is successful in between 50 and 75 percent of cases, compared to a 3 percent success rate for those given dummy pills or no acupuncture.

TABLE 10.2: ALCOHOL CONTENT

Type	Alcohol content
Beer (12 oz.)	5 percent
Wine cooler (12 oz.)	5 percent
Wine (6 oz.)	15 percent
Hard liquor (1.5 oz.)	40 percent

Getting help for someone else

If you're worried about a woman you know who's an alcoholic, there are ways you can intervene to try to get the person to acknowledge that she has a problem and needs help. An alcoholic can't be forced to get help except under certain circumstances, such as if the police are called in following a violent incident. This doesn't mean, however, that you have to wait for a crisis to make an impact. Alcoholism treatment specialists recommend taking the following steps to help an alcoholic accept treatment:

1. Stop all "rescue missions." Family members often try to protect an alcoholic by making excuses to others about her drinking or by getting her out of alcohol-related jams. Instead, the alcoholic needs to fully experience the harmful effects of her drinking so she'll be more motivated to stop.

2. Time your intervention. Plan to talk with the drinker shortly after an alcohol-related problem has occurred (such as an alcohol-related accident). Choose a time when she's sober,

when you're both calm, and when you can speak privately.

3. Be specific. Tell her that you're concerned about her drinking and want to help. Give examples of how her drinking has caused problems for both of you, including the most recent incident.

4. State the consequences. Tell her that until she gets help, you'll need to protect yourself from the harmful effects of her drinking. You may refuse to go with her to any alcohol-related activities, for example, or move out of the house (if you live together). Don't make any threats you aren't prepared to carry out.

5. Be ready to help. Get information ahead of time about local treatment options. If she's willing to get help, call right away for an appointment with a treatment program counselor. Offer to go with her on her first visit to a treatment program and/or Alcoholics Anonymous (AA) meeting.

Unofficially...
Once they do get help, studies have shown that women who abuse alcohol seem to respond better than men to treatment, especially if they are treated in a medically oriented alcoholism facility with a smaller proportion of female clients.

6. Call on a friend. If she still refuses to get help, ask a friend to talk with her (ask her to use the steps above). A friend who's a recovering alcoholic herself may be particularly persuasive, but any caring, nonjudgmental friend may be able to make a difference. The intervention of more than one person, more than one time, is often necessary to persuade an alcoholic to seek help.

7. Try a group approach. With the help of a therapist, some families join with other relatives and friends to confront an alcoholic as a group. While this approach may be effective, it should only be attempted under the guidance of a therapist who is experienced in this kind of group intervention.

8. Get support. Whether or not the person in need gets help, you may benefit from the encouragement and support of other people in your situation.

Support groups—Working the steps

Many women benefit from 12-step support groups such as AA, an informal society of more than 2,000,000 recovering alcoholics in the United States, Canada, and other countries. These men and women meet in local groups, which range in size from a handful in some localities to many hundreds in larger communities. Currently, women make up 35 percent of the total membership.

Support groups for family members offered in most communities include Al-Anon, which holds regular meetings for spouses and other significant adults in an alcoholic's life, and Alateen, for children of alcoholics. These groups help family members understand that they aren't responsible for an alcoholic's drinking and that they need to take steps to take care of themselves, regardless of whether the alcoholic family member chooses to get help. For meeting locations, call your local Al-Anon chapter (check your phone book under the heading "alcoholism") or call the following toll-free numbers: 800/344-2666 (United States) or 800/443-4525 (Canada).

Bright Idea
For information on local support meetings run by Alcoholics Anonymous, call your local AA chapter, call 212/870-3400, or visit the AA Web site at www.alcoholics-anonymous.org.

Legal and illegal drug abuse

The term "drug abuse" may conjure up visions of a streetwise heroin dealer or an inner city crack house—but it can also mean the habitual reliance on legal substances, such as prescription drugs or even over-the-counter products. In fact, prescription drugs like minor tranquilizers, painkillers, and diet pills are much more often abused by women than alcohol or street drugs.

Who's at risk?

Some women are at higher risk for developing a problem with drugs than others. You're more likely to abuse drugs if you

- Have a close family member who is a substance abuser.
- Started using drugs or alcohol when you were young.
- Have been prescribed a tranquilizer, antidepressant, or sedative.
- Smoke.
- Have an eating disorder.
- Were the victim of incest, rape, or molestation during childhood, or have otherwise been physically abused.

About 5 percent of all women admit abusing drugs (compared to 8 percent of men); women who abuse drugs are most often of childbearing age. Women who abuse drugs run the risk of a range of physical and mental health problems, including

- Poor nutrition and below-average weight.
- Low self-esteem.
- Depression.
- Physical abuse.
- Pre-term labor or early delivery.
- Sexually transmitted diseases (STDs).

AIDS is now the fourth leading cause of death among women of childbearing age in the United States. Substance abuse compounds the risk of AIDS for women, especially for women who are injecting drug users and who share drug paraphernalia, because HIV/AIDS often is transmitted through shared needles or syringes.

In addition, under the influence of illicit drugs and alcohol, women may engage in unprotected sex, which increases their risk for contracting or transmitting HIV/AIDS. From 1993 to 1994, the number of new AIDS cases among women increased 17 percent; as of June 1995, the Centers for Disease Control and Prevention had documented almost 65,000 cases of AIDS among adolescent and adult women in the United States. Of these cases, nearly 66 percent were related either to the woman's own injecting drug use or to her having sex with an injecting drug user; of these, almost half acquired HIV/AIDS by having sex with an injecting drug user.

Prescription drugs

Most legal drugs abused by women are prescription mood-altering drugs (especially sedatives and minor tranquilizers). In this country, women are far more likely to be diagnosed with anxiety and depression than are men, more likely to seek help for psychological problems—and more likely to be prescribed medications when they might be better treated with therapy or social support. Statistics show that these prescription drugs are prescribed more often and at an earlier age for women than for men.

Diet pills are another medication that can be abused by women, mostly because of society's pressure for women to be thin. Chronic use of amphetamines can permanently damage the heart and blood vessels, especially since toleration quickly develops so women must take more and more for the same effect.

Watch Out!
It's a myth that using cocaine in late pregnancy will make your labor shorter and less painful. Instead, cocaine can cause the pregnant woman's sudden death, premature labor, and stillbirth.

Illicit drugs

Illicit drug use is a common problem in this country, not just for men but also for women. Of the nearly 60 million women in this country, more than 5 million use marijuana or cocaine monthly. The abuse of illicit drugs during pregnancy can pose even more serious problems for the unborn child. Both cocaine and heroin use can lead to premature delivery and stillbirth. If you use drugs during your pregnancy, your baby can be born with an addiction and show signs of withdrawal soon afterwards.

Treatment

Research indicates that more than 4 million women need treatment for drug abuse. Unfortunately, there are some important reasons why many women don't get help.

Many drug-using women don't seek treatment because they are afraid—they fear not being able to take care of or keep their children, they fear reprisal from their spouses or boyfriends, and they fear punishment by authorities. Many women report that their drug-using male sex partners introduced them to drugs and then sabotaged their efforts to quit using drugs.

Research indicates that women can become addicted quickly to certain drugs, such as crack cocaine, even after casual or experimental use. Therefore, by the time a woman enters treatment, she may be severely addicted and may require treatment that both identifies her specific needs and responds to them. These needs will likely include addressing other serious health problems, such as STDs and mental health issues.

There are a range of treatment possibilities for substance abuse, but studies have found that women receive the most benefits from drug treatment programs that provide comprehensive services for meeting basic needs, including

- Access to food, clothing, and shelter.
- Transportation.
- Parenting training.
- Family therapy.
- Child care.
- Social services.
- Social support.
- Assertiveness training.
- Family planning services.

Traditional male-oriented drug treatment programs may not be appropriate for women because those programs may not provide these services. Research also indicates that, for women in particular, a continuing relationship with a treatment provider is an important factor throughout treatment.

Any individual may experience lapses and relapses as expected steps of the treatment and recovery process; during these periods, women particularly need the support of the community and encouragement of those closest to them. After completing a drug treatment program, women also need services to assist them in sustaining their recovery and in rejoining the community.

Where to get help...

To find a drug treatment center, ask your doctor or look in your local Yellow Pages under "Drug Abuse Treatment" (or in the White Pages for Narcotics Anonymous). You can find out more about substance abuse and treatment by contacting any of the substance abuse information organizations listed in Appendix A.

Just the facts

- If your immediate family members have a problem with substance abuse, you're more likely to have a problem, too.
- Lung cancer—often the result of nicotine use—is now the leading cause of cancer deaths in women (surpassing breast cancer).
- Don't smoke if you're using a nicotine patch; it could be fatal.
- Women respond better than men to alcoholism treatment, especially in medically oriented facilities with a smaller proportion of women clients.
- Most legal drugs that women abuse are prescription mood-altering drugs (especially sedatives and minor tranquilizers).

PART IV

Symptoms, Diagnoses, and Treatments

GET THE SCOOP ON...
How to find a great skin care specialist ▪ The newest acne treatments ▪ Is it acne or rosacea? ▪ How to tell if it's really skin cancer ▪ Is "safe" tanning possible? ▪ Which sunscreen is best? ▪ Which drugs cause skin sensitivity

Keeping Your Skin Healthy

Fifty years ago, there wasn't much that you could do about the skin you were born with. Dermatologists couldn't control acne, remove old acne scars, or treat sun-damaged skin. Skin cancer wasn't a serious risk—in fact, no one thought much about it at all.

Today, many women are discovering it's possible to significantly improve their skin conditions, either by themselves or with the help of a skin care professional. But to do that, you need the latest, most up-to-date information you can get to help you sift through the hype and the controversy.

How to find a great skin care specialist

When looking for a good dermatologist, many women use the Yellow Pages as a sort of medical dart board, closing their eyes and picking a name at random. Others choose a skin specialist by the sound of the name or the size of the person's ad. And some women don't bother with a dermatologist at all, figuring they can get all the skin care advice they need from their general practitioner.

While it's true that most family doctors can certainly tell the difference between a pimple and a mosquito bite, other more serious skin conditions can be much more difficult for nonspecialists to diagnose. For example, dry skin, eczema, and dermatitis all look very much alike—so much so that it can take a specialist to tell the difference.

Choosing a dermatologist

Dermatologists are physicians who specialize in diagnosing and treating skin problems. They are also trained to offer a wide range of cosmetic treatments as well, including chemical peels to remove age spots and acne lesions, laser resurfacing, and cosmetic surgery.

All dermatologists spend at least one year after medical school in a hospital in general medicine, and then go on to complete at least three years of advanced training in dermatology. They are skilled in treating all skin-related manners, so if you've been noticing more hair in your drain than on your head, a dermatologist is the one to call. Ditto for that pesky nail fungus or sty on the edge of your eye. In addition, dermatologists are carefully trained to understand how diseases of the skin can be related to many other medical conditions.

The best way to start your search for a good dermatologist is by getting a recommendation from a doctor, relative, or friend who's had good experience with the person. But that's not always possible, especially if you're new to an area—in that case, you've got to do your own investigating.

Unofficially... If you're looking for something more drastic—say, a face lift—then you should be shopping for a cosmetic or plastic surgeon, not a dermatologist. You can get a referral by calling the American Board of Plastic Surgery at 800/635-0635.

The first thing you want to make sure of is that the dermatologist you choose is board certified (that is, has fulfilled certain requirements and passed an exam by the American Board of Dermatology).

Once you've narrowed down your search to board-certified dermatologists, you still need to find out which dermatologists are most experienced in the procedures or conditions in which you're interested.

Remember, not all dermatologists are alike. For example, many dermatologists perform some cosmetic surgery (they can remove moles, destroy small capillaries on the face, and remove brown spots, for instance). Some inject collagen or fat to smooth out facial creases and wrinkles. Others have extra training in the surgical management of skin cancer, and limit their practice to the treatment of this disease. While many dermatologists have some experience with laser surgery, some are more experienced than others. Other dermatologists spend most of their time resurfacing skin using chemical peels and dermabrasion.

If you have a specific procedure in mind, you may be able to tell from a phone book ad what sorts of techniques a particular dermatologist offers. When you call for an appointment, ask the dermatologist's staff what types of procedures make up the majority of the practice.

What to expect from a good dermatologist

If you're interested in having a certain procedure such as laser resurfacing, make an appointment to interview the dermatologist before any work is done. (You may have to pay for this appointment, but it'll be well worth it.)

Timesaver
Instead of searching through the phone book to find a dermatologist, check out the "where to find a dermatologist" section at the American Academy of Dermatology's Web site at www.aad.org.

Ask the doctor how many procedures he or she has performed. Ask to see "before" and "after" pictures of patients the doctor has treated, ideally with the "after" picture taken at least six months beyond the treatment date. Request phone numbers for at least three patients the doctor has treated—and make sure you call them. If what you want is a fairly new procedure, find out where the doctor learned the new technique. With the very latest technology (such as laser resurfacing), it's best for a doctor who is new to the procedure to have participated in a preceptorship—observing an experienced physician and then treating several patients under that doctor's supervision.

Although you may feel awkward asking these questions, remember: It's your skin and your body. You have a right to ask these questions. If a dermatologist balks at any one of these questions, leave and find another doctor.

Once you've found a dermatologist you can feel comfortable with, you'll be able to visit this specialist to take care of a wide range of potential skin conditions. One of the most common is acne, which we'll talk about in the next section.

Acne

When it comes to skin diseases, acne is probably the most common problem a woman will experience. In fact, acne is the most common skin disease in the United States, and accounts for up to 25 percent of all visits to dermatologists. This very common inflammatory reaction in the oil-producing follicles is most common during adolescence, but it can affect anyone from infancy to middle age.

We think of acne as a teenage problem lasting for only five or six years. In fact, many women suffer from the recurrent problems of acne for 20, 30, or more years. Because it most commonly affects the face and can lead to permanent scarring, acne can have profound and long-lasting psychological effects in addition to the physical traces it leaves behind.

Myths: Chocolate, french fries, and more...

To a surprising degree, many women still believe in the myths of acne regarding what causes it and what to do about it. The simple truth is that heredity and hormones are behind most forms of acne. In addition, poor hygiene, poor diet, and stress can aggravate acne, although they clearly don't cause it. Although there is an association between the severity of acne and the amount of oil a person's skin produces, not all people with oily skin have acne, and some people with dry skin do.

Despite what your mother told you, acne is not caused by

- Chocolate.
- Greasy foods.
- Dirt.
- Shellfish.
- Nuts.
- Oily hair and skin.

So what does cause acne?

Among girls, acne most often starts at around age 11 when sebaceous (oil) glands in the hair follicles of the skin begin to produce too much sebum, an oily substance that keeps hair and skin lubricated. At the same time, dead skin cells mix with the sebum to form a plug that clogs the follicle opening or pore. This blockage is known as a *blackhead*. If you

Unofficially...
In one study, 65 people ate chocolate bars every day for a month, but although the bars contained 10 times the normal amount of chocolate, the subjects experienced no worsening of blemishes.

have a blackhead, the dark surface of the plug is visible within the pore (in a whitehead, the follicle wall bulges but does not rupture).

As the follicles fill up and bacteria multiply, blackheads or whiteheads form on the skin's surface—a condition called noninflammatory acne. If the follicle wall ruptures under pressure and sebum leaks into nearby tissue, the result is a pustule (or inflammatory acne). If you also have a bacterium called *Propionibacterium acnes,* the pustule can become infected and inflamed; once this happens, the infection can penetrate deep into the skin and create cysts, which can rupture and leave temporary or permanent scars.

Hormones play a large part in acne. Androgens (male sex hormones) kick in at puberty, stepping up production of sebum, the substance that lubricates skin and helps it retain moisture. After puberty, boys produce 10 times as much androgen as girls, and so it's not surprising that more boys than girls develop severe teenage cases of acne.

In women with acne, these glands also appear to have an exaggerated reaction to the body's usual hormonal signals. Tiny hair follicles, especially those on the face, neck, chest, and back, can become plugged with sebum. Androgens are also responsible for the abnormal, excessive shedding of dead skin cells that contribute to clogged pores.

Despite the normal increase in androgen levels during puberty, some researchers believe that flare-ups of acne have less to do with your androgen levels than with how your skin responds to an increase in sebum production.

The bacteria *Propionibacterium acnes* and *Staphylococcus epidermidis* are found naturally in

Unofficially... Hormonal changes during menstruation or when taking or stopping oral contraceptives also can cause skin to break out. Some studies have shown that up to 70 percent of women notice their acne worsening the week before their periods.

healthy hair follicles. However, if bacterial levels build up in plugged follicles, they may produce too much of an enzyme that breaks down sebum, triggering localized inflammation. Some women are more sensitive than others to this reaction, so that sebum levels that might cause a pimple or two in one woman may cause severe outbreaks in another.

Other things that can cause acne, or make it worse, are certain drugs, such as those used to treat epilepsy or tuberculosis; exposure to industrial oils, grease, and chemicals; and stress and strong emotions (which may account for the big date breakout). Oily cosmetics and shampoos can sometimes trigger acne in people who are prone to get it.

The over-20 acne myths

If you've successfully maneuvered through the teenage acne minefield, you may be horrified when you suddenly break out in pimples during your late 20s, 30s—or even beyond. Adult acne can be very frustrating for women who may be confronted by very stubborn skin conditions years after their teenage years. Indeed, although acne remains largely a curse of adolescence, about 20 percent of all cases occur in adults. In addition, women are more likely than men to have mild to moderate forms into their 30s and beyond, and are somewhat more susceptible to a related skin condition known as rosacea.

Can you prevent acne?

Dermatologists agree that the time to treat acne is before a young girl starts breaking out. However, because of acne's association with fluctuating hormone levels and possible genetic influences, there may be no way to completely prevent the problem.

Bright Idea
According to the American Academy of Dermatology, it's a good idea for acne sufferers to check with a dermatologist to ensure their skin condition really is acne. Rashes from other sources, such as makeup and oral medicine, can create acnelike symptoms.

Watch Out!
There is some concern about what happens when skin treated with benzoyl peroxide is exposed to the sun. Research done so far hasn't shown the combination to be harmful, but the FDA plans to review other studies currently in progress.

Good general hygiene and sensible skin care are especially important during adolescence, including

- A daily bath or shower.
- Washing with unscented or mildly antibacterial soap.
- Not using cosmetics regularly.

Treat yourself or see a dermatologist?

If the above prevention strategies alone don't work, you may want to try one of the over-the-counter acne medicines that can be applied directly to the skin. These contain a variety of compounds such as benzoyl peroxide, sulfur, resorcinol, or salicylic acid, all of which the U.S. Food and Drug Administration has found effective for treating mild acne.

First try a cleanser or astringent containing salicylic acid to help unclog pores. If that doesn't work, try a 10-percent benzoyl peroxide gel or cleanser, which kills bacteria and dries your skin. These drugs are known as peeling agents—products which irritate and dry the skin, helping to loosen plugs and shed dead cells. The drugs also can keep bacteria from forming, which reduces the fatty acids that contribute to acne.

There are, however, several situations in which you should seek help from a dermatologist for acne:

- If your acne doesn't respond after a few months of trying the above over-the-counter remedies
- If you have severe acne which produces cysts under the skin and persistent pimples that may become infected
- If you're over age 30 and your skin becomes abnormally flushed around your cheeks and nose

Hot off the press: Newest treatments

Fortunately, dermatologists really can help almost all cases of acne, according to a review of the latest treatments in the April 17, 1998, issue of the *New England Journal of Medicine*. New medications and a better understanding of the disease's underlying causes have greatly improved treatment in recent years.

Conventional medicine favors drug therapies that slow down sebum production, limit bacterial growth, or encourage shedding of skin cells to unclog pores. The choice of treatment also depends on the types of skin problem you have. If you have mostly blackheads, your doctor will probably suggest topical agents to control abnormal skin growth. These include

- Retin-A and Renova (tretinoin). Renova is an antiaging cream that contains the active ingredient retinoic acid. Retinoic acid has been sold for years under the brand name Retin-A. Retin-A is a prescription drug used for the treatment of acne. The FDA has now approved the use of retinoic acid sold under the name Renova for the treatment of sun damaged skin.

- Azelex (azelaic acid), a recently-approved drug that affects skin turnover and seems to have an antibacterial effect against *P. acnes*.

- Differin (adapalene), another recently-approved retinoid.

- Sulfur products: Novacet and other sulfur products have antibacterial, peeling, and drying actions and are used topically to treat acne and oily skin.

If you have inflammatory acne (infected lesions), your doctor will probably prescribe either oral or topical antibiotics, such as clindamycin or erythromycin. (Often antibiotic treatment is combined with a topical retinoid.) One of the oldest and most successful oral antibiotics for acne is tetracycline, which is safe, effective, and inexpensive. If your condition isn't so easy to treat, your doctor may suggest oral minocycline.

Women with deep, cystic acne usually require systemic treatment geared to reducing sebum. The latest treatment in this category is the oral contraceptive Ortho Tri-Cyclen, which was recently approved by the FDA for this use in women. However, most gynecologists believe that most oral contraceptives can have a beneficial effect (to date, Tri-Cyclen is the only brand that has submitted evidence of this). If a woman is starting the Pill to control acne, it makes sense to choose Tri-Cyclen. If she is already on a birth control pill, there is no evidence to suggest that changing to Tri-cyclen will improve her acne.

Unofficially... Studies show that compared with a placebo, birth control pills improve acne, probably by reducing the effects of androgens (male sex hormones). However, not all women see an improvement in their acne; in some it gets worse, and in some it has no effect.

The other main choice for reducing sebum production is Accutane (isotretinoin), which is also derived from vitamin A and is usually reserved for women with deep, nodular acne. This oral medication has a 70 to 80 percent cure rate after five months of therapy, but it should be used with caution in women of child-bearing age since it causes birth defects if used during pregnancy.

Accutane is approved by the FDA for treating severe cystic acne for women whose skin condition doesn't sufficiently improve with other treatments, including oral antibiotics. However, because of the serious risk of birth defects, your doctor should not prescribe Accutane for you if you are still menstruating unless you have severe, disfiguring cystic acne that doesn't improve with standard treatment. If you're still of childbearing age, before prescribing Accutane your doctor should give you an information sheet that includes statements about the drug's ability to cause birth defects. You'll be asked to initial these statements and to sign an authorization for treatment. If you're a minor, a parent's or guardian's initials and signature are required.

Other common side effects include dry and cracked lips; itching; thinning hair; dry and flaky skin; aching muscles, joints, and bones; increased lipid levels; and (rarely) liver damage. Currently, Accutane is given for four to five months for the first treatment; after treatment has stopped, the condition may continue to improve for at least two more months and sometimes for as long as a year. About one-third of patients need a second course of the drug, which should be given only after a six-month hiatus. Typically, doctors recommend that women wait for one to two months after the medication is stopped before getting pregnant.

All reputable dermatologists require a negative pregnancy test prior to starting accutane, as well as use of a reliable contraceptive. Most will require women on Accutane to also be on birth control pills, Depoprovera, or Norplant (unless she has been sterilized previously).

Retin-A and Renova both are also derived from vitamin A, but are applied to the skin, not taken by mouth; there have been no reports of birth defects related to their use.

Don't give up!

Although there are now more options for treating adult acne than ever before, finding a treatment that works requires a lot of trial and error. Some

Watch Out!
Acne treatments can have potent side effects. Tretinoin and benzoyl peroxide can leave skin reddened, dry, and sensitive to sunlight. Benzoyl peroxide may inhibit the healing effects of tretinoin, so never apply them at the same time.

women respond better to some products than others, and some women object to side effects such as skin irritation or dryness. Because improvement isn't usually evident for at least six to eight weeks, you have to be patient.

However, if you're not getting better after a few months, you should probably see your doctor for a reevaluation. You may need to alter the dose, add a drug, or try a different drug.

Help for acne scars

There are new treatments for women who have scars or pitted skin from cysts or deep pimples that were scratched or severely infected. Two relatively aggressive surgical procedures can improve the skin's appearance: Dermabrasion, in which a dermatologist essentially sandpapers frozen skin, and chemical peeling.

Both procedures remove the scarred surface and expose unblemished skin layers. Before considering such treatment, however, discuss the procedures, necessary precautions, and likely results with at least two dermatologists.

Is it acne or rosacea?

If you're over 30 and you've noticed a reddening across your face, you could have a condition known as *rosacea*, which affects the nose, cheeks, chin, or forehead with redness, pimples, pustules, and dilated blood vessels. Sometimes it can be hard to tell the difference between acne and rosacea; that's why you need a dermatologist's opinion.

In rosacea, pimples aren't usually associated with blackheads and whiteheads, and while the condition usually appears in adults over age 30, occasionally it has been diagnosed in teenagers. Rosacea also can occur around the eyes (known as rosacea blepharitis). This can be a severe problem, since the swelling can affect the eyes and eyesight.

Who gets it?

Rosacea can affect anyone, but women are three times more likely than men to develop the problem. It occurs more often in fair-skinned women with a history of blushing often and easily. It may affect members of the same family, and it appears especially among Irish Americans and others of Celtic descent. It's not associated with alcoholism, although alcohol may worsen the condition.

Rosacea usually develops slowly and most of the time, it will get worse unless it's treated. In most women, the condition comes and goes for no apparent reason. The typical "red face" is caused by enlarged blood vessels under the skin that make you look like you're always blushing; gradually, the color becomes permanent and more noticeable. As the redness worsens, pimples may also appear, and snakey red lines (they're really blood vessels) may appear on your face.

You'll notice certain things make the condition worse, including

- Alcohol.
- The sun.
- Vigorous exercise.
- Hot liquids.
- Spicy foods.
- Wind.
- Endocrine disturbances.
- Heat and cold.
- Emotional stress.

- Prolonged application of fluorinated corticosteroids.

Is it in your genes?

Genetics do play a role in rosacea, although specific genes haven't been identified. It appears as though some gene triggers an increased sensitivity to a specific set of conditions. This could be due to one or several related genes that may control flushing and reddening of the face. Many experts believe more women get rosacea than men because of hormonal changes experienced during menopause (remember, rosacea usually appears during middle age).

Treatment: The newest info

Rosacea can be treated very effectively if it's detected in an early stage. While there is no cure, treatment with topical and oral drugs can control redness and reduce pimples.

Bright Idea
If you have rosacea, use only mild cleanser, wash your face gently, use a sunscreen of SPF 15 or higher, apply high-quality moisturizer after your topical medication has dried, and avoid skin care products with alcohols like menthol or isopropanol.

Topical antibiotics such as metronidazole (Metrogel) is often the first medication your doctor will try; often, a combination of topical and oral antibioitic (such as a tetracycline) are effective. No drug will work immediately, however; it usually takes several weeks before you'll notice a lessening of the symptoms. It's also important to avoid "triggers" such as heat, spicy food, and alcohol.

Short-term, mild topical steroids are sometimes used to help control redness, but long-term use of these drugs isn't recommended. In addition, your dermatologist may recommend specific moisturizers, soaps, sunscreens, or other products to improve the condition of your skin.

In more severe cases, surgery, dermabrasion, electro-cautery, and laser treatments are used to try to control the condition. The laser in particular has been effectively used to treat the red spidery facial veins found in more advanced cases of rosacea.

Skin cancer

While acne and rosacea can be profoundly upsetting and disfiguring for women, they are not life threatening. One of the most serious skin conditions that send women to see a dermatologist is the suspicion of skin cancer.

In 1930, a person had a 1 in 1,500 lifetime chance of getting skin cancer. As of 1998, that risk rose to 1 in 82; by the year 2000, it's estimated that it will be 1 in 75.

Today, skin cancer strikes one out of every five Americans. It occurs in one of three types—squamous cell carcinoma, basal cell carcinoma, or malignant melanoma—and it's the most common of all malignancies, affecting more than 600,000 Americans each year. However, it's also the easiest cancer to cure, if it's diagnosed and treated soon enough. That's a big "if."

Check your skin monthly

While most women have gotten the message that self breast exams are crucial to their health, most don't regularly check their bodies for suspicious growths on the skin. And yet a woman's risk of getting skin cancer is higher than her risk of getting breast cancer.

If you've been a sun worshiper all your life, it's especially important for you to do a monthly "skin check" because 90 percent of all skin cancer is related to sun exposure, according to the American Academy of Dermatology. The trick to doing a skin exam is to check your entire body thoroughly (remember that some melanomas can crop up in places where the sun doesn't shine!).

Skin cancer can look many different ways—warty, lumpy, bumpy, or just "funny." Some women who have been diagnosed with skin cancer have explained the growth as nothing more serious-looking than a mosquito bite.

The most common sign of skin cancer is a change on the skin, such as a growth or a sore that won't heal. Sometimes there may be a small lump. This lump can be smooth, shiny, and waxy looking, or it can be red or reddish brown. Skin cancer may also appear as a flat red spot that is rough or scaly. Not all changes in your skin are cancer, but you should see your doctor if you notice changes in your skin of any kind.

To do your "skin check," stand in front of a full-length mirror in a brightly lit room and perform the following exam:

- Examine your body front and back, and then inspect your right and left sides with arms raised.
- Bend your elbows and look at your forearms, upper underarms, and palms.
- Check the backs of your legs and feet (including between your toes and your soles).
- Examine the back of your neck and scalp using a hand mirror; part your hair and check that area as well.
- Check your back, buttocks, vulva, and perineum with a hand mirror.

The warning sign of skin cancer could be any spot that

- Changes color.
- Gets bigger or thicker.
- Changes in texture.

- Has an irregular outline.
- Is bigger than a pea.
- Appears after age 21.
- Constantly itches, hurts, crusts, scabs, erodes, or bleeds.
- Doesn't heal.
- Looks pearl-colored, translucent, tan, brown, black, or multicolored.

Mole or cancer—can you tell the difference?

Many women have moles, but that doesn't mean they've all got skin cancer. Moles and skin cancer may both qualify as skin growths, but they really don't look much alike—you should be able to tell the difference yourself. To remember what features to look for, think of "A-B-C-D" (asymmetry, border, color, and diameter). Go to a dermatologist to check out any mole that is

- Asymmetrical.
- Has uneven borders.
- Changing color.
- Bigger than a pea (larger than ¼ inch).
- Bleeding.

What to expect with skin cancer

If a lab test reveals skin cancer, your dermatologist and oncologist will determine the best treatment, depending on the stage and location of the disease. The primary lesion will be removed, and you may be given other treatment including radiation, immunotherapy, or chemotherapy.

Basal cell carcinoma

Basal cell carcinoma usually looks like a small shiny bump and that is almost certainly the result of sun

Unofficially... Studies have shown that every inch of hat brim cuts your risk of skin cancer by about 10 percent, since two-thirds of all skin cancers appears on the face and neck, according to the American Academy of Dermatology.

exposure. Fortunately, these skin cancers can be treated if discovered early enough.

More than 90 percent of basal cell carcinomas are found on the face (often at the side of the eye or the nose or other exposed area). Basal cell carcinoma may be

- An open sore that bleeds or oozes for three or more weeks.
- A red patch or irritated area on shoulder, chest, arms, or legs that may itch or hurt.
- A smooth growth with an elevated, rolled border and indented center that develops tiny blood vessels on the surface.
- A shiny bump that is pearly or translucent (often pink or white, tan-black, or brown).
- A scar with poorly defined borders, looking shiny and taut.

Your doctor will diagnose basal cell carcinoma after a physical exam and a biopsy; if tumor cells are found, the growth will be removed or destroyed by radiation. (Treatment is based on your age and health, but whichever it is, it's usually an outpatient procedure.) Your doctor will use local anesthetic and you won't feel much pain.

When removed early, basal cell carcinoma is easily treated—but the larger the growth, the more extensive the treatment. This type of cancer almost never spreads, but it can destroy surrounding tissue.

Remember: If you've been diagnosed with one basal cell carcinoma that's been successfully removed, that doesn't mean you're home free. You've got a higher chance of developing it elsewhere on your body in the future. It may even reappear in the same place where the original was removed, usually within two years. That's why it's imperative to continue those monthly skin self-exams in addition to continuing follow-up with your dermatologist.

Squamous cell carcinoma

Squamous cell carcinoma is the second most common skin cancer, affecting more than 100,000 Americans each year. This type of cancer begins in the upper layer of skin and may be found on all areas of the body (including the mucous membranes) and usually appears as a red, scaly patch that grows slowly and eventually becomes crusted and eroded. Most often, you can find these lesions on parts of your body that were exposed to the sun.

Squamous cell carcinoma can spread to underlying tissues if not treated; rarely, it can spread to internal organs, which can be fatal. Those squamous cell cancers that do spread usually begin from a chronic inflammatory skin condition, or on the mucous membranes, lips, or ears.

Suspect squamous cell carcinoma if you have

- A persistent scaly red patch with irregular borders that crusts or bleeds.
- An elevated growth with a central depression that may bleed.
- A warty crust that may bleed.
- An open persistent sore that bleeds and crusts.

Your doctor will diagnose squamous cell cancer after removing and examining a piece of tissue. This is usually an outpatient procedure. Most often, a doctor will cut away the entire growth and an additional border of normal skin as a safety margin; the site is then stitched closed, and the tissue sent to a lab to determine if all malignant cells have been removed.

When removed early, squamous cell carcinomas are easily treated, but the larger the growth the more extensive the treatment.

If you've been diagnosed with one squamous cell cancer, you'll have a higher chance of developing more in the future. No matter how carefully your doctor removes a tumor, another can develop in the same place. If the cancer recurs, your doctor may use a different type of treatment the second time.

Malignant melanoma

Malignant melanoma is the most deadly of the three types, usually beginning as a small brown, black, or multicolored patch with an irregular outline. Melanoma is much more dangerous because it has a tendency to spread quickly to internal organs. One in five patients with this type of cancer will die.

Genes, rather than sunburns, may be a stronger determinant of melanoma. Those at highest risk have a family history of the disease, many moles (more than 100), fair skin, light hair, and blue-green or gray eyes. Recently, scientists have identified a defective gene that appears to cause an inherited tendency to this type of deadly skin cancer.

Nevertheless, researchers found that sun worshippers had two times the melanoma risk as people who spent little time in the sun. But the most sensitive people—those who burn easily and have fair hair and light-colored eyes, or people with many moles—had six times the risk of melanoma than the least sensitive people.

Melanoma usually begins as a pigmented growth on the skin, with many shades of color from white to black. It usually has an irregular outline, and may be larger than an ordinary mole. The spot may crust, bleed, or itch, or it may develop within an ordinary mole.

There are usually a variety of treatment possibilities, from excision to radiation and chemotherapy, depending on the type of tumor, size, location, and other factors.

Unofficially... Studies at the Stanford Medical School showed that women with malignant melanoma live longer after a course of group therapy.

Skin cancer quiz

The following quiz can help determine your risk for developing skin cancer. After you add up your points, match your score to the chart to find your risk level.

WORKSHEET 11.1: SKIN CANCER QUIZ*

Hair Color Blond/red (4); brown (3); black (1)	___
Eye Color Blue/green (4); hazel (3); brown (1)	___
When exposed to one hour of summer sun, you... Burn and sometimes blister (4); burn and then tan (3); tan (1)	___
Do you have freckles? Many (4); some (3); none (2)	___
Where is your job? Outdoors (4); mixed (3); indoors (2)	___
Has anyone in your family had skin cancer? Yes (5); no (1)	___
Where in the U.S. did you live most before age 18? South (4); Midwest (3); North (2)	___
TOTAL	___

RISK LEVELS	
10–15	Below-average risk
16–22	Average risk
23–25	High risk
26–30	Very high risk

*Reprinted with permission of the American Academy of Dermatology

Sun safety: Help keep skin cancer at bay

Recently, the idea that sunscreen alone can prevent all types of skin cancer has become less clear, since one recent study suggested that sunscreens may not protect against malignant melanoma, the most virulent type of skin cancer. Still, everyone agrees that while you can't change your skin type or your family history, you can control your sun safety habits and take precautions for protection.

What that means is staying out of the sun when possible, covering up when you can't avoid the sun, and using sunscreen of at least SPF 15, every day.

Whenever you're out in the sun, remember the following sun safety tips:

- Always cover up with a hat and dark clothing when outdoors.
- Put on a shirt and hat after swimming.
- Consider wearing a T-shirt while swimming.
- Choose tightly woven clothing to filter the sun and reflect heat.
- Wear dry clothing (many materials can lose up to half their SPF ability when wet).

Watch out for the UV Index, as well. The UV Index is a number from 0 to 10 that indicates the amount of ultraviolet radiation reaching the Earth's surface during the hour around noon. The higher the number, the greater your exposure to UV radiation if you go outdoors.

The National Weather Service forecasts the UV Index daily in 58 U.S. cities, based on local predicted conditions. The index covers about a 30-mile radius from each city. Check the local newspaper or TV and radio news broadcasts to learn the UV Index

Watch Out! Sun tanning became fashionable in the 1930s after fashion trendsetter Coco Chanel returned from a beach vacation with a dark tan. Since then, the rate of malignant melanoma in the United States has increased 18-fold.

in your area. It also may be available through your local phone company and is available on the Internet from the National Weather Service at www.cpc.ncep.noaa.gov/products/stratosphere/uv_index/bulletin.txt.

Screening the sun

If you can't avoid the sun, you should apply a broad spectrum sunscreen to your skin to protect against the sun's harmful ultraviolet radiation. When applied to the skin, sunscreen lotions, creams, ointments, gels, or wax sticks absorb, reflect, or scatter some or all of the sun's rays.

When it comes to sunscreen, you need protection against both types of ultraviolet radiation (UVA and UVB) since both are now known to be harmful.

Most sunscreens today are called "broad spectrum" products and are designed to protect against both UVB light—the type of radiation that causes sunburn—and UVA (the "tanning rays"). Sunscreens which provide UVA protection may contain avobenzone and/or microfine zinc oxide. Check the ingredient list to be sure.

In the past, UVA was considered less dangerous because it didn't directly damage skin by causing sunburn—but new research suggests UVA can indeed damage the skin and may play a role in malignant melanoma, the deadliest form of skin cancer.

However, keep in mind that while all sunscreens block UVB rays, no product screens out all UVA rays. Some may advertise UVA protection, but there's no system yet for rating UVA protection. Even when you use a sunscreen with a high SPF number, there's no way to know how much UVA protection you're getting.

Bright Idea
If you're applying sunscreen and moisturizer to your skin, apply the sunscreen first. It should be as close to your skin as possible.

Watch Out!
You can still develop sun-induced aging and skin cancer even if you don't get a sunburn. The only way to completely protect yourself against aging and skin cancer is to avoid the sun.

In the past, lifeguards smeared white zinc oxide paste on their noses for maximum protection—today, it's available in a clear form which has broad sun-blocking power. Because zinc oxide sits on top of the skin and isn't absorbed, it doesn't cause any allergic reactions. (This is important if you have sensitive skin or if you're using a sunscreen every day.)

The American Medical Association and the American Academy of Dermatology recommend using a broad-spectrum sunscreen (which means it shields against both UVB and UVA rays) with an SPF of at least 15. But remember, when you reach for that bottle of sunscreen, you don't need to choose a stratosphere-level of SPF. In fact, higher SPFs don't indicate a higher degree of UV protection, as some people believe. Higher numbers offer protection for a longer period of time, but above 25, there is no appreciable difference. The actual time you're burn-free depends upon your skin type.

If you turn into a lobster at noon after 20 minutes of exposure without sunscreen, putting on an SPF 15 sunscreen beforehand means you can sit out 15 times longer (about five hours) before you burn. If you have very fair skin, you might burn in less than 20 minutes, and so the same sunscreen would protect you for less time. On the other hand, if your skin is dark, you'll probably take longer to burn, so an SPF of 15 would protect you longer than five hours.

Sunscreen tips

Don't be fooled by cloudy skies. Clouds block only as much as 20 percent of UV radiation, and since UV radiation also can pass through water, don't assume you're safe from UV radiation if you're in the water and feeling cool. Also, be especially careful on the

TABLE 11.1: HOW LONG CAN YOU SAFELY SUNBATHE USING SUNSCREEN?

PROTECTION FACTOR	4	8	15
Skin type	Safe exposure time		
Fair	10 minutes	40–80 minutes	1.5–2 hours
Medium	50–80 minutes	2–2.5 hours	5–5.5 hours
Dark	1.5–2 hours	3.5–4 hours	all day
Black	4 hours	all day	all day

Unofficially...
The higher the altitude, the quicker you will develop sunburn—and the risk gets greater faster with increasing altitude, according to a study at the New York University School of Medicine.

beach and in the snow because sand and snow reflect sunlight and increase the amount of UV radiation you receive.

For the best protection, here's the inside scoop on sunscreens:

- Don't skimp on the amount (an average-size woman should use about an ounce per application—about the size of a shot glass).
- Repeat applications every two hours after you've been in the sun or the water, even if the sunscreen claims to be waterproof.
- Try to avoid the sun between 10 a.m. and 2 p.m.
- Put sunscreen on with your kids; you'll be a good role model and you'll also be protected.
- Make sure your hat brim is at least four inches wide.
- Waterproof or water-resistant sunscreens can be applied less often, but if you're not sure whether your sunscreen is still working, apply some more.
- Apply even in cloudy weather (80 percent of the sun's rays break through the clouds).
- Apply on eyelids and around the eyes, too, even if you're wearing sunglasses (sunglasses prevent

> To reduce the risk of skin cancer, [it is recommended] that people limit or avoid exposure to the sun, cover as much skin as possible when outdoors, and use a sunscreen with a SPF of 15 or higher.
> —American Cancer Society, 1998

UV rays from getting into the eyes; they won't help protect the skin around them).

Waterproof sunscreens are a good choice if you're swimming—but also if you're active, since they protect better while you're sweating. The only exception is women with acne—the waterproof brands may make you break out. If you have acne, choose a regular sunscreen and simply apply it more often.

Regarding creams versus gels, one type of sunscreen isn't inherently any better than another, but many dermatologists recommend that you use a cream for your face, since gels contain alcohol and may sting. (On the other hand, some women find lotions easier to apply.) If you have acne, a heavier sunscreen can make you break out; instead, try a light texture sunscreen first, but apply a thick layer.

Protect your eyes, too!

Sunglasses can help protect your eyes from sun damage. The ideal sunglasses don't have to be expensive, but they should block 99 to 100 percent of UVA and UVB radiation. Check the label to see that they do. If there's no label, don't buy the glasses. And don't go by how dark the glasses are because UV protection comes from an invisible chemical applied to the lenses, not from the color or darkness of the lenses.

Drugs and the sun—which ones don't mix

It's called photosensitivity—a toxic skin reaction to the sun that can be caused by a number of substances, including certain drugs, dyes, chemicals in perfumes, parsnips, and mustard, and fruits such as limes and lemons.

Studies show the combination of ultraviolet rays and some medicines, birth control pills, cosmetics, and soaps may accelerate skin burns or produce painful adverse skin reactions, such as rashes. However, some products are more likely to cause reactions than others, and not everyone who uses the products will be affected.

Before going out in the sun, it's a good idea to check with your doctor to see if any of the medications you're taking are likely to cause problems and decide how to best avoid such reactions. Read the labels of over the counter (OTC) drugs and note if they may be photosensitizing.

If you get symptoms after being out in the sun, you may want to consider what drugs and chemicals you are using and contact your doctor immediately for advice. Drugs are the most common culprits and may include

- Acne medicines.
- Antibiotics (tetracycline, griseofulvin, and so forth).
- Antihistamines.
- Antiarrythmics.
- Antidepressants (tricyclics, St. John's wort).
- Nonsteroidal anti-inflammatory drugs, such as naproxen sodium.
- Oral contraceptives containing estrogen.
- Sulfa drugs.
- Tranquilizers (Librium, Thorazine).
- Diuretics.

A wide range of other products also may react to the sun in sensitive people, including

- Deodorants.
- Antibacterial soaps.
- Artificial sweeteners.

Watch Out!
In recent years, "suntan accelerators" have appeared on the market. Manufacturers claim that these products enhance tanning by stimulating and increasing melanin formation. The FDA recently concluded that these suntan accelerators are actually unapproved drugs, and the agency has issued warning letters to several manufacturers of these products.

Bright Idea
Make sure there's a tube of sunscreen in the car, for last-minute sun activities.

- Fluorescent brightening agents.
- Mothballs.
- Petroleum products.
- Cadmium sulfide (a chemical injected into the skin during tattooing).

Photoreactive products can also aggravate existing skin problems like eczema, herpes, psoriasis, and acne, and can inflame scar tissue. They can also trigger or worsen autoimmune diseases such as lupus erythematosus and rheumatoid arthritis, in which the body's immune system mistakenly destroys itself. Women infected with the HIV virus are more susceptible to photosensitive disorders and should take special care in the sun.

You may get reactions ranging from exaggerated sunburnlike skin conditions, eye burn, mild allergic reactions, hives, abnormal reddening of the skin, and eczema-like rashes with itching, swelling, blistering, oozing, and scaling of the skin. Chronic effects from long-term exposure include premature skin aging, stronger allergic reactions, cataracts, blood vessel damage, a weakened immune system, and skin cancer.

The degree of photosensitivity varies among women; not everyone who uses medications containing photoreactive agents will have a problem. In fact, a person who has a photoreaction after a single exposure may not react to the same product again. On the other hand, if you're allergic to one chemical, you may develop photosensitivity to another related chemical.

Indoor tans

In our search for the perfect tan, many women have turned to tanning beds to maintain that golden glow, even in the middle of winter. The most popular device used in tanning salons is a clamshell-like tanning bed; you lie down on a Plexiglas surface as lights from above and below bake your skin.

Many older tanning devices used light sources that emitted shortwave ultraviolet rays (UVB) that actually caused burning; aware of the harmful effects of UVB radiation, salon owners began using tanning beds that emitted mostly long-wave (UVA) light sources.

While some salons still claim this type of tanning is safe (UVA rays are less likely to cause burning than UVB rays), they are suspected to have links to malignant melanoma and immune system damage. Tanning indoors damages your skin because indoor tanning devices emit ultraviolet rays; tanning occurs when the skin produces additional pigment (coloring) to protect itself against burn from ultraviolet rays. Overexposure to these rays can cause eye injury, premature wrinkling of the skin, and light-induced skin rashes, and can increase your chances of developing skin cancer. Exposure to the UV radiation from sunlamps adds to the total amount of UV radiation you get from the sun during your lifetime, further increasing your risk of cancer.

In spite of all this, if you insist on tanning with the aid of a tanning device, ask whether the manufacturer or the salon staff recommend exposure limits for your skin type. Set a timer on the tanning device that automatically shuts off the lights or somehow signals that you've reached your exposure time. Remember that exposure time affects burning, as does your age at the time of exposure.

Be sure that you wear goggles while you tan; the Food and Drug Administration requires tanning salons to have you wear protective eye goggles. This

Watch Out!
Women who have lupus or diabetes, or who are susceptible to cold sores, should know that these conditions can be worsened after exposure to ultraviolet radiation from tanning devices, sunlamps, or natural sunlight.

is because studies show that too much exposure to ultraviolet rays, including UVA rays, can damage the retina. Overexposure can burn the cornea, and repeated exposure over many years can change the structure of the lens so that it begins to cloud, forming a cataract.

Closing your eyes, wearing ordinary sunglasses, and using cotton wads don't protect the cornea from the intensity of UV radiation in tanning devices. Make sure the goggles fit snugly. Check to see that the salon sterilizes the goggles after each use to prevent the spread of eye infections.

Remember, too, that your skin may be more sensitive to artificial light if you use certain medications (for example, antihistamines, tranquilizers, or birth control pills). If your tanning salon keeps a file with information on your medical history, medications, and treatments, make sure you update it as necessary.

Just the facts

- Acne is affected by heredity and hormones, not greasy food and chocolate.
- There's no such thing as a safe tan.
- Use a sunscreen of at least SPF 15 every time you go into the sun.
- Some drugs can cause sun sensitivity; check labels and ask your doctor.
- Check for skin cancer using the A-B-C-D method (asymmetry, border, color, and diameter).

GET THE SCOOP ON...
Your real odds for having breast cancer ▪ Your chances of surviving breast cancer ▪ Breast cancer genes ▪ How to find the best mammography ▪ Newest Pap tests for cervical cancer

Reducing the Risk for Cancers

Cancer can strike women in many different forms, but it's always characterized by the uncontrolled growth and spread of abnormal cells. Yet, despite intensive study over the past 50 years, scientists still aren't sure just what triggers the sudden uncontrolled growth of malignant cells.

The cells in your body are constantly renewing themselves by dividing and growing as old tissues are replaced with new ones and injuries are repaired. When things are working normally, your body has ways to control this cell division so it doesn't spiral out of control—but for some reason, cancer cells break free of these controls, wildly subdividing without restraint, competing with healthy cells for nutrients. As these cancerous groups of cells continue to grow, they begin to invade nearby areas of the body; eventually they can spread to the far corners of the body, invading other organs and forming new tumors. If they are not caught and removed, or killed with drugs, eventually, they can be fatal.

This doesn't mean that a cancer diagnosis is an automatic death sentence. Recent advances in cancer treatment mean that, on average, 50 percent of women are free of disease at least five years past diagnosis. In some types of cancer, the survival rate is much better than that. What's clear is that with any type of cancer, the earlier it can be detected, the better your chances of a cure. This chapter will focus on several types of cancer that only affect (or, in the case of cancer of the breast, generally) women.

Early detection

Because it's so important to uncover these errant cells before they begin their deadly spread to other parts of your body, a wide range of screening tests have been developed to watch for these uncontrolled cellular storms. To do your part in cancer surveillance, you should examine your skin and breasts each month for lumps, thickening, discharge, or pain. In addition, there are a number of other important screening tests you shouldn't overlook:

Bright Idea
You should examine your breasts at the same time each month in your cycle, or the same day of each month if you're postmenopausal, because your breasts change throughout your cycle.

- Pelvic exam: Every year after age 18 (or as soon as sexual activity begins) to detect cancers of the cervix, ovary, or uterus.

- Pap smear: Every year after age 18 (or as soon as sexual activity begins) to detect cancer of the cervix.

- Mammography: Every one to two years between ages 40 and 49; every year afterward: Note—women at high risk should have an annual mammogram after age 40. The American Cancer Society recently changed its recommendations to yearly mammograms after age 40; other experts still recommend a mammogram every one or two years between ages 40 and 49.

- Fecal occult blood test: Annually after age 40 to detect blood in the stool, which may be a sign of colon or rectal cancer.

- Sigmoidoscopy: Every three to five years after age 50 to detect changes in the colon or rectum that could indicate cancer.

Leading a low-risk life

Many women seem to feel that cancer is almost an inevitable part of life, but it doesn't have to be. In fact, 80 percent of all cancer seems to be related to lifestyle choices that we could moderate: The things we eat, drink, and smoke, and the air we breathe.

You are what you eat

Many studies throughout the world have linked a high-fat diet with many kinds of malignancies, including cancer of the rectum, colon, and ovaries. While scientists don't understand exactly how the two are related, they agree that eating a varied diet high in fiber while limiting saturated fats (such as animal protein) and cholesterol is a good start. If you eat fresh fruits and vegetables every day, you may slash your risk in half; at the same time, boosting your intake of foods containing vitamins A, C, and E (the antioxidants) may help protect you.

Dietary consumption of vitamin A, beta-carotene, and fruits and vegetables appears to reduce the risk of breast cancer in premenopausal women, particularly those already at increased risk due to family history or alcohol consumption, according to new findings from the Harvard Nurses' Health Study. The benefits of vitamin A, beta-carotene, and fruits and cruciferous vegetables like broccoli and cauliflower were even stronger in premenopausal women at higher risk of breast

Watch Out!
Seven warning signs of cancer are a change in bowel or bladder habits; a sore that doesn't heal; an unusual bleeding or discharge; a thickening or lump in the breast or elsewhere; indigestion or problems swallowing; an obvious change in a wart or mole; and a nagging cough or hoarseness.

cancer—especially those with a family history of the disease and who drank the equivalent of at least 15 grams of alcohol a day. Unfortunately, the nutrients didn't seem to offer much help to postmenopausal women.

Alcohol

Even the most moderate drinking may increase a woman's risk of breast cancer (scientists suspect this is because of alcohol's interaction with estrogen). The risk of breast cancer increases when a woman drinks as little as one ounce of alcohol a day. Moreover, some studies suggest that the risk for breast cancer exists for even occasional consumption of alcoholic beverages, although the results aren't clear. Clearly, alcohol and hormones are interrelated, since alcohol abuse can also lead to fertility problems and early menopause.

Hormones

Every woman produces estrogen and a range of other hormones that protect her from developing osteoporosis and heart disease. However, estrogen has been linked to a number of different cancers, especially breast cancer and endometrial cancer, which grow faster when exposed to estrogen. In fact, one recent study found that women over age 65 who had the highest blood levels of estrogen and testosterone were three times more likely to develop breast cancer three years later.

In addition to the natural stores of estrogen in a woman's body, you can be exposed to excess estrogen if you take birth control pills or hormone replacement therapy (HRT). After exhaustive studies, scientists have been unable to link birth control pills to cancer risk in most women, and the pills may

Bright Idea
If you regularly drink more than two glasses of wine or mixed drinks a day, you should think about trying to cut back; women with a history of breast cancer in their family, and certainly women who have had breast cancer, should consider eliminating alcohol completely.

in fact protect against some types of cancer. However, if you're postmenopausal, taking estrogen-only HRT (ERT) will put you at higher risk for developing endometrial cancer. For this reason, postmenopausal women with a uterus add the hormone progesterone to their ERT regimen, which effectively counters the estrogen-related risk of endometrial cancer.

For every 100,000 women on hormone replacement, about 5,000 lives will be saved from heart disease and about 500 from complications of osteoporosis—compared to about 18 additional cases of breast cancer. In addition, it's important to note that the women who do get breast cancer while on HRT tend to have earlier, lower stage, more easily curable disease.

Tobacco

By now, most women know that smoking is a major cause of lung cancer, but it also contributes to the risk of cancers of the cervix, mouth, throat, esophagus, pancreas, bladder, and, possibly, the stomach. It's not easy, but if you quit smoking as soon as you can, your risk of cancer will begin to decrease immediately.

Heredity

Scientists don't fully understand why, but certain kinds of cancers (especially breast, ovarian, colon, and skin) seem to run in families. Depending on the type of cancer in question, your risk is higher if your mother, father, sister, or brother had cancer. Breast cancer is primarily carried on the maternal side, but there is still some risk from paternal relatives. Ovarian cancer likewise is primarily carried on the maternal side. Colon and lung cancer risk can be traced to either side.

Breast cancer

Breast cancer is the most common form of gynecological cancer in American women, and the second major cause of cancer death after lung cancer. A report from the National Cancer Institute (NCI) estimates that about one in eight women in the United States will develop breast cancer during her lifetime.

What too many women at risk don't realize is that the statistic refers to the risk of developing breast cancer at some point in your lifetime, assuming that you live to be 95. Let's look at this statistic in another way: If you're an average 30-year-old white woman, you have only a 1 in 5,900 chance of getting breast cancer this year.

Charting your true risk

Breast cancer is not inevitable. (In fact, as a group, women are far more likely to die of heart disease than of breast cancer.) Even if you were at very high risk for breast cancer, you're still more likely not to get the disease. It's true that one out of eight women develops breast cancer in her lifetime. That means that the average woman has a 12.6 percent total lifetime risk—which also means that she has an 88 percent risk of not ever getting breast cancer.

The most prevalent risk factor is age: 80 percent of women with breast cancer are over age 50. Other risk factors include

- No children.
- Having a first child after age 30.
- A family history of breast cancer.
- Beginning menstruation before age 12.
- Completing menopause after age 55.

Unofficially... Women between ages 70 and 74 are 56 times more likely to get breast cancer than women aged 25 to 29, regardless of family history, pregnancy history, age at first menstruation, or any other risk factors that have been identified so far.

- Being overweight.
- Drinking alcohol.

More than 70 percent of women who get breast cancer have no known risk factors, however, and while having several risk factors may boost your chances of having breast cancer, the interplay of factors is complex. The best way to assess breast cancer risk is by seeking a risk assessment consultation at one of the many breast cancer centers located throughout the United States.

If you have a family history

If your mother or your sister has been diagnosed with breast cancer, you may be at a higher risk, but that doesn't mean you'll automatically inherit breast cancer—this is true even if your family has something called "cancer syndrome" (a family pattern characterized by several different kinds of cancers occurring early and running through generations).

In a recent Harvard University study of 2,389 women aged 30 to 50 who got breast cancer, only 215 of them had a family history of the disease. The reason why all first-degree relatives of a woman with breast cancer are considered to be at higher risk is because, at the moment, doctors can't tell which cases of breast cancer are genetic and which aren't, so all first-degree relatives of breast cancer patients are considered "at risk," although most won't get breast cancer themselves.

Of the women who do inherit a vulnerability for breast cancer, some of the cases seem to be caused by a defect in a gene known as BRCA1. Every woman has two copies of the BRCA1 gene, one inherited from her mother and one from her father. In most people, both BRCA1 genes function normally. But

Unofficially...
Your risk of getting breast cancer goes up by 1.9 percent every year past age 20 that you put off having your first child. This means that if you got pregnant for the first time at age 25, you would multiply 5 by 1.9 to get your risk factor: Your risk would be 9.5 percent higher if you had your first child at age 25 instead of age 20.

in some women, one copy carries an error. This error can occur anywhere along the BRCA1 gene, but some of the errors can raise your risk of developing breast or ovarian cancer.

Scientists suspect that BRCA1 is a "tumor suppressor" gene; that is, it supplies the blueprint for a protein "brake" that can stop cellular growth. A healthy BRCA1 would make sure cells don't become malignant and begin growing out of control. But a woman who inherits one normal and one mutant BRCA1 gene would remain free of breast cancer only as long as the healthy gene directs the production of the cellular brake. If something (such as an environmental toxin) damaged the normal gene, the breast cell would lose that brake. Unprotected, the cell would begin proliferating at will, generating a malignant tumor.

A woman with the BRCA1 mutation has up to an 87 percent risk of getting breast cancer and up to a 60 percent risk of getting ovarian cancer by age 70. The risk associated with a second, related gene, known as BRCA2, is similar in women, but men with this mutation have a higher risk of breast cancer also.

Fortunately, as far as we know, the mutant BRCA1 and BRCA2 genes are fairly rare, accounting for only about one-half of inherited breast cancer (or five percent of all breast cancers). Still, scientists suspect that at least 600,000 American women may carry the defective genes and many have no idea of their inherited risk. Moreover, these genes are quite complex, which means that there may be many different types of mutations that could occur along their length, making it hard to devise an effective, inexpensive screening test.

Most women who develop breast cancer have normal BRCA1 genes, so testing negative for an alteration in BRCA1 doesn't mean you're home free, either. There could be other genes that may increase your risk of breast and ovarian cancers that haven't yet been identified.

On the other hand, just because you carry the BRCA1 alteration doesn't mean that you will definitely develop breast or ovarian cancer. Certainly you'd be at high risk, but there are other factors scientists don't yet understand that affect the development of cancer.

Short of screening for the BRCA1 and BRCA2 genes, there are some clues that a family's breast cancer is genetic:

- Two close relatives (such as mother and sister) with the disease
- Separate malignancies that appear in both breasts
- Diagnosis at an early age, especially well before menopause (the older a woman is when she gets breast cancer, the less likely it is that her disease is inherited)

As you can see, your own risk of inherited breast cancer is based on a wide variety of variables. If your mother got breast cancer, how old was she when she was diagnosed? If she was diagnosed before menopause, your risk increases. If she had unrelated bilateral breast cancer (separate cancers in each breast), your risk is higher. In fact, the more relatives who got breast cancer early or in both breasts, the higher your risk.

Still, these variables are only clues—not guarantees. Even if two of your relatives developed breast

Unofficially...
New research has found that one error in BRCA1 occurs more often among some Ashkenazi Jews. The NCI and the National Center for Human Genome Research will soon begin another research study of this group to determine how common this is and how it's related to breast and ovarian cancer.

cancer early in their lives, it doesn't necessarily mean the disease runs in your family. Everyone has cancer in her family, and the larger the family and the longer she lives, the more cancer the family's going to have. Most likely, scientists say, no one will ever find just one cause for breast cancer. Certainly, they do know that inherited cases of breast cancer are in the minority.

Genetic risk: What you can do

Most women with breast cancer in their family believe that they have close to a 100 percent chance of getting the same disease—but it's just not so. Nevertheless, some are so profoundly distressed that they choose prophylactic mastectomy (removal of healthy breasts) rather than wait to develop malignant tumors.

What many women don't understand is that your true inherited risk is not nearly as great as most people think. While most daughters and sisters of patients estimate their risk at 100 percent, in actuality, a woman whose mother has breast cancer has only a 21 percent risk of getting cancer herself. And if your mother and sister both had breast cancer, your own risk rises only to about 25 percent, which still means you have a 75 percent risk of not having breast cancer. Only the presence of BRCA1 brings the risk up above 85 percent.

If you're at risk because of your family history, the first thing you need to do is get accurate information about your risk factors, together with information that helps you take control of your own health. This way, you'll know what to fear and what not to fear, when to ask questions and when to seek second opinions.

Nowhere is a woman's search for this information more difficult than in the area of breast cancer, where the facts are so often either disputed or unclear. If you think you're at risk because of your family history, there are several things you can do to ease your worries:

- Make an appointment with a risk assessment program at a comprehensive cancer center or medical center near you.
- Seek genetic counseling.
- Begin an intensive preventive program of breast self-exams.
- If two of your immediate relatives had the disease (or one developed it well before menopause or in both breasts), you may want to start yearly mammograms at age 40.
- If you have an extremely strong family history with many breast cancers striking early, some experts recommend yearly mammograms beginning at five years younger than the age at which cancer was diagnosed in the previous generation.
- Consider a generalized screening for the BRCA1 and BRCA2 genes, comparing blood samples from afflicted family members with yours.
- Discuss preventive tamoxifen (a medication that seems to help prevent the onset of breast cancer) with your health care provider.
- Discuss joining the national experimental trials of tamoxifen-raloxifene with your health care provider.

Take the test: BRCA1 and BRCA2
It's possible to have genetic testing to see if you carry the gene mutation for breast cancer. While this testing has been commercially available since 1996, its complexity and cost mean it is not a tool for every

Moneysaver
While any doctor can order the BRCA test for you, you may be able to have the test done for free if you're part of a clinical trial—and your confidentiality will be guaranteed.

woman. Testing should only be considered by those women with a risk of carrying the gene mutation.

Moreover, if you're considering genetic testing, you need to also consider the tremendous emotional impact that goes along with finding out that you are BRCA-positive. Unless the test is done as part of a confidential research study, it may have an impact on your ability to get life or health insurance. This test should not be taken—in the literal sense—lightly.

On the horizon...

Scientists are busy studying ways that may be used someday to help screen for breast cancer:

- Hair analysis: A new Australian study suggests analyzing a strand of hair could provide a simple breast cancer screen, since hairs from cancer patients are structurally different. Hair from women testing positive for BRCA mutations have rings of intensity not seen in other women's hair.

- Blood test: Tests of levels of estrogen and testosterone in women over age 65 may someday reveal breast cancer risk, since one study found high levels of these hormones at this age were linked to breast cancer.

Warning signs...

There are a number of changes in the breast that may be a sign of breast cancer. These include

- Lump or thickening in breast or armpit.
- Changes in a nipple (thickening, pulling in, bleeding, or discharge).
- Dimpled or reddened skin.
- Swelling.
- Change in color or texture.

- Bulging, irregular veins.
- Pain.
- Change in size or shape.
- Spot on a mammogram.

Your breasts are always changing during different periods of your life. Some of your symptoms may be linked to your menstrual cycle, pregnancy, breast feeding, or menopause. Often the lump turns out to be a harmless cyst (fluid-filled sac), and not a cancerous tumor at all. Most of these cysts will disappear on their own. But on the slight possibility that your symptoms could be a sign of cancer, it's important to report any changes to your health care provider, who will check out your symptoms and do a breast exam. A mammogram (an X-ray of the breast) may be ordered to take a closer look at the inside of your breast. Other tests might be ordered to help diagnose the problem:

- Ultrasound (sound waves that create a picture of the inside of your breast) to find a lump and tell whether or not it is a solid tumor
- Aspiration (using a needle to draw fluid from the breast to check the cells)
- Biopsy (surgical removal of all or part of a breast lump)

Getting a good mammogram

A mammogram is an X-ray film of the breast that can detect breast cancer when it is in its earliest, most treatable stage, up to two years before a lump can be felt. More than 90 percent of all breast cancers are detected this way.

Despite the controversy about the cost-effectiveness of mammograms for women in their

Moneysaver
If you can't afford a mammogram, the Breast and Cervical Cancer Early Screening Program provides them, as well as Pap smears, at low to no cost for women in financial need.

40s, most doctors agree with the current American Cancer Society guidelines that recommend screening mammograms every year or two for women between 40 and 49, and every year after age 50. Women with a history of breast cancer may want to have a mammogram every year after age 40.

If anything irregular is detected, such as a mass, changes from earlier mammograms, abnormalities of the skin, or enlargement of the lymph nodes, an ultrasound, a biopsy, (needle sampling) or consultation with a breast surgeon may be ordered.

Things to know before scheduling a mammogram

There are also things you should do to prepare before having a mammogram:

- Don't use deodorant, perfume, powders, or ointments of any sort in the underarm area or on the breast on the day of the exam—these products may cause shadows to appear on the mammogram.

- Wear a blouse with a skirt or slacks (not a dress), to the mammography facility, since you'll have to undress above the waist for the exam.

- Schedule a mammogram in the first several days after a menstrual period, since that is when hormone levels are lowest and are least likely to show a hormonally induced lump. The exam should not be outright painful, although the compression of the breast during the exam may cause some discomfort.

Your mammogram rights

Until recently, you could go to a mammography facility and have no idea if the machine was 20 years old or whether the person who positioned you for the test or interpreted the X-ray findings was well trained.

Today, as a result of the Mammography Quality Standards Act, the nation's mammography facilities must meet high standards for technical quality, safety, and staff training—or lose Food and Drug Administration (FDA) certification (and it's illegal for these facilities to operate without being certified). The new rules also guarantee that you will get an easy-to-read report on the results of your mammogram rather than having to wait for the results to be sent to your referring doctor. The Act gave you the right to see your own results because too many reports of malignancies that were sent to a woman's referring doctor were misplaced and not reported to the patients in time.

Bright Idea
To help you find an FDA-certified facility closest to you, call 800/4-CANCER, or check the FDA Web site at www.fda.gov/cdrh/faclist.html.

Ultrasounds versus mammograms

Mammograms work well in a breast made up of mostly fat, but in many younger women with "dense breasts," the ducts, glands, and tissue can hide a tumor. In fact, mammograms miss at least 10 percent of cancerous tumors, while between 75 and 80 percent of the lesions that do appear on a mammogram turn out to be harmless. As a diagnostic tool, high-resolution ultrasounds are very good at determining whether something found by palpation or by mammogram is benign or malignant.

Needle and tissue biopsies: What to ask

If a solid mass does show up on a mammogram or ultrasound, your doctor will need to do a biopsy to check for malignant cells. In the past, these needle biopsies could be quite painful and unpleasant, especially if the lump was deep within the breast tissue.

Today between 40 and 50 percent of hospitals in the United States can get the same data with a simple, quick procedure called minimally invasive breast biopsy (MIBB) or stereotactic biopsy. After application of a local anesthetic and while guided by a digital X-ray camera, the doctor aligns the needle mechanically until it's precisely over the lump; with one flip of the switch, the needle is sent into the mass and painlessly withdraws some tissue.

However, minimally invasive procedures are not appropriate in all cases. For example, when a lump is palpable, doctors may be concerned that the small sample of tissue might miss a cancerous spot. Moreover, many women prefer the entire lump to be gone so that they don't continue to feel it every month.

There are a number of questions you can ask your health care provider if you need a biopsy of a suspicious lump:

- What type of biopsy will I have? Why? Will the entire lump be removed or just part of it?
- Can the fluid be drained with a needle?
- How long will the biopsy take?
- Will I be awake during the biopsy and can it be done on an outpatient basis?
- Does the hospital do MIBB?
- If I do have cancer, what other tests should I have?
- Will estrogen or progesterone receptor tests be done on the biopsied tissue you remove? What will these tests tell you? Will other special tests (flow cytometry and other markers for tumor aggressiveness) be done on the tissue?
- Will you do a two-step procedure? (In a two-step procedure, you would be informed of treatment options after the biopsy results are available. Any further surgery is done separately.) These

days, laws generally require specific consent either authorizing a one-step or two-step procedure.

- How visible will the biopsy scar be?
- Are there any after-effects of biopsy?
- After the biopsy, how soon will I know if I have cancer or not? Will you call me with the results?
- After a biopsy, if cancer is found, how much time can I take to decide what type of treatment to have?

If your tests are positive...

If your biopsy comes back positive, you'll need to make some important decisions about the next steps. You do have options. Ask your health care provider these questions to help you decide:

- What kind of breast cancer do I have?
- What tests will I have before surgery to see if the cancer has spread to other organs?
- What are my treatment options? What procedure are you recommending for me and why?
- What are the potential risks and benefits of these procedures?
- Will estrogen and progesterone receptor tests be done on the tissue removed during surgery? What will these tests tell you? Will other special tests be done on the tissue?
- What is your opinion about breast-conserving surgery (lumpectomy) followed by radiation therapy? Am I a candidate for this type of treatment?
- Will I need additional treatment with radiation therapy, chemotherapy, or hormonal therapy

following my surgery? If so, can you refer me to a medical oncologist?

- Can breast reconstruction surgery be done at the time of the surgery, as well as later? Would you recommend it for me? What potential risks and benefits are involved?

- If I choose not to have reconstruction, what can you tell me about breast prostheses?

- How long do I have to make a treatment decision?

- Is there a clinical trial that is enrolling patients with my type of breast cancer? If so, how can I learn more?

- Could you recommend a breast cancer specialist for a second opinion?

- Can you give me a referral to a comprehensive cancer center?

What about a clinical trial?

Before you start treatment for breast cancer, you may want to think about taking part in a clinical trial, a study that looks at innovative treatments to care for patients. Clinical trials are undertaken to find new and better ways to help cancer patients. If clinical trials show that the new therapy is better than the treatment currently being used, the new treatment may become standard.

Before joining a clinical trial, however, find out as much as you can about the risks and benefits. Think long and hard before joining a trial in which you may be given a placebo (in other words, a "dummy" treatment) instead of a medication that may well help treat your cancer.

Bright Idea
If you live near a comprehensive cancer center, consider getting treatment there. A facility like this can offer you a coordinated "team" approach to cancer care and access to the latest in experimental and innovative treatments.

Finding the best treatment

The type of surgery you have depends on the type of breast cancer, whether the cancer has spread, your age, and your health. If your tumor is small, you and your doctor may decide to do a lumpectomy. Studies have shown that this type of conservative treatment offers the same odds of survival as does a total mastectomy in someone with a small breast tumor that has not spread into the nearby lymph nodes. New studies suggest that after lumpectomy, a combination of chemotherapy and radiation offers the best chance of long-term survival.

During a lumpectomy, your doctor will remove and test a few of your lymph nodes to see if there are any cancer cells there. Find out if your doctor is trained to do a "sentinel node biopsy"—a new version of an older process in which up to 30 lymph nodes had to be removed to test breast cancer spread. In the new method, doctors inject the tumor with a radioactive tracer and then massage the breast to spread the tracer outward through the lymph vessels; this way, doctors can see which node the cancer cells would reach first. If this "sentinel" node is cancer free, doctors can assume the cancer hasn't spread. Only 10 percent of surgeons were trained to perform it in 1999, but within a few years it's expected to be widely available.

If the tumor is larger, your doctor may suggest a simple mastectomy, or a modified radical mastectomy if the tumor is large or has spread, or if there is a chance the cancer might return otherwise. This more drastic surgery can be combined with breast reconstruction, either right away or later on. If you are interested in having breast reconstruction, tell

Bright Idea
To find out more about clinical trials for your kind of cancer, you can call the NCI's cancer information service at 800/4-CANCER (TTY 800/332-8615). The call is free and a trained information specialist will talk with you and answer your questions.

your doctor before surgery. Having breast reconstruction could change the way your doctor does the operation. If the cancer has spread to the muscles in the chest, most doctors believe a radical mastectomy is the best choice. Today, this operation is used only when the cancer has spread to the chest muscle.

However, no matter how careful your surgeon, the surgery won't catch cancer cells that may have already spread through the lymph glands or into your blood. This is why other treatments (such as radiation therapy, chemotherapy, and/or hormonal therapy) may be used.

After surgery
Once the cancer has been removed, the doctor may recommend radiation to destroy or shrink any remaining breast cancer cells. Radiation works because it kills rapidly dividing cells like cancer cells. Unfortunately, it will also affect other rapidly dividing cells, such as those of the skin, hair, and nails. This is why radiation can sometimes cause skin problems and hair loss.

Even if no cancer is found in any lymph nodes, a lumpectomy is always followed by radiation therapy. Breast cancer surgery also may be followed by chemotherapy in even the earliest stages. While this can reduce the risk of recurrence, the side effects can be difficult—and there's no guarantee that the breast cancer won't return. If a breast tumor does spread, your chance of surviving for five years falls to 22 percent.

If chemotherapy will be used, your doctor may suggest using stem-cell treatment to make the therapy more effective. By first removing a woman's stem cells from her bone marrow or blood, the doctor can use very high doses of chemotherapy or radiation to kill cancer cells. Because this also kills healthy white blood cells, leaving the woman vulnerable to infection, the stem cells are then replaced, where they restore the body's ability to fight infection.

The growth of some breast cancer cells may be slowed by giving a type of "anti-estrogen," which is usually administered in the form of the drug called tamoxifen. Tamoxifen treatment lasts at least two years, and often as long as five.

Research over the past 15 years has shown that the drug tamoxifen has reduced the chance of a second, unrelated breast cancer in women who have had one breast cancer. Side effects of tamoxifen may include a slightly higher risk of endometrial cancer (cancer of the lining of the uterus). The risk increases if the drug is taken for more than five years. Other side effects include menopause-like symptoms of weight gain, hot flashes, mood swings and so on.

Surviving breast cancer

Many women at risk feel doomed, not just because they expect to get breast cancer, but because they are positive that they will die from it. In fact, most women diagnosed with breast cancer do survive, not just for five years, but 10 years, 20 years and more. About two-thirds of all women who are diagnosed with early-stage breast cancer are still alive 10 years later. For those whose tumors were smaller than 1 cm, 80 percent survive at least 10 years. And the American Cancer Society estimates that half of all the women diagnosed with breast cancer more than 25 years ago are still living today.

Unofficially...
A new cancer drug may improve the odds of breast cancer recurrence: Herceptin is a medication that seems to interfere with the spread of cancer. When combined with other types of chemotherapy, Herceptin improved the response rate over chemotherapy alone.

TABLE 12.1: APPROXIMATE SURVIVAL RATE WITH BREAST CANCER

Stage	Five-year survival	10-year survival
I (early)	80 percent	65 percent
II	60 percent	45 percent
IIIa	50 percent	40 percent
IIIb	35 percent	20 percent
IV and inflammatory breast cancer	10 percent	5 percent

Your chance of recovery and choice of treatment depend on the stage of your cancer (the size of the tumor and whether it is just in the breast or has spread to other places in the body), the type of breast cancer, certain characteristics of the cancer cells, and whether the cancer is found in your other breast. Your age, weight, menopausal status (whether or not you still have periods) and general health can also affect your prognosis and choice of treatment.

Prevention: From tamoxifen to mastectomy

As a matter of routine, you should check your breasts every month, go for an annual breast exam by a health care provider, and have a mammogram performed every one to two years. These measures will increase the chance of discovering breast cancer early. When detected and treated at an early stage, chances for survival will increase and there will be more options for treatment. But for some women at high risk for breast cancer, that's not good enough.

Breast cancer can't be reliably prevented other than by having both healthy breasts removed before cancer strikes (prophylactic mastectomy). Even this may not prevent breast cancer from appearing in the chest wall beneath the breast, however. This controversial procedure is sometimes recommended for women who are at very high risk of developing breast cancer and who are extraordinarily worried about that risk. But the American Cancer Society has "great concern" about this procedure, since it is still possible that cancer cells could grow in the chest wall.

The only other way that women at high risk can effectively protect themselves is by taking the drug tamoxifen, which, in a large study in 1998, was shown to cut the risk of breast cancer in half in healthy, high-risk women. Researchers had intended to follow the 13,000 women in the study for five years, but after four years, the rate of invasive breast cancer was 49 percent lower among the women taking tamoxifen than among those getting the placebo. Researchers interrupted the study, and the FDA allowed Zeneca Pharmaceutical to sell tamoxifen (Nolvadex) as a breast-cancer preventive.

Unfortunately, tamoxifen increases the risk of blood clots and uterine cancer in some women—and although it reduces the risk of breast cancer, studies haven't shown whether it lowers the death rate from the disease.

An even newer drug called raloxifene (Evista), manufactured by Eli Lilly, may offer better protection for the breast without the risk of uterine cancer, although the link is not yet clearly proven. The FDA has approved it as a way to prevent bone loss in postmenopausal women, but new studies suggest it also cuts the risk of invasive breast cancer by 63 percent over three years. Side which include hot flashes, leg cramps, and blood clots, effects are less annoying as well. In 1999, the federal government launched a new study comparing raloxifene and tamoxifen, but results won't be available until at least 2004. The

Bright Idea
One recent study found that exercising four hours weekly can reduce your risk of breast cancer by 50 to 60 percent.

advantages of raloxiphene over tamoxifen are no increase in endometrial cancer and prevention of osteoporosis and heart disease.

For more information...

You can find information about breast cancer support groups at

- The social service office of your local hospital.
- The local office of the American Cancer Society.
- The Cancer Information Service (800/4-CANCER).
- The National Alliance of Breast Cancer Organizations (www.nabco.org).
- The Community Breast Health Project (www.med.stanford.edu/CBHP).
- The Breast Cancer Information Clearinghouse (nysernet.org/bcic).
- The American Cancer Society (www.cancer.org).

See Appendix A as well.

Ovarian cancer

One out of every 70 women can expect to develop ovarian cancer at some point in her life—it's the second most common cancer of the female reproductive tract (after endometrial cancer). While your lifetime risk is only 1 in 57, and only 25,000 women are diagnosed each year, 15,000 of those diagnosed will die.

The mortality rate is so high because ovarian cancer is truly a silent disease—a woman has no symptoms to tip her off to her condition until the disease has progressed far beyond modern medicine's ability to treat it. This is unfortunate, since, if the disease is caught early, the five year survival rate is 93 percent—but only a quarter of cases are caught early. Far too often, the cancer isn't caught until it has spread; half of ovarian cancers aren't found until stage III, when a woman has only a 20 percent chance of surviving for five years. At stage IV, the survival rate is much lower than that.

This type of cancer starts in the ovaries and spreads quickly to the pelvic organs, the peritoneum, lymph nodes, and liver. Unfortunately, the prognosis for most women with this type of cancer is hardly much better than it was 50 years ago. Research has shown, however, that taking birth control pills can decrease a woman's chance of ovarian cancer by up to 80 percent.

If you are considered to be at very high risk with a strong family history of ovarian cancer, you may wish to discuss your situation with your health care provider. Some women with a very strong history elect to have their ovaries removed (prophylactic oophorectomy) if they are sure they don't want to get pregnant.

Charting your risk

You can develop ovarian cancer any time, but your risk rises as you get older. There are a number of risk factors that contribute to the development of ovarian cancer, including the number of times you've ovulated, your family history of cancer and your diet.

The most important of these risk factors appears to be how many times you've ovulated. Every time an egg is released, it ruptures the surface of an ovary. Cells must repair this damage, and each time they do, there's a greater chance that a cancer-causing mutation will occur. Therefore, the more times the ovaries rupture, the higher the chance of problems. Puberty before age 12, menopause after age 50, first pregnancy after age 30, or no pregnancies all contribute to higher risk.

Because pregnancy, breast feeding, and the Pill all meddle with ovulation, this is why all three lessen the risk that you'll develop ovarian cancer. In fact, women who are on the Pill for five years slash their risk by half. This also may be why fertility drugs, which boost the number of eggs released during ovulation, seem to be associated with a higher risk of ovarian cancer, although the link remains unproven.

Unfortunately, there's very little information about risk factors for this type of cancer, and fewer than 7 percent of affected women have any family members with the condition. If you want to assess your risk for ovarian cancer, consider the following risk factors:

- Hereditary cancer syndromes: If your family is vulnerable to one of the ovarian cancer syndromes, your risk rises to a 50 percent chance of developing this cancer some time in your life. Markers for this syndrome are family members across several generations who have had breast, endometrial, or colorectal cancers, in addition to those who have developed ovarian cancer at an unusually young age. Scientists believe that these cancer syndromes are caused by a mutation in one or more "control" genes that regulate other genes, causing brain, blood, bone, and breast cancers.

- Family history: A relative with ovarian cancer boosts your risk; if your mother or sister has ovarian cancer, you've got a slightly higher chance of developing this type of cancer, compared with women in the general population.

- Diet: A diet high in unsaturated fat seems to be linked to ovarian cancer, according to a range of studies from around the world.

Screening breakthroughs

The poor prognosis for ovarian cancer is directly related to the fact that the only available diagnostic test gives so many false positives and false negatives that it's about as accurate as a coin toss. The test, known as the CA-125 blood test, checks for a substance called CA-125 that is found in many ovarian tumors.

Studies have found that CA-125 is higher in 80 percent of women with ovarian cancer, but it's also high in about 2 percent of healthy women. It's also higher in women with benign conditions of fibroids, endometriosis, infection, or menstruation. At the same time, the test misses 20 percent of women who do have ovarian cancer. For these reasons, most doctors believe that CA-125 is not a reasonable screening test for ovarian cancer.

Fortunately, there is at least one new diagnostic screening test on the drawing board: A measure of the level of a chemical in the body called lysophosphatidic acid (LPA), a substance that stimulates the growth of ovarian cancer cells. High levels of LPA indicate that you may have ovarian cancer. According to one new study, the test is more than 90 percent accurate in detecting the disease—much more precise than CA-125. Unfortunately, the LPA still isn't as specific as doctors would like. While high levels of LPA can indicate ovarian cancer, it could also mean you have endometrial or cervical cancer instead.

Hereditary cancer syndrome

Hereditary cancers account for about 10 percent of all ovarian cancers, and ovarian cancers associated

Unofficially... British researchers say they've discovered the defective gene that makes ovarian cancer unresponsive to chemotherapy. This could help scientists develop a test to screen ovarian cancer patients for the genetic basis of their tumors to find out if they will respond to chemotherapy.

with BRCA1 or BRCA2 mutations are most likely to occur after age 60. Because these hereditary cancers are quite rare under age 40, the study suggests that women with the gene mutation may be able to delay prophylactic oophorectomy until about age 35. The study also found that women with BRCA-associated hereditary ovarian cancers seem to remain disease free after chemotherapy much longer than those with cancers not associated with BRCA mutations. In advanced ovarian cancer, the disease does recur, but it appears that the BRCA mutation actually helps chemotherapy work.

Treatment

If cancer is limited to the ovaries, the surgeon will remove them, along with the uterus, fallopian tubes, and nearby lymph nodes. Tissue samples are also taken from nearby areas in the abdomen to check for cancer cells there. If the cancer has spread, portions of the stomach, intestines, or urinary tract may also need to be removed.

After surgery, almost all women will receive chemotherapy (or, less often, radiation). Chemotherapy often only works for a limited amount of time; more surgery may be needed in a year or so to see if different drugs should be used. About half of ovarian cancers seem to respond to another round of chemotherapy, but only for a limited time.

In the future: New treatments

So far, surgery, chemotherapy, and radiation have not been overwhelmingly effective in the treatment of advanced ovarian cancer. But new treatments that target a type of "suicide gene" may help. The gene, which would be inserted into cancer cells, would cause them to self-destruct. Scientists are also studying other brands of this sort of viral warfare in mice, in which genetically programmed herpes viruses are directed to seek out and destroy ovarian cancer cells.

Endometrial cancer

Unofficially... Studies show that having many children or taking the Pill dramatically lowers the risk of endometrial cancer.

The uterus is a large organ with the cervix at one end, and an inner layer called the endometrium. Endometrial cancer is the most common cancer of the reproductive organs in the United States, affecting 2 or 3 out of every 100 women each year. If detected and treated early, however, it's highly curable; about 95 percent of women with stage one, grade one endometrial cancer will survive for at least five years after diagnosis and hysterectomy and oophorectomy, but only 10 percent of women with the most advanced cases survive that long.

Endometrial cancer begins when malignant cells start to wildly reproduce in the lining of the uterus. If undetected, however, the malignant cells may invade the wall of the uterus, the cervix, and eventually the bladder, bowel, and other organs farther away.

Risk factors

The biggest risk for the development of endometrial cancer (which usually appears after menopause) is exposure to high levels of unopposed estrogen. This means that you're at higher risk for this type of cancer if you've had or been

- Early menstruation.
- Late menopause.
- Any source of unopposed estrogen.
- One or no children.

- An increase in the number of normal cells lining the uterus.
- Obese, since fat tissue contains an enzyme that converts other hormones to estrogen.

In addition, you're at higher risk because of estrogen exposure if you have already had breast cancer, or you've had breast cancer and are taking the drug tamoxifen to prevent a recurrence. Women who have liver disease are also at higher risk for endometrial cancer, since the liver is responsible for destroying excess estrogen. Obese women are also at greater risk, since fat cells raise the level of estrogen.

Watch Out! Women who are 21 to 50 pounds overweight have triple the risk of developing endometrial cancer.

Do you have endometrial cancer?

The most common symptom of endometrial cancer is bleeding after menopause—but any unusual bleeding (extra-heavy flow, spotting between periods, etc.) may be a sign of this type of cancer. You also may notice a watery discharge that can indicate malignancy. You'll only have pain or discomfort in more advanced stages of endometrial cancer, however.

Tests your doctor may do

There are several tests to detect endometrial cancer, usually beginning with a pelvic examination. During the examination, your health care provider will feel for any lumps or changes in the shape of the uterus. Next comes a Pap smear—if any endometrial cells are picked up outside of the cervix in a postmenopausal woman, the doctor will suspect endometrial cancer.

If your health care provider suspects cancer, an endometrial biopsy will usually be performed to check out the uterine cells. While sometimes uncomfortable, it's usually an outpatient procedure done without anesthesia.

If all these tests are negative but your bleeding doesn't stop (and because cancer of the endometrium begins inside the uterus and doesn't usually show up on a Pap test), your health care provider may next schedule a dilation and curettage (D&C). During a D&C, the opening of the cervix is stretched with a spoon-shaped instrument and the walls of the uterus are gently scraped to remove any growths. This tissue is then checked for cancer cells. Alternatively, a hysteroscopy may be done to evaluate the endometrium, after which a biopsy of any abnormal areas is performed under direct visualization. Then the endometrium is curetted.

Watch Out!
All women who have had endometrial cancer should probably avoid ERT no matter how severe their postmenopausal symptoms are; discuss this with your doctor.

Treatment

If malignant cells are discovered, you'll be referred to an oncologist to do more tests to assess how far the cancer has spread. Once the diagnosis has been made by biopsy or D&C, a hysterectomy with removal of the ovaries is scheduled. The findings at the hysterectomy determine the stage and the need for any adjuvant therapy. Radiation and chemotherapy may be scheduled afterward, depending on your history and the extent of disease. In advanced cancer, hormonal therapy using a form of progesterone may be attempted. In 3 out of 10 women, this slows the growth of cancerous cells by interfering with estrogen.

Cervical cancer

Cancer of the cervix usually grows slowly over a period of time. Before cancer cells are found on the cervix, the tissues of the cervix go through changes in which cells that are not normal begin to appear. A Pap smear can reveal early a precancerous but highly treatable condition called dysplasia, in which normal cells are damaged and grow unchecked.

While any woman can develop cervical cancer, you're at higher risk for developing cancer of the cervix if you

- Have had sex before age 16.
- Have had more than two sexual partners.
- Smoke.
- Have genital warts.
- Have other sexually transmitted diseases (STDs).
- Have other genital tract cancers.
- Have had many children.
- Have used oral contraceptives for a long time.
- Don't eat well.
- Have a current or past sexual partner who has had multiple partners; the more sexual partners a man has had, the higher his current partner's risk of developing cervical cancer.

While some studies have suggested a link between oral contraceptives or a vitamin deficiency of A and C and cervical cancer, no sure link has yet been found. Most of these studies have been explained away because the women using oral contraceptives were not using any form of barrier contraception that was protective against cervical cancer. However, there is a fairly definite link between a deficiency of folate (a B vitamin) and an increased risk of cervical cancer.

HPV and genital warts

The sexually transmitted human papillomavirus (HPV) can cause changes in the cells of the cervix and trigger the growth of warts on the outside of the genitals. A history of this infection is a risk factor for cervical cancer. Still, not everyone with genital warts is going to get cervical cancer. Several million men and women are infected with the virus, but only 15,000 cases of cervical cancer are reported each year. But particular high-risk types of genital HPV are the primary cause of 95 percent of cervical cancers. In addition, infection with the human immunodeficiency virus (HIV) also increases your risk of developing abnormal cellular changes in the cervix, which can lead to a more aggressive form of cancer.

Unofficially...
Cervical cancer occurs almost twice as often in younger black women than in white women in the same age group; over age 65, black women get cervical cancer three times more often than white women.

Early warning signs

Cervical cancer can develop without any warning signs; once it has become more advanced, you may notice abnormal bleeding or vaginal discharge (especially after sex). More than 9,000 American women die each year from cervical cancer, yet, if caught early, it's highly curable.

You should see a doctor if you have any of the following problems:

- Bleeding after intercourse not related to menstruation
- Difficult or painful urination
- Pain during intercourse
- Pain in the pelvic area

Fortunately, cervical cancer is highly treatable because precancerous changes in the cervix itself can be found by a variety of tests such as the Pap smear; if caught early, the problem can be treated before the cells become malignant. Annual Pap smears can decrease the chance of dying from cervical cancer from 4 in 1,000 to 5 in 10,000.

A Pap smear is performed using a piece of cotton, a brush, or a small wooden stick to gently scrape the outside of the cervix to pick up some cells that can be examined under a microscope. You may feel some pressure during the test but you usually do not feel pain.

The DNA-based test for HPV recently approved by the FDA can detect about 90 to 95 percent of cervical cancers, compared with 70 to 80 percent of cancer cases detected via a Pap smear, according to its manufacturer. The Hybrid Capture II test is said to be able to detect all key HPV cancer-causing types (there are 13 strains of HPV that account for essentially all cases of cervical cancer).

What does your pap smear mean?

It's important to take responsibility for your own health care. Ask to have a copy of your Pap smear results sent to you, so you can see the results.

TABLE 12.2: DECIPHERING YOUR PAP SMEAR RESULTS

If it says...	It means...	What to do
Inadequate sample	The scraping was not thorough or cells were obscured by blood or inflammation	Have another test in 3 months; best time: mid-cycle
Typical squamous	Results are not normal, but not necessarily precancerous	Your ob/gyn will another test in 3 months
High- or low-grade squamous intra-epithelial lesion (HGSIL or LGSIL)	HGSIL indicates dysplasia (a precancerous condition); LGSIL is not as likely to progress to cancer	Your ob/gyn will probably suggest colposcopy
Suspicious for cancer	Cancer cells have been found	See your ob/gyn right away and schedule a colposcopy

If cervical cancer is detected during a routine pelvic exam and Pap smear and is treated early, 99 percent of women survive the disease—but if it's undiagnosed before it reaches the most advanced stage, only 7 percent of women survive. The incidence of cervical cancer is highest between the ages of 35 and 55. Thanks to early detection and treatment, deaths from cervical cancer have plummeted by about 70 percent in the past 40 years while the number of women at risk for developing it has increased 500 percent.

New treatments: What you should know

If cancer is detected early in the cervix (Stage I or II), the malignancy can be surgically removed or treated with radiation; the combination of surgery and radiation is seldom (if ever) indicated. New research suggests that chemotherapy with cisplatin be combined with radiation in treating cervical cancer, a double-barreled approach that can significantly improve the survival rate of women with cervical cancer. The recent findings were endorsed by the NCI. (Traditionally, cervical cancer has been treated with radiation or surgery, with varying degrees of success.) This new method should be "strongly considered," according to the NCI.

Coping with cancer

A diagnosis of cancer can be devastating. Gynecological cancers usually strike at parts of a woman's body that are often an important part of self-image, involving feelings of femininity, sexuality, love, and nurturing. As a result, cancer can trigger feelings of anxiety, anger, and depression. As with any serious illness, you must face the possibility that you might die. If you have had a mastectomy, it's common to feel vulnerable, guilty, shocked, and helpless. Some women have problems with sexuality or family relationships after surgery.

If you feel sad, upset, or seriously depressed, it can help to talk to a counselor or therapist to assist you in dealing with uncomfortable feelings after your treatment ends. There are many different kinds of treatment from a variety of different types of mental health providers that include psychiatrists, psychologists, social workers, psychiatric nurses, and pastoral counselors. Check with your local mental health association listed in the Yellow Pages for referrals.

Just the facts

- Diet, hormones, smoking, alcohol, and chemicals have all been linked with cancer.
- One in eight women will develop breast cancer in her lifetime—if she lives to age 95.
- Some breast cancers are linked to a defect in genes known as BRCA1 and BRCA2.
- Ovarian cancer is hard to detect and difficult to treat in advanced stages.
- Cervical cancer is highly treatable when detected early, which is easy to do with a Pap smear.
- The most common symptom of endometrial cancer is bleeding after menopause.

GET THE SCOOP ON...
The unique symptoms of heart attacks in women ▪ How to be sure your heart symptoms are taken seriously ▪ What a "mini stroke" can tell you ▪ LDL and HDL cholesterol ▪ Eating your way to heart health

Cardiovascular Disease

Breast cancer tops the list of most women's health fears, but it's cardiovascular disease that kills twice as many women as all other cancers combined. In fact, in 1996, about half a million women died of heart problems—but only 44,000 will die from breast cancer. It's even more deadly than you may realize: Cardiovascular disease (including heart attacks and strokes) kills more women than the next 16 causes of death combined. If current rates continue, a third of all women now under age 40 will develop heart disease sometime during their lives.

One in ten American women aged 45 to 64 has some form of heart disease; this statistic rises to one in four women over age 65. At least 300,000 American women have a congenital malformation of the cardiovascular system. And each year, nearly 2.5 million American women are hospitalized for cardiovascular disease. Another 1.6 million women have had a stroke. Women are also more likely than

Watch Out! Taking the "anti-aging hormone" DHEA may increase your risk of heart disease, according to Baylor College of Medicine researchers. After six months of taking the hormone, the women's bloodstream levels of HDL ("good") cholesterol dropped by 13 percent.

men to have a "silent" heart attack, a condition that causes little or no pain but that damages the heart muscle nonetheless. And according to a Yale University study, women heart patients under age 75 are almost twice as likely to die in the hospital as men are.

Despite these alarming statistics, very little research has been conducted on the best ways to diagnose, treat, and prevent cardiovascular disease in women, and there have not been any large studies on how the condition affects women in their everyday lives. As a result, far too many women—and their health care providers—think of heart disease, heart attacks, and stroke as a man's problem. Moreover, most people don't know that heart attacks tend to be more severe in women, and that women are more likely to die from a first-time heart attack.

Often, women and their health care providers don't recognize heart disease symptoms in women. Recent surveys show that less than a third of women say their practitioners even discuss heart disease with them.

In most hospitals, women with symptoms of heart disease (such as chest pain) are less likely to receive diagnostic interventions such as stress electrocardiograms, and women usually have to present with more severe symptoms before they're referred for angiograms, the tests that indicate whether major arteries are narrowing. And since women don't get angiograms that reveal these problems, they're less likely to have either an angioplasty to open those arteries, or bypass surgery to reroute blood flow. In fact, an Alabama study found that women were 31 percent less likely than men to undergo angioplasty to open clogged arteries, and also were less likely to receive clot-dissolving drugs to minimize the damage from a heart attack.

Symptoms to take seriously

If you want to get the best care, it's vital that you know about and can recognize the symptoms of heart disease. Unfortunately, when we think of heart disease, we think of crushing chest pain radiating up into the jaw or down the left shoulder and arm, together with nausea and sweating. What most people don't know is that those are the symptoms of heart problems in men.

Women may have these signs, but they are just as likely to have completely different symptoms, many of them vague. Because of these confusing and often-mild symptoms, it often takes a woman longer to call an ambulance during a heart attack—a wait that can be fatal, since clot-breaking drugs only work if they are administered within six hours of the beginning of an attack. Call your health care provider if you notice any of the following symptoms and you're at risk for heart disease:

- Stomach or abdominal pain that may feel like heartburn
- Nausea or dizziness
- Fatigue and shortness of breath after light exertion
- Numbness or tingling in arms or jaw
- A sensation of anxiety or unease

The following symptoms of heart disease are common in both men and women:

- Uncomfortable pain or squeezing, pressure or fullness in the center of the chest lasting longer than a few minutes
- Pain radiating to the neck, shoulders, or arms

- Chest discomfort with lightheadedness, fainting, sweating, nausea or shortness of breath

Types of heart problems

Some kinds of heart problems are present at birth, but others develop later and are influenced by both genetics and poor lifestyle choices. Most of the time, you won't have any clue that heart problems are beginning to take root, as your cholesterol and triglyceride levels rise, your arteries silently plug up, narrow and harden, and your blood pressure builds. Some women even have "silent" heart attacks and have no idea their heart muscles have been damaged.

Atherosclerosis

One out of every two Americans who die this year will succumb to disease caused by blocked arteries—a disease characterized by the build-up of fatty plaques in stiffened, hardened arteries. Once considered a "man's disease," we now know it's an equal opportunity killer—in fact, women have a higher risk of dying from blocked arteries than from breast cancer. But if you're like most Americans, you know very little about the disease that has a 50-50 chance of ending your life prematurely.

As you get older, your arteries thicken and harden, clogging with fatty deposits that build up until they completely block an artery. As the arteries narrow, the heart has to work harder to pump blood throughout the body; blood clots break free and can travel to the heart or brain, causing a heart attack or stroke. This slow process of deposit-building begins as early as childhood, and is worsened by smoking, poor diet, infection, and any other form of irritation. Most coronary heart disease is due to this problem.

What scientists realize today is that the process of artery blockages can begin very early in life, as long

Watch Out! Some infections can affect the heart (especially viruses accompanied by a high fever). If you've ever had such an illness and now you're having heart symptoms, contact your health care provider.

ago as adolescence. In fact, new research shows that girls as young as 15 develop streaks of fat on the walls of their arteries, and some have as many fat deposits as men three times their age.

At first, these fat streaks aren't a threat to a young girl's health, but the streaks are the foundations of plaque—the thick fatty deposits that can clog arteries and cause a heart attack later.

Fortunately, most women are protected from heart disease despite these early fat deposits, at least until they reach about age 55, because of the hormone estrogen, which helps keep blood vessels open and cholesterol levels down. But once they enter menopause, unless they begin hormone replacement therapy (HRT), their lower estrogen levels can no longer protect their heart, and their own arteries will begin to deteriorate.

Coronary heart disease

When one of the arteries supplying blood to the heart becomes completely blocked, it causes coronary heart disease, one of the most common types of heart conditions.

If the blood supply is temporarily reduced, you'll experience chest pain (angina)—a symptom that your heart isn't getting enough blood. This may happen during exercise, when more is asked of your heart and it can't get enough oxygen to do its job. Angina is often a warning sign that something is wrong with your heart. If the blood supply becomes completely blocked, you'll have a heart attack. When the heart is deprived of oxygen, part of the muscle dies, resulting in permanent heart damage.

Predicting a stroke

Just as a blocked artery leading into the heart can cause a heart attack, a blocked artery leading to the

Unofficially...
When women take estrogen replacement after menopause, their risk drops to half that of women not taking hormones. HRT raises "good cholesterol" and lowers "bad cholesterol" while helping to keep blood vessels relaxed.

Bright Idea
Scientists are studying a new treatment involving an intravenous mixture of glucose, insulin, and potassium (GIK) designed to minimize the danger of a heart attack. One study found that patients who were given GIK within 24 hours of a heart attack slashed the risk of death in half.

brain can lead to a stroke, one of several disorders that occur if the blood supply to the brain is interrupted. When a part of the brain loses oxygen, even for a brief time, it dies, which then affects the part of the body that it controlled.

You may be able to predict an impending stroke if you have a transient ischemic attack (TIA), a temporary halt in the blood supply to the brain. More than a third of people who've had one or two TIAs go on to have a stroke at some point. Since prompt medical attention may be able to stop a stroke or at least reduce the damage, go to the emergency room immediately if you notice any of the following symptoms:

- Weakness or clumsiness in the arm, leg, side of the face, or body
- Numbness in the arm, leg, or side of the face
- Speech problems or difficulty understanding speech
- Dizziness
- Double vision
- Staggering gait
- Dimness or loss of vision (especially in just one eye)

Are you at risk for stroke?

The older you are, the higher your risk for stroke; the chances double for each 10 years after age 35. Risk factors include

- High blood pressure.
- Diabetes.
- Atherosclerosis.
- Smoking.

- Family history.
- Migraines.
- Abnormally high cholesterol levels.
- Obesity.
- Periodontal disease.

In addition, certain types of heart disease (such as a recent heart attack) are associated with strokes. In younger women with mitral valve prolapse (it's three times more common in women), discussed below, the risk of stroke is four times higher.

There are other health conditions associated with strokes. Women with gum disease are twice as likely to have a stroke caused by blocked arteries, according to a University of Buffalo study released in June 1999. Scientists suspect that gum disease increases the stroke risk because bacteria and other poisons get into the bloodstream from the infected gum pockets, triggering inflammation; bacteria also may directly attack the blood vessels.

Did you have a stroke?

You may notice symptoms for a few hours or as long as a day or two. The symptoms of a stroke depend on where in the brain the damage occurred, but common symptoms include

- Dizziness.
- Confusion.
- Sudden loss of consciousness.
- Rapid loss of senses (vision, speech, and so on).
- Weakness or paralysis on one side.
- Headache.
- Vomiting.
- Difficulty swallowing.

Unofficially...
Strokes affect men more often than women, but when a woman does have a stroke, she's twice as likely to die. This could be because women tend to have strokes later in life, when they are more frail.

If your health care provider suspects a stroke, he or she will do a detailed neurological exam and blood tests in order to tell the difference between a stroke and other conditions, such as infections, seizures, drug-related confusion, multiple sclerosis, high or low blood sugar or tumors. A CT scan will try to locate a hemorrhage; if no blood is found, other tests will try to locate a heart problem that could have caused a clot. It's important to have any of these symptoms checked out right away so that any existing clots can be treated immediately.

Mitral valve prolapse

This form of structural heart disease keeps the heart from working efficiently. As the flaps of the heart's valve become enlarged, thickened, or stretched, they don't close smoothly when the heart beats. Blood leaks backward, causing a murmur.

You may not have any symptoms with this problem, or you may have stabbing chest pain or skipped heartbeats. You may be at risk for bacterial endocarditis—which would mean you'd need to take antibiotics before any type of surgery or dental procedure. Most of the time, this condition isn't serious, but you need to be sure to see a health care provider regularly to make sure any problems are identified and treated.

Congestive heart failure

Almost five million Americans suffer from congestive heart failure, a condition in which the heart can't pump enough blood to meet the body's demands because of past heart damage. As the blood backs up into the lungs, fluid collects and makes it hard to breathe.

In severe cases, blood backs up in the right side of the heart so that the veins become congested or swollen in the ankles and legs as the body tries to get blood back into the heart. While most cases can be treated with medications or surgery, about 20 percent of patients die within one year of being diagnosed with the disease, and 50 percent die within five years. In severe cases, a heart transplant may be required.

There is now good news for women with this problem—a new study finds that women live twice as long as men with this condition. Experts believe that hormonal differences between men and women affect the way they respond to heart failure.

Unofficially... Women who undergo heart transplants are more likely than men to start rejecting their donor organ within a year of surgery. In order to avoid rejection, they usually require extra treatment with immune-suppressing drugs.

Heart rhythm disturbances

Any irregularity in the way your heart beats is called an "arrhythmia," which can interfere with the heart's regular rhythm, causing it too beat too fast or too slow. If your heart skips beats, you'll notice this during periods of stress, when it feels like your heart is fluttering or jumping. It may be possible to control this rhythm disturbance with medication, but you should also try to lessen or manage stress and avoid stimulants such as caffeine.

If your heart doesn't beat fast enough (bradycardia), you'll feel dizzy, tired and faint because your body isn't getting enough oxygen. Your health care provider will want to find out the underlying reason for the slow heartbeat (such as thyroid disease) so it can be treated, which will then alleviate the rhythm problem. Otherwise, you might need to have a pacemaker implanted under the skin to transmit a signal, triggering the heart to beat more normally.

Other women have the opposite problem: Racing heartbeat, also known as tachycardia. Rapid heartbeat can produce sensations of palpitations, fluttering, dizziness, and feeling faint. If your heart is beating too fast, it can't fill up with blood, so it's not able to circulate the blood around your body efficiently. Most of the time, this condition can be treated with medications.

One of the most serious of the arrhythmias occurs when the upper or lower chamber of the heart starts to quiver instead of beat; this is known as "fibrillation" (either "atrial" or "ventricular," depending on the part of the heart that's quivering).

If you have atrial fibrillation (the most common heart rhythm disorder), you have a less serious problem since your heart, in most cases, can still fill up with blood (although the problem can trigger blood clots). Atrial fibrillation is often associated with high blood pressure and affects between 5 and 10 percent of everyone over age 60. While it's not as serious as ventricular fibrillation, women are more likely to be disabled by this condition than are men, either by being more troubled with symptoms or interpreting their symptoms more seriously.

The other type of heart quivering disorder is known as ventricular fibrillation, which is potentially life threatening if not quickly treated. Fortunately, normal heart rhythms can often be restored by using a "defibrillator," a device that delivers an electrical shock to the heart—provided you can get emergency help in time.

Risk factors for heart disease

It's especially important for women to know their risk factors for heart disease because, if you can explain why you're at risk for cardiovascular problems, you'll have a better chance at getting the treatment you need.

Unofficially... Another new class of drugs, called glycoprotein IIb/IIIa inhibitors, slow blood clotting when given intravenously after a heart attack. One day, a pill version of this drug could be given after a heart attack to stave off future incidents.

Despite the ominous statistics at the beginning of this chapter, it's important to remember that, while all women go through menopause, not all women go on to develop heart disease.

Heart problems are caused not just by loss of hormones, but also by lifestyle, personal habits, and family history. You'll be more likely to develop heart problems if you have the following risk factors, and the more risk factors you have, the higher your risk:

- You smoke.
- Have high blood pressure.
- Have high blood cholesterol.
- Are overweight.
- Are sedentary.
- Have diabetes.

Bright Idea
You can decrease your risk of heart disease in just a few months by not smoking, eating five or more servings of fruits or vegetables daily, exercising for at least 30 minutes at least three times a week, and treating your high blood pressure or high cholesterol.

Why are women at higher risk?

The rate of heart disease in women is low during their reproductive years, when only 1 in 1,000 women between 35 and 44, and only 4 in 1,000 between 45 and 54, develop heart problems. Before entering menopause, hormones such as estrogen are at their peak, which is probably why women are protected against heart problems during this time.

However, as the level of estrogen begins to drop, the risk of heart disease and stroke in women increases until it equals the risk in men. After menopause, a woman's risk of heart disease almost triples. Most experts think that this is because lower estrogen levels encourage atherosclerosis in the arteries that supply the heart.

Experts don't really know why, but it's true that a woman's heart and coronary arteries are smaller and lighter than a man's, which may have some affect either on the hardening of the arteries or on treatment. Medications that work well in men don't always succeed in women.

For example, while clot-destroying drugs work equally well in men and women, women are more prone to serious bleeding complications after taking them. In addition, certain types of surgery do not work as well in women, including balloon angioplasty, a technique that stretches the arteries with an inflatable balloon in order to clear them—another technique that removes plaque from arteries—and coronary bypass operations, in which vessel detours are created around blocked arteries. Although long-term survival rates after these operations are about the same in men and women, women do have more complications after surgery and are twice as likely to keep on having symptoms of heart disease several years later.

It's also possible that social factors influence the poor prognosis in women with heart conditions. In general, women are older than men when they develop heart conditions, and they may be less likely than men of the same age to have a spouse still living who urges them to seek medical care or who helps with household duties when they leave the hospital. This may also explain why so many women who are referred for rehabilitation programs don't go as often as men do.

Moreover, women are more likely to experience anxiety and depression after heart problems, which may be because they are, in fact, sicker than men with similar conditions and less able to "get back to normal" after their surgery. It's true that women seem to take longer to recover after heart attacks, losing more days from work; many more women don't return to the job at all after surgery or a heart attack.

Questions to ask your cardiologist

If you suspect that you may have some heart problems, you'll need to see a cardiologist. The recent spurt of studies looking specifically at women and heart disease have made it much easier for a woman who suspects she has heart problems to be taken seriously. Still, women need to learn how to speak up and ask for the health care they need, especially when it comes to heart disease. Before your appointment

- Write down your concerns.
- Keep a diary of symptoms so you can describe them clearly.
- Write down any past treatments.
- Bring along any drugs you're taking.

During the office visit

- Be open and honest.
- Describe your symptoms: When they started, how often they happen and if they've been getting worse.
- Note any stress in your life.
- Ask questions.
- Be sure you understand what your health care provider says; ask for explanations of any unfamiliar terms.
- If medicine is prescribed, make sure you understand the instructions (when to take it; what to do if you forget; what foods or drugs to avoid while taking it; what side effects may occur).

Watch Out!
Use a cloth tape measure to measure your waist and then the distance around your hips. Divide the first number by the second. If your waist-to-hip ratio is above 0.88, you have a three times higher risk for heart disease than if your ratio is lower, even if you're not overweight.

- Take notes.
- Bring a friend or relative to help listen and understand.
- If you think you'll have trouble following a treatment regimen, say so.
- If your health care provider seems to shrug off your concerns about your heart, ask him or her to take a closer look at your heart, and to give you an exercise stress test (a baseline electrocardiogram [EKG] is a good idea at about the age of 40).
- If you're approaching menopause, discuss hormone replacement (see Chapter 18); the decision to take HRT is yours, but you'll need to get all the information about benefits and risks.

If a diagnostic test is ordered, ask

- Why you're having the test and what you can learn from it.
- When the results will be ready.
- What the test will involve and how to prepare for it.
- If you'll need help driving afterward.
- If the test poses any danger of side effects.
- What the risks and benefits are.

If you need a special procedure, ask

- Whether you'll be hospitalized, and, if so, for how long.
- What other kind of doctor you'll need to see (and get a referral).
- Whether there will be any pain or discomfort.
- How long the recovery period will last and what it involves.

High blood pressure

High blood pressure ("the silent killer") is often considered to be a disease in itself, not just a symptom. It can make your heart work harder and lead to heart disease, stroke, heart failure, kidney problems, and other conditions.

An estimated 25 percent of white women and 30 percent of African-American women have high blood pressure, most of the time from unknown causes. Most American women over age 60 do have high blood pressure, and nearly 80 percent of black women over age 60 have it.

If you smoke, you're two to six times more likely to have this problem. Your risk increases with the number of cigarettes you smoke each day. If you quit, however, the risk to your heart drops right away, no matter what your age.

If your blood pressure is consistently above 140/90, you have high blood pressure—but readings even slightly under that can still put your heart at higher risk. Most women don't know that they have high blood pressure because, at first, it doesn't cause any symptoms. If symptoms do appear, they may include headaches, tiredness, dizziness, shortness of breath, anxiety, or insomnia.

Still, high blood pressure doesn't have to increase with age—you can prevent it, and thereby lower your risk of having that first heart attack. To lower your blood pressure, you should lose excess weight, be physically active, choose foods low in salt, and limit alcohol. Limit stress, too, and if you can't limit stress, then practice relaxation techniques or meditation (see Chapter 9). In fact, stress is a very important component of high blood pressure.

Watch Out! Your heart rate and blood pressure rise every morning just before you wake and your medication may not be giving you enough protection. Take your pressure early in the morning to see; if your pressure's too high, talk to your health care provider about taking your medicine more often.

One new study has found that mild psychological stress can temporarily raise the blood level of a chemical (homocysteine) associated with the development of heart disease. Homocysteine is a dietary by-product of animal protein that is normally broken down in the blood by folic acid and the B vitamins. If you don't have enough folic acid or B vitamins in your blood, your levels of homocysteine will rise, making you at risk for heart problems.

If you can't control your blood pressure, your health care provider can prescribe medications that will.

Tips for taking blood pressure

Your blood pressure isn't static; it changes all the time, depending on how you move, talk, sit, or stand. Here are some tips to make sure you get a good reading:

- Don't smoke or drink caffeinated beverages 30 minutes before the test.
- Sit for five minutes with your feet flat on the ground before the test, with your arm resting on a table at the level of the heart.
- Wear short sleeves so your arm is exposed.
- Don't chew gum or speak during the test.
- Get two readings at least two minutes apart and average the results.
- If the two readings differ by more than 5 mm Hg, you should have more readings taken.

Measuring cholesterol

Cholesterol is the fatty substance in the cells of your body and blood. Your liver produces about 1,000 mg a day of cholesterol from saturated fat; another 400 to 500 mg come from the food you eat, including

Unofficially... According to a June 1999 study, women who had a family history of high blood pressure were at more than twice the risk of developing high blood pressure later in life. But those who had a family history who also showed strong responses to stress in college had more than seven times the risk of developing high blood pressure later on.

eggs, meat, fish, and dairy products. You do need some cholesterol for some bodily functions, but too much cholesterol can lead to blocked arteries and coronary heart disease.

There are two types of fat in the food you eat: saturated and unsaturated fat. Saturated fat is found in red meat and is one of the big causes of high cholesterol. Unsaturated fat (found in foods such as canola oil) can be either poly- or mono-unsaturated. If you eat too much saturated fat, your liver will crank out too much cholesterol, which means you'll have too much cholesterol circulating in your blood, where it will eventually build up in your arteries.

You can either measure total cholesterol in your blood (the way we used to do it) or measure LDL ("bad") and HDL ("good") cholesterol separately. A total cholesterol measure of more than 260 means you're at twice the risk of a heart attack as someone with a total cholesterol level of under 200. (But remember, in women the link between high cholesterol and heart attack is not as strong as in men.) If you're healthy, you'll want low LDL and high HDL cholesterol.

Ask your health care provider for a lipid profile, which will measure both types of cholesterol and also the level of triglycerides, another type of dietary fat that can clog arteries. A lipid profile is much better than having a total cholesterol count done. Here's what the readings mean in women (and remember, with HDL, the higher the better):

- An HDL cholesterol reading (in milligrams per deciliter, or mg/dL) of 55 is ideal.

- A reading of 45 or less is considered a low reading (undesirable).

Bright Idea
If you have a problem with blood pressure, you may want to measure it yourself at home, where the reading is likely to be more accurate because you're less stressed. Be sure you understand how to use the device correctly.

Bright Idea
To keep the two "cholesterols" straight, remember that you want "<u>L</u>DL" cholesterol to be Low and "<u>H</u>DL" cholesterol to be High.

- A reading of 70 or more is deemed a high reading (desirable).

For every 10 mg/dL increase in HDL, you'll slash your heart attack risk by 50 percent.

The National Cholesterol Education Program recommends that women over age 20 should have their levels checked every five years; you should have more frequent checks if you're at risk for heart disease, you've gained or lost a lot of weight, or you've been ill.

Triglycerides

Scientists don't really know what role triglycerides play in heart disease other than that there is a link between high levels and heart conditions. If you have low HDL and high LDL cholesterol levels, you probably have high triglycerides, too. But even if your cholesterol levels are normal, you need to have a triglyceride reading. For this test, you'll need to fast for 12 to 14 hours before giving blood.

TABLE 13.1: TRIGLYCERIDE TEST

Level (in mg/dL)	What it means
Less than 200	Good
201–239	Borderline
240 or above	High

If your triglycerides are above 200, you need to be concerned about your diet and the state of your heart—and a reading of more than 240 means you should immediately consult with your health care provider and try to alter your diet to lower the levels. You can lower your levels by eating less sugar, losing weight, getting more exercise, and avoiding alcohol.

General heart-smart strategies

You can't change some of your heart risk factors, such as your age, your race, and your genes. That's why the things you can change are so important—lifestyle changes like your diet, exercise, weight, and so on. It's never too late to change, even if you've already had a heart attack. There are a number of things you can do to keep your heart healthy, no matter what your age:

- Don't smoke: Women who smoke have a higher risk of heart attacks than men who smoke, according to a recent Danish study. But if you kick the habit, you can cut your risk of heart problems in half within the first year of quitting, and by 80 percent by the second year.

- Exercise: Working out can boost your level of HDL ("good") cholesterol—even low-to-moderate activities such as walking, gardening, or climbing stairs have a benefit.

- Have a salad: A recent study found that eating olive oil-and-vinegar salad dressing five or six times a week can lower the risk of fatal heart diseases. Fat-free salad dressings may not provide the healthy types of fat the body needs.

- Eat healthfully: Fruits and vegetables have a range of chemicals that may protect you from heart disease. Heart-healthy foods include lean meat, low-fat diary products, whole-grain cereals and legumes, corn, broccoli, red beets, grapefruit, and orange juice.

- Fiber first: Eating foods high in dietary fiber (especially breakfast cereal products such as oatmeal) can help protect against cardiovascular disease in women.

Bright Idea
For a healthy heart, eat foods high in folic acid, such as grapefruit, broccoli, corn, red beets, wheat germ, and orange juice.

Bright Idea
You should eat at least 22 grams of fiber a day to protect your heart; you'll get 30 grams if you eat a high-fiber bran cereal for breakfast, an apple for a snack and an ear of corn and a carrot at dinner.

- Eat fish: Get one or two weekly servings of fatty fish, such as tuna, salmon, herring, and bluefish, or shellfish (such as shrimp). These are good sources of omega-3 fatty acids, which help cut your cholesterol levels.

- Try nuts: If you eat just five ounces of peanuts, almonds or walnuts a week, you can lower your cholesterol and reduce the risk of heart problems.

- Use soy: Soy foods (tofu and soy milk, for example) may help lower cholesterol and help to keep blood vessels clear.

- Test your cholesterol: You want to have a total cholesterol level of 200mg/dL or less. And the higher your HDL and the lower your LDL levels, the lower your risk of heart disease. You'll want your LDL level to be below 130.

- Watch your blood pressure: Aim for a reading of 120/80 or below; anything higher and you run the risk of heart disease.

- Social support: A strong social support system can lower your risk of heart attack and stroke, according to Swedish researchers; women with the weakest social ties had more than twice the risk of having severely narrowed arteries, compared with women who had a network of support.

- Acupuncture: This ancient Chinese treatment can activate the endorphin system to lower blood pressure and treat some types of heart disease, according to a team of researchers at University of California, Irvine. Acupuncture treatments have lowered blood pressure in some patients and, in some instances, have effectively treated cardiac ischemia, a condition caused by a poor supply of blood to the heart muscle cells. The disorder can be quite painful and can lead to more serious heart problems.

- Promensil: This natural isoflavone-based dietary supplement, derived from red clover, helps women maintain estrogen levels and cardiovascular health during menopause, according to a new study in the *Journal of Clinical Endocrinology and Metabolism*. While natural, isoflavones still act in the body exactly like estrogen.

- If you're having a hysterectomy and it's not medically necessary to remove your ovaries, talk to your health care provider about retaining them. The estrogen they may continue to produce until menopause will protect you from heart disease.

Bright Idea
For more information about Promensil, visit the Novogen Web site at www.novogen.com, or call 888/NOVOGEN.

Checking out your heart

There is a wide range of special tests you can take to assess the strength and health of your heart. Some, like the treadmill test, are very basic (and aren't a good way to assess a woman's heart problems). Because most of these tests were standardized in studies using men as patients, it's important that your health care provider interpret the findings based on your gender:

- EKG: The basic EKG makes a graphic record of the heart's electrical activity. It can show abnormal heart beats, muscle damage, blood flow problems, and heart enlargement.

- Holter monitor: Everyday stress can affect your heart rhythm, and this device can measure how well you deal with life. Your health care provider may suggest you try a Holter monitor if you've been noticing fast or slow heartbeats, palpitations or irregular beats. The monitor includes a miniature EKG with a small recording device that you wear for 24 hours to find out how well your heart responds to stress.

- Stress test (treadmill): This test joins the EKG with exercise (usually on a treadmill or exercise bike) because some heart problems only appear when the heart is stressed. The test can be stopped at any time if you feel any discomfort, and it's safe when performed under medical supervision. The classic treadmill test used by cardiologists to diagnose potential heart disease isn't as accurate in diagnosing coronary artery disease in women as it is in men. You may find that your test reveals EKG abnormalities that aren't caused by narrowed blood vessels. Some newer tests may be better for women, such as nuclear perfusion imaging or echocardiology.

- Stress echocardiography: This test uses sound waves to create pictures of the heart during exercise. During exercise, the test can reveal heart motion and its response to stress, and can help diagnose the presence of coronary artery disease. It's much more accurate for women (although it's more expensive than a simple treadmill test).

- Ultrafast CT scan: Another promising test takes up to 35 X-ray cross-section views of the heart in a few seconds. This scan can find any accumulation of calcium, a component of plaque, which can help experts predict potential heart problems in women as young as 40 or 50, even if they have no signs of cardiovascular disease.

Experts believe this test, which is today available in only about 50 medical centers in the country, will one day be as common a test to screen for heart disease as a mammogram is for breast cancer.

- Blood test for C-reactive protein: Yet another early-warning screening test for a heart attack measures C-reactive protein, a substance released into the blood when vessels leading into the heart become damaged. Abnormally high levels of this protein can signal an impending heart attack. A very sensitive version of this test can even predict a heart attack three to four years before it occurs, even among those at low risk for heart problems.

- Nuclear scan (perfusion imaging): This test assesses heart muscle contractions as blood flows through the heart using a radioactive material injected into a vein and scanned with a camera. If your blood flow during exercise is sluggish, that could mean you have narrowed blood vessels to the heart. Some of the newer tracers (such as technetium 99-m sestamibi) perform better in women than some of the older tracers (such as thallium).

- Coronary angiography: Also called arteriography or cardiac catheterization, this test measures blood flow problems and blocks with a fine tube threaded through an artery into the heart; a fluid that shows up on X-rays is injected and the blood vessels are filmed as the heart pumps. This test, which can reveal narrowed arteries, is the standard against which all other tests are matched.

Just the facts

- Fatty deposits can begin to build up in the arteries as early as the teenage years.
- About half a million American women die of heart problems each year, compared with 44,000 who die from breast cancer.
- Women often don't have the "typical" symptoms of heart attacks that men do, don't respond the same way to diagnostic tests, and often experience a poorer recovery after treatment.
- Symptoms of a "mini stroke" can often be used to predict a later stroke.
- For heart health, HDL ("good") cholesterol should be high and LDL ("bad") cholesterol should be low.

GET THE SCOOP ON...
Figuring your risks ▪ Newest treatments ▪
Decoding your bone density test ▪ Bone-friendly
exercises ▪ Calcium choices you can live with ▪
What to expect in the future

Osteoporosis

You may think your bones are hard, unchanging structures—but in fact, bone is complex, living tissue. Bone growth is affected by the food you eat and how much exercise you get, by your hormone levels, your family history, and your lifestyle.

Throughout our lives, our bones constantly undergo "remodeling." Until about age 35, your body efficiently creates new bone and dissolves old bone. Specialized cells, called osteoclasts, break down bone, while other cells, called osteoblasts, lay down new bone. The balance between breaking down and building up is dramatically shifted at menopause. As you get older, your bones begin to break down faster than new bone can be formed. Bone loss then occurs, leading to weakened and brittle bones, and the increased risk of fracture. This damaging process speeds up as you enter menopause because your ovaries stop producing estrogen—a hormone that helps maintain bone density because it is required for adequate calcium absorption.

As you age, if you aren't able to replace and store enough bone, your bone mass begins to decrease, and you become susceptible to osteoporosis ("porous bones"), a disease that progressively weakens the bones of your entire skeleton. This condition causes formerly strong bones to gradually thin and weaken, leaving them susceptible to fractures (especially in the hips, spine, and forearms).

The hard truth about weak bones

By age 60, one in four women will have developed osteoporosis; by age 65, one out of every two women will fracture a bone as a result of the disease. Today, 28 million people are affected by osteoporosis, but doctors expect this number to increase as baby boomers get older. If women don't take adequate preventive measures, the number of osteoporosis sufferers is predicted to swell to 41 million by 2015.

Some bone loss is considered to be a natural part of aging, but osteoporosis—a severe form of bone loss—affects women much more drastically than men. Some women may lose up to 30 percent of bone density by age 70, while men typically lose only about 10 percent. Experts believe women are more susceptible because their bones tend to be lighter and thinner, and because of the hormonal changes after menopause that appear to accelerate the loss of bone mass. In men, osteoporosis is uncommon until after the age of 70.

It's an insidious disease. Your bones may gradually be weakening and weakening every year, but you won't have any symptoms—until suddenly, one day you fracture a bone simply by coughing too hard, or by bumping into a piece of furniture. An easy way to check on your bone health is by measuring your height on a yearly basis. Your gynecologist should do this for you.

The most typical sites of fractures related to osteoporosis are the hip, spine, wrist, and ribs, although the disease can affect any bone in the body. The rate of hip fractures is two to three times higher in women than men.

Hip fractures in elderly women in particular can be hard to treat and may result in hip replacement. They are especially dangerous for elderly women because the prolonged immobility needed during the healing process often leads to blood clots or pneumonia. It's so dangerous that about a third of elderly women with hip fractures die within six months after their accidents and up to 50 percent die within a year.

Unofficially... Women who followed a vegetarian diet for at least 20 years lost only 18 percent of their bone mineral density, while women who didn't eat a vegetarian diet lost an average of 35 percent by the time they reached age 80, according to one study published in the *American Journal of Clinical Nutrition*.

What causes osteoporosis?

A combination of genetic, dietary, hormonal, age-related, and lifestyle factors all contribute to this condition. Research into what causes calcium loss is ongoing, but scientists know now that there are several things acting together to trigger osteoporosis:

- Couch-potato lifestyle: The less physical exercise you get, the more quickly your bones will weaken as you age.

- Menopause: Estrogen helps maintain bone density by interfering with the cells that break down bone. When the ovaries stop producing estrogen, these bone-damaging cells are no longer held in check. Men don't suffer from osteoporosis to the same degree as women do because testosterone contributes to bone strength and most men have more bone mass. At the same time, women live longer, have less

> While there is increased awareness about the importance of calcium nutrition for skeletal health ... data suggest that deficient vitamin D levels should be of concern to women with hip fractures.
> —*Journal of the American Medical Association* (Brigham and Women's Hospital researchers, Boston, April 28, 1999).

dense bones to begin with, and suffer estrogen deprivation beginning in their 30s.

- Diet: A poor diet (especially one low in calcium, or high in protein), can lead to osteoporosis. Various studies show that diets that are high in protein (particularly animal protein) trigger the loss of calcium through the urine.
- Lack of sunlight: Sunlight helps the body use vitamin D, which boosts your ability to absorb calcium. Vitamin D levels drop during the winter, when the skin is exposed to less sunlight, causing the body to take calcium from the bones to compensate for deficient calcium intake.

Got milk?

The best time to start boning up on calcium is during childhood—certainly no later than adolescence. Calcium intake may be most important in young adults, beginning many years before most people even think about osteoporosis. Concern about calcium intake and bone density should start decades before menopause.

Since parents of young children are able to control how much milk their youngsters drink, most kids get enough calcium. But once those children enter adolescence, it can be much harder to make sure they get enough calcium. In fact, teens average just one eight-ounce glass of milk a day, and half of all teenage girls don't drink any milk at all. Instead, teenage girls (and boys) drink twice as much soda as they do milk.

The health of your daughter's bones for her entire lifetime is pretty much determined by how much milk she drinks between the ages of 9 and 18. To be sure their bones are getting enough calcium, teenage girls should drink four eight-ounce glasses of milk every day (for a total of 1300 mg of calcium daily).

If you're lactose intolerant or you just don't like drinking that much milk, you might want to consider a calcium supplement—try Tums! Many experts today recommend starting at age six with five Tums per day. Tums are rich in calcium, have few calories, are cheap, and come in several flavors. Other foods high in calcium include vegetables like broccoli, turnip greens, and kale. Canned fishes such as salmon and sardines are good because they have calcium rich bones in them. Also try tofu, cornbread, eggs, and, of course, the already fortified fruit juices.

Are you at risk?

Certain people are more likely to develop osteoporosis than others. To find out if you're at risk for developing this disease, consider the following risk factors and see how many apply to you:

- Family history of osteoporosis
- Thyroid problems
- Thin or small frame
- Race (Caucasian, Hispanics, and Asians are at higher risk; African Americans have denser bones)
- Cigarette use
- Alcohol abuse
- Lack of exercise
- Lifelong low-calcium intake
- Menopause before age 45
- A previous broken bone from a minor injury
- Use of glucocorticosteroids or anticonvulsants

- Absence of menstrual periods (amenorrhea) lasting more than three months (if not pregnant)
- Eating disorders (anorexia nervosa or bulimia)
- Low body weight

Symptoms of osteoporosis

Osteoporosis is often called the "silent disease" because bone loss occurs without symptoms. You may not know that you have osteoporosis until your bones become so weak that a sudden strain, bump, or fall causes a fracture or a vertebra to collapse. Many experts recommend being checked for osteoporosis each year after age 40 and immediately if you have at least two of these osteoporosis symptoms:

- Severe back pain
- Height loss
- Curving spine
- Broken bone (especially from a minor fall)
- History of broken bones
- Stooped posture

Diagnosis and monitoring

The good news is that you're not destined to succumb to osteoporosis. You can prevent and even reverse bone loss, and thanks to better diagnostic tools, you don't have to wait until you fracture a bone to find out your bone status.

Routine X-rays can't detect osteoporosis until it's quite advanced (you'd have to lose about 25 percent of your bone density before an X-ray would pick it up), but other radiological methods can determine the strength of your framework. The FDA has approved several kinds of devices that use various methods to estimate bone density; most require far less radiation than a chest X-ray.

The best device for measuring brittle bones (or estimating your risk of fracture) is a bone mineral density test (BMT). There are several types of these tests, all of which use sophisticated X-rays or ultrasound to read bone density:

- DEXA (dual energy X-ray absorptiometry)
- dual-photon absorptiometry
- CT scans (osteo CT or QCT) of bones in the spinal column, wrist, arm, or leg
- ultrasound of the heel

These reliable, painless tests can usually be finished within 30 minutes. In many testing centers, you don't even have to change out of your clothes. Bone density tests can measure bone density in various sites of the body to

- Detect osteoporosis before a fracture occurs.
- Predict your chance of having a fracture.
- Determine your bone loss rate.
- Monitor the effects of treatment, if the test is conducted at intervals of a year or more.

Here's how to decode your bone scan results:

- 1 or less: Safe
- Between 1 and 2.5: Could indicate a risk for the disease
- 2.5 or higher: The definition of osteoporosis— a bone loss of 25 percent or more

These numbers are standard deviations of bone density compared to maximum bone density in young, healthy women. In other words, a score of 2 means that your bone density is 2 standard deviations less than maximum. Results are reported as a "T-score"—greater than negative 1 is normal; between negative 2.5 and negative 1 is considered to be "low bone mass"; less than negative 2.5 is osteoporosis. The "minus" or negative is important—a result of 1.5 would indicate great bone mass, while negative 1.5 means low bone mass.

Bone density tests: All you need to know

The dual energy X-ray absorptiometry (DEXA) test is the most accurate among the new generation of machines, and is also the most widely available method. In much the same ways as a baseline mammogram is used, this test can establish a basic reading for your bone health, against which your doctor can measure future tests. The DEXA can help show whether you're building or losing bone mass, or just staying the same. Most insurance plans will cover the cost for the test if certain risk factors apply to you. Although DEXA uses X-rays, the radiation dose during the test is less than the radiation exposure during a New York to California airline flight.

Measurement of bone mineral density with the DEXA is painless, so you don't need any shots or invasive procedures, sedation, special diet, or other advance preparation. During a DEXA exam, you'll lie in your clothes on a padded table while the machine scans one or more areas of bone (usually the lower spine or hip). The entire exam typically takes just a few minutes to complete.

Your bone density is compared against two "normal" readings, known as "age matched" and "young normal." The age-matched reading compares your bone density with what would be expected for someone of your age and size. The "young normal" reading compares your bone density with the estimated peak bone density of a healthy young adult woman. Generally, the lower your bone density, the higher your risk for a fracture.

Bone densitometry also can be used to monitor a patient's response to treatment for osteoporosis. However, because evidence of a good response to treatment may not show up on a DEXA scan for nearly one to two years after treatment has started, patients are only scanned every one or two years during treatment. Women at high risk of rapid bone loss (for example, patients taking steroids) may receive bone densitometry scanning more often.

Ultrasound densitometry

Your doctor may suggest a method of measuring osteoporosis that involves the use of ultrasound to measure the bone mineral density of your heel. This test, recently approved by the FDA, takes about a minute to perform.

It uses a smaller, less expensive system than traditional DEXA to measure peripheral sites, such as the heel, but ultrasound densitometry may not be as sensitive as other techniques that measure the spine or hip. This is because the heel may be normal in bone density, even when central sites, such as the hip or spine, are already significantly abnormal.

Because density changes in the heel occur much slower than in the hip or spine, ultrasound densitometry should not be used to monitor your response to treatment. The main value of the heel test is as a screening tool; if it's abnormal, a full DEXA is indicated. The new ultrasound densitometry systems will, however, allow many more people access to bone densitometry—and potential diagnosis of osteoporosis before a traumatic fracture occurs.

Unofficially...
A woman's risk of hip fracture is equal to her combined risk of getting breast, uterine, and ovarian cancer.

Urine tests

Laboratory tests that measure the amount of collagen in urine samples can indicate bone loss, but the value of these tests is controversial. They aren't as sensitive or accurate as DEXA scanning. These tests may also be used in conjunction with DEXA or other methods of bone densitometry to diagnose osteoporosis.

Do you need to be tested?

Generally speaking, everybody loses bone as they age—your race, size, lifestyle, and gender will influence how strong your bones are and how great your risk of osteoporosis is (and therefore, how great your need to be tested).

Not every woman needs a bone density test. For example, it won't reveal much bone loss to most women in their 30s, unless they were experiencing early menopause. New guidelines make specific recommendations for diagnosing and treating osteoporosis, and are based on identifying risk factors for the disease. Osteoporosis experts say that the following women should receive a bone density test:

- Women over age 65
- Postmenopausal women under age 65 with one or more risk factors
- Postmenopausal women who have had bone fractures
- Pre-menopausal women with any risk factors should get a doctor's advice about having a scan
- Women who take corticosteroids
- Women who have had cracked or fractured vertebra detected on X-ray
- Women with hyperparathyroidism

Medicare guidelines for bone densitometry are as follows:

- Women with low levels of estrogen who are at risk for osteoporosis
- Women with vertebral abnormalities
- Women receiving (or planning on taking) long-term glucocorticoids
- Women with hyperparathyroidism
- Women being treated for osteoporosis who need to be monitored to see if they are responding to drug therapy

Medicare will reimburse you only if the bone-mineral tests are ordered by the primary health care provider. The insurer will cover bone mineral density testing once every two years. The benefit applies to all Medicare patients, including managed care program patients. (Non-Medicare insurers may have different guidelines.)

If you think you meet these guidelines and you'd like to know the status of your bone strength, ask your doctor for the test. But keep in mind that some doctors may not be as aware of the problem as they should be. In fact, 80 percent of low bone mass and osteoporosis goes undiagnosed. If you have any risk factors, you need to take responsibility for your own bone health, according to the National Osteoporosis Foundation. Insist on having a baseline test. If your doctor seems reluctant to order the test, take along this list of risk factors to explain why you want the exam.

Bright Idea
To find the nearest bone density testing center, call the National Osteoporosis Foundation Action Line: 800/464-6700.

Treating osteoporosis the natural way

If your bone scan shows your bones are as brittle as a porcelain teacup, don't panic! You can treat osteoporosis the same way you can prevent it: By boosting your calcium intake through supplements and a proper diet, getting plenty of exercise and avoiding cigarettes and too much alcohol.

Using these methods, you can reduce (or even halt) the rate of bone loss. Women at particularly high risk, or those who already have significant bone loss, may want to consider hormone replacement or other drugs (discussed below) to boost their bone strength.

Is your diet calcium-friendly?

It's obvious to most people: If calcium builds bones, and your bones are weak, it follows that taking in more calcium should help. Dairy products are the best sources of dietary calcium. But calcium can also come from nondairy, calcium-fortified foods, such as cereals and orange juice, or from supplements, if a doctor recommends them.

You should eat a range of healthy foods that are rich in calcium, such as

- Low-fat dairy products, such as cheese, yogurt, and milk.
- Canned fish with bones you can eat (salmon and sardines, for example).
- Dark green vegetables (such as kale, collard greens, and broccoli).
- Breads made with calcium-fortified flour.
- Tofu (soybean curd).
- Legumes (peas and beans).
- Lime-processed tortillas.
- Seeds and nuts.

Of course, many women are also trying to watch their weight, and many diary products are considered to be high-fat no-nos. While dairy products do pack a calcium wallop, they needn't be high fat. Use one percent or skim milk instead of whole milk or cream, and choose lower-fat cheeses (parmesan and other hard cheeses, for example), yogurt, frozen yogurt, and ice cream substitutes.

Calcium supplements: If you need more

If you suspect you aren't getting enough calcium from your food, you might think about taking a calcium supplement. (Always check with your doctor before taking any dietary supplement, of course.) Calcium supplements have been shown to be more effective at strengthening bone than simply drinking milk.

In one recent study, researchers divided 60 postmenopausal women into three groups: One group drank four glasses of milk a day, one took 1,000 mg of calcium carbonate a day, and one group took a placebo (sugar pill) a day. The three groups took their prescribed allotments for two years. The placebo group lost three percent of bone mineral density in the two years of the study. Women who drank milk had some bone mineral loss—but women who took calcium supplements suffered no bone loss at all.

A total intake of 1,500 mg per day is about the average amount of calcium required to keep a postmenopausal woman in calcium balance. This intake is probably two or three times what most adult women in the United States actually get.

If your diet is rich in protein (more than four ounces per day of meat, poultry, or fish), you should be getting between 1,500 and 1,800 mg of calcium per day; this figure is for all women, including those on hormone replacement therapy (HRT), discussed later in this chapter.

Note ➡
These guidelines are based upon calcium from the diet, plus any calcium taken in supplemental form. Adequate vitamin D is essential for optimal calcium absorption.

TABLE 14.1: OPTIMAL DAILY CALCIUM INTAKE REQUIREMENTS[1]

Age	Mg of calcium
Birth to 6 months	400
6 months to 1 year	600
1 to 5 years	800
6 to 10 years	800 to 1,200
11 to 24 years	1,200 to 1,500
25 to 50 years	1,200 to 1500
Pregnant and lactating women	1,200 to 1,500
Postmenopausal women over 50 years	1,500
on estrogens	1,000
not on estrogens	1,500

[1] Source: National Institute of Health.

It's never too late...

Even if you already have significant osteoporosis, it's not too late to start taking calcium supplements. Reductions in fracture rates can occur within 18 months of starting calcium supplementation, no matter how far along the osteoporosis continuum you are.

Unofficially...
One recent study of 48,000 women found that only 38 percent of postmenopausal African-American women suffered significant bone loss, compared with 50 percent of Caucasians, Hispanics, and Asians.

Can vitamins help?

Unfortunately, calcium doesn't work alone; you also need vitamin D to help your body absorb the calcium supplements. Aim for between 400 and 800 international units (IU) of vitamin D daily. Being out in the sun for even a short time every day (15 minutes of natural sun a day will trigger adequate vitamin D production) gives most people enough vitamin D. You can also get this vitamin from supplements, as well as from cereal and milk fortified with vitamin D.

Postmenopausal women who have been treated for hip fractures are likely to have low levels of vitamin D, an important vitamin in bone development, according to researchers at Boston's Brigham and Women's Hospital. Additionally, women who suffered hip fractures had higher levels of parathyroid hormone, which is responsible for maintaining calcium levels in the body.

According to the National Institutes of Health, these are the current vitamin D recommendations:

- Adults, aged 51 to 70: 400 IU of vitamin D daily
- Adults over age 70: 600 IU of vitamin D daily

Bright Idea
In addition to taking a calcium supplement, make sure you eat a diet rich in calcium, which should include milk products, green leafy vegetables, citrus fruits, and shellfish.

Magnesium: Slowing and preventing loss

Taking magnesium supplements daily may help reduce and prevent bone loss and osteoporosis, according to researchers from the Veterans Administration Medical Center in Loma Linda, CA. About half of the magnesium found in the body is contained in the bones. When you don't get enough magnesium in your diet, your body begins to draw the mineral from the bones resulting in bone weakening.

The recommended dietary allowance (RDA) of magnesium is 350 mg. Some calcium tablets are sold in combination with magnesium; if yours isn't, some good sources of dietary magnesium include

- Milk and other dairy products.
- Whole grains.
- Nuts.
- Legumes.
- Leafy green vegetables.

Watch Out!
Since vitamin D levels can drop in the winter when the skin is exposed to less sunlight, researchers say you need 800 IU of vitamin D daily, plus calcium, to counteract wintertime bone loss and reduce fractures.

Exercise

Exercise builds bone strength and helps prevent bone loss; it also helps older women stay active and mobile. Regular weight-bearing exercises, such as walking, jogging, and playing tennis, are best in helping to prevent osteoporosis. Weight-bearing and strengthening exercises have been shown to improve coordination, and may even increase bone density, but always check with your doctor before starting an exercise program.

Because osteoporosis weakens vertebrae, making them prone to collapse and fracture, women with osteoporosis gradually become shorter and develop a stooped posture. Therefore, while you're doing weight-bearing exercises, don't neglect exercises that strengthen your back muscles. Strong back muscles may help prevent fractures in, and improve the posture of, women with osteoporosis, according to a recent study by Mayo Clinic scientists.

Women with osteoporosis would likely benefit from simple, back-strengthening exercises, provided they aren't so frail that the effort puts too much strain on their bones, says Mehrsheed Sinaki, MD, a professor of medicine and rehabilitation at Mayo Clinic, who led the new study. Exercise causes the muscles to pull against their attachment to the bone, making the bone strengthen itself by taking in and holding more calcium and other bone-strengthening chemicals. Because of the risks involved, Dr. Sinaki advises women to check with their doctors before trying the exercises.

To strengthen your back:

1. Sit in a chair with your back straight.
2. Squeeze your shoulders together at the back; hold five seconds and release.
3. Repeat 10 to 15 times, four times a week.

A second back strengthener:
1. Lie face-down on the floor.
2. Lift your torso slightly off the floor by arching your back.
3. Hold the position for five seconds and then release.
4. Repeat 10 to 15 times, four times a week.

Drug treatments

There are some women whose bone loss has progressed to the point that simply taking calcium and vitamin supplements and getting more exercise may not be enough to prevent fractures. For women with advanced disease, medications are available that can slow bone loss, increase spinal bone density and help prevent fractures. Your doctor can recommend treatment based on the results of your bone density test.

There are several drugs (some new, some not-so-new) that can stop—even reverse—bone loss that has already begun. They do it not by building new bone, but by slowing down your body's tendency to shed old bone cells. What happens, then, is that new bone cells fill in. These drugs can help your body add between two and three percent a year in better bone mass—not a lot, but enough to prevent fractures.

To meet FDA guidelines, drugs to treat osteoporosis must be shown to preserve or increase bone mass and maintain bone quality in order to reduce the risk of fractures. Before 1996, the only choices were calcium supplements, estrogen or injectable calcitonin.

Since then, however, some new products have been added to the arsenal in the war against osteoporosis. Today, there are four medications approved

Unofficially...
CAT scans have shown that tennis players have stronger bones in their playing arm than in their non-playing arm. The larger, stronger bone in the playing arm is due to the added force applied to the bone from swinging the racket repeatedly.

by the FDA for postmenopausal women, to prevent and/or treat osteoporosis. (Each is discussed in the following sections.) These are

- Alendronate (Fosamax): This drug can strengthen bone and cut your fracture risk in half—and it's a good option if you can't, or don't want to, take hormones. You'll see an effect within three months, and the benefits may continue as long as you keep taking it.

- Estrogens: Approved for both the prevention and treatment of osteoporosis. Recent studies suggest that very low doses may be enough to strengthen bones and lower the risk of fractures, without boosting breast cancer risk.

- Calcitonin (Miacalcin): This drug inhibits bone resorption, but it may be less effective than HRT or other drugs. The dynamics of bone involve constant interaction between osteoblasts (builders) and osteoclasts (demolishers). Bone is constantly being remodeled (resorbed) and then replaced.

- Raloxifene (Evista): This selective estrogen receptor modulator (SERM) can decrease the risk of osteoporosis, and provides many of the benefits of estrogen and boosts the health of bone and cardiovascular systems—but there are no data about memory, colon cancer, and other documented estrogen benefits, and it has some of the same side effects as estrogen. Raloxifene increases the risk of blood clots in large veins (deep vein thrombosis), blood clots in the lung (pulmonary embolism), and possibly stroke. Its effect on the uterus is still being studied. Most physicians recommend raloxifene for women who for some other reason (high risk for breast cancer, previous breast cancer, endometrial cancer) can't take estrogen.

Alendronate

While calcium supplements, vitamin D, vigorous exercise, a healthy diet, and estrogen replacement therapy may still be the first choice, there are some women who are looking for a non-hormone drug to help prevent bone breakdown.

Alendronate (Fosamax) is that drug, blocking the resorption of bone by inhibiting the activity of osteoclasts. Since its introduction, it has been used to treat osteoporosis and a chronic bone disease called Paget's disease. Doctors consider alendronate a good second choice for the treatment of bone loss, especially for women who can't, or don't want to, take estrogen and who have begun to lose bone. Overall, alendronate appears to be a safe and effective nonhormonal option for preventing osteoporosis. It was approved in 1997 by the FDA for the prevention of osteoporosis in postmenopausal women at risk for osteoporosis.

Two new studies on menopausal women under age 60, most of whom did not yet have osteoporosis, show that daily alendronate tablets not only prevent bone loss, but help build bone, as well. One study, published in the February 15, 1999 *Annals of Internal Medicine,* showed that among 265 women who took at least 5 mg of alendronate daily for two years, bones in the lower spine and hip became more solid. In the control group, women taking placebo lost bone density. The second study (published in the February 19, 1999 *New England Journal of Medicine*) found that bone density increased in 445 women who took 5 mg of alendronate a day for two years, and decreased in women taking a placebo. Alendronate was only slightly less effective at building bone than a combination of estrogen and progestin.

Alendronate is considered to be a good anti-osteoporosis medication because it doesn't induce the side effects or carry the same risks that estrogen therapies might, including an increased risk of breast cancer. However, experts stop short of suggesting that every woman should take alendronate. Here's why:

- Not all women are destined to get osteoporosis, which means many would be taking a drug for a condition they may never develop.

- Although many women can tolerate the drug, it can irritate the lining of the esophagus if it's not taken as directed.

- It should be used with caution by women with upper gastrointestinal disease. It should not be taken at all by women with disorders of the esophagus that delay emptying; those who can't stand or sit upright for at least 30 minutes; women with low levels of calcium in the blood or who have severe kidney disease; or those who are pregnant or nursing.

- Just as with estrogen, alendronate must be taken indefinitely—and once the drug is stopped, bone erosion begins again. Scientists don't know the long-term effects of alendronate in healthy menopausal women, although this type of drug has been used safely to treat Paget's disease for more than 20 years.

Watch Out! Some women notice gastrointestinal irritation while taking alendronate (Fosamax). You must take it on an empty stomach, with a full glass of water (6 to 8 ounces), first thing in the morning, and stay in an upright position for at least 30 minutes afterward. You should wait at least a half hour (preferably one hour) before the first food, beverage, or other medication of the day.

Hormone replacement therapy

Since estrogen is so important for maintaining bone density in women, physicians often prescribe hormone replacement therapy (HRT) or estrogen replacement (ERT) for women when they begin menopause. HRT is a type of hormone replacement that includes estrogen and progesterone (and sometimes testosterone) and is given to women who have not had a hysterectomy. Adding progesterone to estrogen is necessary in women who have not had a hysterectomy in order to protect the uterine lining from the effects of estrogen. Women who have had a hysterectomy do not need to worry about getting cancer of the uterus from estrogen alone, and so can be given ERT without progesterone or other hormones.

HRT is one of the best ways to protect bone during the years of rapid bone loss that immediately follow menopause. When started later in life, estrogen is also effective in preventing hip fractures. In fact, together with a proper diet and exercise, HRT can lead to a 50 to 80 percent decrease in vertebral fractures and a 25 percent decrease in nonvertebral fractures after five years of use. Hormone treatments are so effective in preventing bone thinning that women on HRT may not need bone densitometry until age 65.

There are other benefits of HRT—deaths from heart disease and stroke (the leading cause of death in postmenopausal women) are cut in half by HRT. There is new evidence that HRT also decreases the incidence of Alzheimer's disease by about one-third. And because vaginal and urinary tract linings are thickened by estrogen, HRT may prevent certain vaginal and urinary tract infections and make intercourse more tolerable for those who previously had pain.

HRT is not without risks, however. Some of the 200 studies looking at the HRT–breast cancer link suggest that some forms of HRT may slightly

Timesaver
The estrogen patch was approved by the FDA in the spring of 1999 for the prevention of osteoporosis. The once-a-week patch is an easy way to treat menopause symptoms and prevent bone thinning. However, it costs more than pills and since it bypasses the intestinal tract and liver, there is some concern that it may not yield all of the beneficial effects of ERT.

increase the risk of developing breast cancer (statistics suggest that if a woman's risk of breast cancer is 10 percent, it will go up to 11 percent with estrogen). As a result, women at high risk for developing breast cancer may need to balance the benefits of HRT in preventing osteoporosis against the possible risks of cancer. Additionally, most women who start hormone therapy stop within a year because of bothersome side effects (such as breast tenderness, headache, fluid retention and bleeding). Because individual circumstances differ, you must discuss the pros and cons of HRT with your doctor.

Raloxifene (Evista)

Raloxifene (Evista), is a drug that mimics estrogen's beneficial effects on bone density in postmenopausal women. It also mimics some of estrogen's beneficial effects on fats in the blood. Unlike estrogen, however, it has been shown to lower the risk for breast cancer and may lower the risk of uterine cancer.

There are several reasons why drug companies are searching for alternatives to ERT. Although it's well established that ERT helps protect against bone thinning and high cholesterol, only one in five postmenopausal women takes ERT. Part of the reason is that oral estrogens stimulate breast and uterine tissue, commonly resulting in bothersome side effects that include vaginal bleeding and breast tenderness and swelling. Oral estrogen also increases the risk of uterine cancer and may increase the risk of breast cancer. (To lower the risk of uterine cancer associated with estrogen replacement, women taking estrogens also take progestin.)

Raloxifene is a type of SERM, a compound that has some estrogen-like effects on some parts of the body. Since estrogen strengthens bones, it's not surprising that raloxifene has been found to cut in half your chances of fracturing your spine. While raloxifene's effect on the spine does not appear to be as powerful as either estrogen's or alendronate's, its effects on the hip and total body are more comparable. Moreover, it's considered to be safer than estrogen. However, raloxifene has two drawbacks—it makes hot flashes worse and it has no positive benefits to the skin, vagina, or libido the way estrogen does. Still, most health care providers consider it to be another option—a very attractive one for women who are at high risk for breast cancer or who are otherwise not candidates for estrogen.

In the body, raloxifene mimics the effects of estrogen in the bones and blood, but blocks some of its effects elsewhere. It's sometimes called an "antiestrogen" because, for a long time, these drugs had been used to counter the harmful effects of estrogen that resulted in breast cancer. (The cancer-fighting drug tamoxifen is an anti-estrogen.) Oddly enough, in other parts of the body, these drugs mimic estrogen, providing estrogen's protection against osteoporosis.

Like estrogen, raloxifene works by attaching to an estrogen "receptor," a certain cell, in the body, much like a key fitting into a lock. When the hormone "key" fits into the receptor "lock," it sends a signal to certain genes in that cell. Preliminary results from a study of more than 12,000 women suggest that raloxifene increases bone density by up to 3 percent.

The nice thing about raloxifene is that it doesn't cause uterine bleeding, bloating, or breast soreness—side effects that prevent many women from using HRT. Moreover, studies of up to three years in length showed no increased risk of breast or uterine cancer. While side effects aren't common, those reported include hot flashes and blood clots.

Calcitonin: The nose has it

Calcitonin is a treatment for women who cannot, or choose not to, take estrogen. In women who are at least five years beyond menopause, calcitonin slows bone loss, increases spinal bone density and, according to anecdotal reports, relieves the pain associated with bone fractures. Calcitonin may reduce the risk of spinal and hip fractures as well, but studies on fracture reduction are ongoing. Because calcitonin is a protein, it cannot be taken orally, as it would be digested before it could work. Calcitonin is therefore available as an injection or nasal spray.

Introduced in 1995, the spray can reduce the risk of spinal fractures by about 40 percent, simply by being sniffed once a day. However, it doesn't work as well in strengthening other bones. This synthetic version of a salmon hormone is the only drug that reduces the long-term pain of existing spinal fractures. It does have some side effects, however, including nasal bleeding and irritation.

Prevention is worth a pound of cure

Osteoporosis is preventable. Preventing bone loss is easier, and far better, for your health than trying to build better bones once they have already become fragile. Begin today to prevent osteoporosis:

- Eat a healthy diet, rich in calcium and vitamin D.
- Don't smoke.
- Don't drink too much alcohol.
- Do plenty of weight-bearing exercises.
- Take five Tums a day for life.

- Get a bone density test and take medication, when appropriate.

Contrary to popular belief, osteoporosis isn't a disease of old people; if you don't take steps to prevent it, bone loss occurs earlier in life, long before symptoms of the disease materialize.

Start young

It's possible to prevent brittle bones later in life as early as childhood if youngsters engage in the right kind of exercise, according to researchers at Oregon State University who studied the impact of exercise on elementary-age kids. After seven months in an exercise program, the kids who spent 15 minutes jumping off a box 100 times, three days a week, had 5 percent more bone (translating into a 30 percent lower risk of hip fracture in adulthood), compared to classmates who had participated in nonimpact exercises.

By about age 20, the average woman has acquired 98 percent of her skeletal mass. Building strong bones during childhood and adolescence can be the best defense against developing osteoporosis later.

Soybeans: The latest preventative

A new Japanese study suggests that consuming soybeans may prevent osteoporosis. Researchers, led by Dr. Kironobu Katsuyama at the Kawasaki Medical School, studied workers at a local health center who ate varying amounts of Natto, a fermented soybean product rich in vitamin K and calcium.

The workers were screened for genetic deficiencies that reduce the body's ability to absorb calcium. People who had a defective gene inhibiting calcium absorption did not suffer calcium loss if they ate

Watch Out! Calcium intake up to 2,000 mg per day appears to be safe for most individuals. Levels above that, however, could cause stomach and intestinal problems.

Bright Idea
Most women receive bone density tests too late to give them the best chance to prevent osteoporosis, according to the Radiological Society of America. Women with risk factors should receive a baseline DEXA test between ages 21 and 35.

Natto, according to Dr. Katsuyama. The findings suggest that the vitamin K found in soybeans may play a vital role in bone formation, and that more research is needed.

Parathyroid hormone

The human parathyroid hormone may help prevent bone loss in women approaching menopause who have low levels of estrogen, say researchers from Massachusetts General Hospital in Boston. In the study, estrogen-deficient women who received a daily dose of the parathyroid hormone over a one-year period showed a higher level of bone mineral density (particularly in the spine), as well as other areas of the body. Estrogen deficiency can be easily determined by a variety of tests.

Parathyroid hormone is produced in two small glands near the thyroid gland in the neck; it controls calcium and, therefore, bone metabolism. It has been used for many years to treat various metabolic bone diseases, but only recently has been tried against osteoporosis in postmenopausal women.

In the future...

With the number of cases of osteoporosis expected to continue to rise, scientists are engaged in a search for new and effective treatments. Among some promising leads you may be hearing about soon are

- Sodium fluoride.
- Vitamin D metabolites.
- Other SERMs, such as idoxifene, currently in development by SmithKline Beecham, which plans to submit the drug to the FDA in 2000.
- Other biophosphonate drugs like Fosamax.

Just the facts

- Your bones are complex, living tissue that is affected by your diet, exercise, and lifestyle.
- Women are at much higher risk for developing osteoporosis than men; by age 60, one in four have the condition.
- Osteoporosis has no symptoms—until your bones are so weak that a slight bump could be enough to cause a fracture.
- You can help prevent osteoporosis by getting enough exercise and calcium, and by limiting alcohol and avoiding cigarettes.
- Bone density tests can predict your risk of fracture, determine your bone loss rate, and monitor how well you're responding to treatment for osteoporosis.
- If your bone loss is severe, medications (such as alendromate or HRT) can strengthen your bones by 2 to 3 percent a year.

GET THE SCOOP ON...
Preventing colds and flu ▪ Preventing urinary tract and vaginal infections ▪ Lyme disease vaccines ▪ Preventing sexually transmitted diseases

Infectious Diseases

Every day, your body is under relentless attack by hordes of living organisms competing for survival in the environment. The air you breathe, the food you eat, the ground you walk on, the water you drink, the buildings you live in, the vegetation that surrounds you—all harbor infectious organisms. They come in all shapes and sizes, from microscopic viruses, bacteria, and protozoa to foot-long parasitic worms that all share a dependence on humans for at least part of their life cycles.

Fortunately, your body isn't defenseless. Because the human environment is biologically hostile, your body has developed wonderfully sensitive ways to react quickly in the presence of infectious organisms. Your skin and immune system are your primary weapons in fighting infection—and when they're intact, they protect you very well. It's only when these barriers break down, or they're affected by another disease, that your body becomes vulnerable to invasion by an array of microorganisms, both mild and deadly.

Preventing colds and flu

It's almost inevitable that you'll catch a cold or flu virus at least once during the winter season, but there are ways to cut down on the number of infections you get.

The best way to prevent a cold is to wash your hands several times a day during cold season, especially if others in your home or work are sick. Most people don't realize that cold viruses are transmitted from hand to nose, not by mouth. This means you won't likely get sick if you kiss a person infected with a cold, but you might if you touch a contaminated door handle and then touch your nose or eyes. In addition to washing your hands often, you should disinfect surfaces that others touch (such as telephones, door handles, and computer keyboards) and don't touch towels, bedding, or used tissues.

Because cold viruses aren't that infectious (as opposed to measles or chicken pox, for example), odds are you won't get sick from spending 20 minutes sitting in your doctor's office—even if you're surrounded by a group of coughing patients—unless someone comes up to you and sneezes right in your face. However, if you spend the day at home with a sick child, picking up used tissues with your bare hands, touching contaminated towels, sheets, blankets, and bedding—and then rubbing or touching your face, eyes, and nose—you can just about guarantee you'll be sneezing in a few days yourself.

If you want to avoid a cold, do everything you can to boost your immune system and stay healthy:

- Get plenty of rest.
- Eat a good diet.
- Drink lots of water.

- Avoid stress (or learn to relax if you can't avoid getting tied up in knots).
- Take 500 mg of vitamin C two to three times a day.
- Wash your hands at least three or four times a day.
- Disinfect household surfaces (phones, faucets, doorknobs, etc.).

Contrary to popular belief, colds are not caused by any of the following:

- Kissing a person who has a cold
- Going outside without your boots or a coat
- Going outside with wet hair
- Sitting beside someone on the bus or train who has a cold (however, sitting in an airplane for long periods of time is a great way to catch a cold, especially since airplane air is recirculated)

Influenza is caused by a different group of viruses than colds—and they are far more infectious than any of the 200 common cold viruses. They can also be deadly—in fact, about 20,000 Americans die each year from complications of the flu. Every so often, extremely virulent strains of flu virus circle the earth during pandemics; the last great flu pandemic in the United States occurred in 1918, killing large numbers of young, otherwise healthy adults.

The best way to prevent infection is by getting a flu shot in the fall. (Don't put this off until the winter, since the shot takes about six weeks to become fully effective.) Flu shots are recommended not just for the elderly, but for anyone with chronic diseases (cancer, diabetes, and so on), heart problems, or respiratory problems (such as asthma), and for

Unofficially... Very soon, a nasal spray loaded with flu vaccine is expected to be introduced so that everyone, including children, can easily be protected against influenza.

pregnant women beyond the first trimester, health care workers, child care workers, and teachers.

Preventing urinary tract infections

There are four parts to the urinary tract—kidneys, ureters (tubes connecting the kidneys to the bladder), the bladder, and urethra (the tube through which the bladder empties). Most often, infections begin in the urethra and move up the urinary tract to the kidneys. Normally, urine is sterile; it contains fluids, salts, and waste products, but it is free of bacteria, viruses, and fungi.

A urinary tract infection (UTI) occurs when microorganisms (usually bacteria from the digestive tract) cling to the opening of the urethra and begin to multiply. Most infections are caused by one type of bacteria—*Escherichia coli (E. coli)*—which normally live in the colon. In most cases, bacteria first begin growing in the urethra and then move on to the bladder, causing a bladder infection (cystitis). If you don't treat the infection right away, bacteria may move up the ureters to infect the kidneys.

Chlamydia and mycoplasma also may cause UTIs, but these infections tend to remain limited to the urethra and reproductive system. Unlike *E. coli,* chlamydia and mycoplasma may be sexually transmitted, and infection requires treatment of both partners.

Any abnormality of the urinary tract that obstructs the flow of urine (a kidney stone, for example) sets the stage for an infection. Catheters are a common source of infection; bacteria on the catheter can infect the bladder, so hospital staff take special care to keep the catheter sterile and to remove it as soon as possible. People with diabetes have a higher risk of getting UTIs because of changes in the immune system—in fact, any disorder that suppresses the immune system raises the risk of a UTI.

In general, women have more UTIs than men because their urethra is relatively short, allowing bacteria quicker access to the bladder. Further, a woman's urethral opening is near sources of bacteria from the anus and vagina. Overall, one in five women develops a UTI during her lifetime. For many women, sexual intercourse seems to trigger an infection, although the reasons for this link are unclear.

Some women suffer from frequent UTIs; nearly 20 percent of women who have one UTI will have another, and 30 percent of those will have yet another. About four out of five women who have a UTI get another in 18 months, but many women have them even more often. If you have three or more UTIs a year, you should ask your doctor about treatment options. (And for those tea drinkers out there—women who drink large quantities of tannic acid [tea] are more prone to bladder infections, as well.)

Watch Out!
Women who use a diaphragm are more likely to develop a UTI than women who use other forms of birth control, according to several studies. And, women whose partners use condoms tend to have growth of *E. coli* in the vagina, which may increase the risk of UTIs.

UTIs during pregnancy

While pregnant women seem no more prone to UTIs than other women, when an infection does occur during pregnancy, it is more likely to travel to the kidneys because of hormonal changes and shifts in the position of the urinary tract during pregnancy. For this reason, many doctors recommend periodic testing of urine. A pregnant woman who develops a UTI should be treated promptly to avoid premature delivery or pyelonephritis, a cause of premature labor.

Do you have a UTI?

Most women with a UTI will have symptoms of the infection, including

- Frequent urge to urinate.
- Painful, burning feeling in the area of the bladder or urethra during urination.
- Fatigue.
- Weakness.
- Uncomfortable pressure above the pubic bone.
- Little urine passed despite constant urge to urinate.
- Milky, cloudy or reddish tint to urine.

If the infection reaches the kidneys, symptoms may involve

- Fever.
- Pain in the back or side below the ribs.
- Nausea.
- Vomiting.

Tests your doctor will order

To diagnose a UTI, your doctor will test a urine sample for pus and bacteria. Although your doctor may begin treatment before the lab report comes back, the lab cultures will confirm the diagnosis and may mean you need to change the prescribed antibiotic. If treatment fails to clear up an infection, your doctor may order a test that makes an image of the urinary tract to identify whether there are structural problems contributing to the infection or getting in the way of treatment.

How to avoid UTIs

It's possible to cut down the rate of UTIs. You can increase your chances of avoiding these infections by doing the following:

- Drinking plenty of water every day
- Urinate when you feel the need; don't resist the urge to urinate

- Wipe from front to back to prevent bacteria from the anal area from entering the vagina or urethra
- Cleanse the genital area before sex or have your partner take a bath before having sex
- Urinate before and after intercourse
- Avoid using feminine hygiene sprays and scented douches, which may irritate the urethra

Bright Idea
To help avoid UTIs, some doctors suggest drinking cranberry juice, which in large amounts inhibits the growth of some bacteria by acidifying the urine. Cranberry juice and blueberries also help prevent bacteria from sticking to the wall of the bladder.

Preventing vaginal infections

You'd likely be astonished at the variety of bacteria and other microorganisms flourishing inside your vagina. Under normal conditions, the acidic environment of the healthy vagina allows the microorganisms to live in balance; it's when that balance is disrupted, allowing one type of bacteria to grow too fast, that a vaginal infection can occur.

It's also possible to develop an infection from bacteria not normally found in the vagina. Although some types of vaginal infections are transmitted sexually, most are not. Instead, the internal vaginal flora may be disrupted by

- Antibiotics.
- Tampon left in too long.
- Birth control pills.
- Douches.
- Perfumed feminine hygiene sprays.
- Topical antimicrobial agents.
- Tight, poorly ventilated clothing and underwear.
- Loose bowel movements.

While vaginal infections are annoying and uncomfortable, most don't pose a risk to your health; untreated, however, a few can lead to more serious problems. The most common vaginal infections are yeast infections (candidiasis) and trichomoniasis.

Your doctor can't be certain of the cause of your vaginal irritation solely on the basis of symptoms or a physical exam; lab tests allowing microscopic evaluation of vaginal fluid are required for a correct diagnosis.

While there are a variety of effective drugs available to treat vaginal infections, it's better to prevent infections before they start:

- Wipe from front to back after using the toilet.
- Keep the genital area clean.
- Thoroughly wash anything inserted in the vagina (whether it's a penis, finger, sex aid, etc.).
- Change condoms between anal and vaginal sex.
- Avoid tight jeans, slacks, pantyhose, or panties.
- Wear white cotton underpants, loose-fitting slacks, and shorts.
- Don't use harsh soaps or douches.
- Avoid scented tampons or pads and scented toilet paper.
- Avoid feminine hygiene sprays.
- Thoroughly clean barrier contraceptive devices.

Yeast infections

Vulvovaginal candidiasis (VVC)—often called, simply a "yeast infection"—is a common cause of vaginal irritation. About 75 percent of women experience at least one episode of yeast infection during their lifetime, caused by an overgrowth of yeast cells (primarily *Candida albicans*) that normally live in the vagina. There is no direct evidence that yeast infections are transmitted during sex; instead, they may be caused by the factors listed above, in addition to pregnancy or uncontrolled diabetes mellitus.

The most frequent symptoms of yeast infection are itching, burning and irritation of the vagina and vulva. Painful urination and/or sex are common. You may not notice any abnormal vaginal discharge, but if you do, it may remind you of cottage cheese (although it may vary from watery to thick).

Yeast infections can usually be cleared up right away with an antifungal cream—many of which are now available over-the-counter. If this is your first infection, however, see your doctor before trying the cream. Also, if your recurrent infection isn't responding to the over-the-counter cream, or if you're not sure if you have a yeast infection, see your doctor.

Bacterial vaginosis

If you've ever noticed lots of water discharge and an unusual fishy odor in the vaginal area, you may have bacterial vaginosis (BV) (previously called non-specific vaginitis). Nearly half the women with clinical signs of BV report no symptoms, however.

This infection can be transmitted during sex, although the organisms responsible also have been found in young women who aren't sexually active. The role of sexual activity in the development of BV is not understood, but experts also believe that intrauterine devices (IUDs) may increase the risk of this type of infection. Your doctor can diagnose BV from symptoms during a physical, and from various tests of vaginal fluid.

If you have BV, you should be treated with antibiotics; your doctor also may recommend an anti-yeast medication. Generally, male sex partners aren't treated, but if your infection doesn't respond to drug therapy, treatment of your partner may help.

Unofficially...
Researchers are investigating the role of BV in pelvic infections that result in infertility and tubal (ectopic) pregnancy, premature birth, and low birth weight infants.

BV during pregnancy has been associated with preterm labor and some studies have shown that early diagnosis and treatment may decrease the incidence of preterm delivery.

Trichomoniasis

Unlike yeast infections or BV, trichomoniasis (or just "trich") is caused by single-celled protozoa not normally found in the vagina. Most of the time, the protozoa gets there during sex. Trichomoniasis, like many other sexually transmitted diseases (STDs), often occurs without any symptoms, but when symptoms do occur (usually within 4 to 20 days), they may include

- Heavy, yellow-green or gray vaginal discharge.
- Discomfort during sex.
- Vaginal odor.
- Painful urination.
- Irritated, itching genitals.
- Lower abdominal pain (this symptom is rare).

Men can have this infection, but they don't usually have symptoms; however, they can transmit the protozoa to their partners at any time, so it's a good idea to treat both partners to eliminate the parasite. A single dose of metronidazole will cure trich. If you take this drug, you shouldn't drink alcohol—mixing the two can cause severe nausea and vomiting.

Preventing pelvic inflammatory disease

The most serious and common complication of STDs among women is pelvic inflammatory disease (PID), an infection of the upper genital tract. PID can affect the uterus, ovaries, fallopian tubes, or other related structures. Untreated, PID can lead to

Watch Out! Recent studies suggest trichomoniasis may increase the risk of transmission of HIV, the virus that causes AIDS, and may cause delivery of low birth weight or premature infants. Additional research is needed to fully explore these relationships.

infertility, tubal (ectopic) pregnancy, chronic pelvic pain, and other serious consequences.

PID occurs when disease-causing organisms migrate upward from the vagina and cervix to the upper genital tract. Many different organisms can cause PID, but most cases are associated with gonorrhea and chlamydial infections. Scientists have found that bacteria normally present in the vagina and cervix may also play a role.

Are you at risk?

There are a number of practices that can put you at risk for developing PID. Women with STDs (especially gonorrhea and chlamydia) are at greater risk of developing PID than other women. Once you've had one episode of PID, you're at higher risk for another because the body's defenses are often damaged during the initial bout.

Sexually active teenagers are more likely to develop PID than are older women; further, the more sexual partners you have or the more sexual partners any of your sexual partners has had, the greater your risk of developing PID. Procedures involving instruments passed into the uterus (IUD insertion, induced abortion, and other procedures) put you at higher risk.

PID symptoms

PID (particularly when caused by chlamydia) may produce only minor symptoms or no symptoms at all, even though it can seriously damage the reproductive organs. If you do have symptoms, they may include some of the following:

- Lower abdominal pain
- Abnormal vaginal discharge
- Fever

Bright Idea
Many women with PID have sex partners who have no symptoms. Because of the risk of re-infection, however, your partner should be treated, even if he doesn't have symptoms.

- Pain in the right upper abdomen
- Painful intercourse
- Irregular menstrual bleeding

Treating PID

Because culture specimens from the upper genital tract are difficult to obtain and because several organisms are usually involved, your doctor will probably give you at least two antibiotics, effective against a wide range of bacteria.

Because you may still have bacteria in your body after your symptoms are gone, it's important to finish taking all of the prescribed medicine. You should see your doctor two to three days after treatment starts to be sure the antibiotics are working to cure the infection. About 25 percent of women with suspected PID must be hospitalized.

Preventing toxic shock syndrome

A new, highly absorbent tampon was the culprit behind an outbreak of a mysterious fatal illness in 1980, eventually diagnosed as toxic shock syndrome (TSS), an infection caused by the bacterium *Staphylococcus aureus*. The illness caused nausea and vomiting, fever, diarrhea, mental confusion, and skin rash, followed in some cases by severe shock and death. The super-absorbent tampon was withdrawn in 1981. Since 1984, there have been 69 reports of death related to tampon use; all but three resulted from TSS.

Just to be sure, you should avoid using tampons with more absorbency than you need and change them every few hours during your period. Some women prefer to use a pad at night instead of tampons for this reason. To help women compare absorbency from one brand to another, the FDA

Watch Out! Never wear a tampon during your period for more than eight hours (or overnight) in order to avoid contamination with deadly bacteria that can cause TSS.

requires manufacturers to use a standard test to measure absorbency and state the findings on the label.

Preventing sexually transmitted diseases

STDs (discussed individually in the in the following sections) are some of the most commonly reported infections, and the incidence has been rising over the past 20 years, despite improved methods of diagnosis and treatment. Once called venereal diseases, STDs are among the most common infectious diseases in the United States today. More than 20 STDs have now been identified, and they affect more than 13 million women and men in this country each year.

Throughout the 1970s and 1980s, women could expect to be cured of any STD they might contract, but by the mid-1980s, doctors began to realize that new sexually transmitted infections, such as herpes, hepatitis B, and AIDS were incurable. STDs are a particular problem for women, who have more severe and frequent health problems as a result of STDs. For example, STDs can spread to the uterus and fallopian tubes, causing PID. Some STDs, such as human papillomavirus infection (HPV), are associated with cervical cancer. Further, STDs can be passed from a mother to her baby before or during birth.

Nevertheless, an STD is certainly not inevitable, no matter how high the numbers of infected people may seem. There is a lot you can do to protect yourself:

- Avoid high-risk sex: Any sexual practice that tears the mucous membranes can make you vulnerable to infection (such as anal intercourse).

- **Condoms:** Use one every time you have sex; other than abstinence, it's the best way to protect yourself against STDs (including AIDS); other forms of birth control won't protect you from viruses and bacteria.

- **Know your partner:** Whenever you have sex, you're also indirectly exposing yourself to everyone your partner has ever had sex with.

- **Get regular pelvic exams:** Your doctor should ask if you want to be tested for gonorrhea and chlamydia at each visit if you're at risk for STDs.

- **Know the symptoms:** Pay attention to any unusual discharge, pain, itching, or burning—and watch for symptoms in your partner.

- **Prevent re-infection:** Both partners should take antibiotics for bacterial STDs at the same time, so you don't pass the infection back and forth.

- **Diaphragms:** These may also help reduce the risk of STD transmission.

If you have multiple partners

If you decide to be sexually active with several partners, there are things that you can do to reduce your risk of developing an STD:

- Use condoms.
- Have regular checkups for STDs, even if you don't have symptoms.
- Learn what the common symptoms are.
- Seek help immediately if any symptoms develop, however mild.

If you've been diagnosed

If you've been diagnosed with an STD, you should

- Notify all recent sex partners and urge them to get a checkup.

Unofficially... Scientists are still evaluating the usefulness of spermicides in preventing STDs to see whether they kill STD organisms.

CHAPTER 15 ■ INFECTIOUS DISEASES

- Follow your doctor's orders.
- Complete the full course of medication prescribed.
- Have a follow-up test to be sure the infection has been cured.
- Avoid all sexual activity during treatment.

Treatment outlook

When diagnosed and dealt with early, almost all STDs can be treated effectively. Some organisms, such as certain strains of gonorrhea, have become resistant to the medications historically used to treat them and now require newer types of antibiotics. The most serious STD for which no cure now exists is AIDS, a fatal viral infection of the immune system, although recent multiple-drug combinations have been improving the long-term outlook for AIDS patients.

Chlamydia

Chlamydia is the most common STD in the United States, infecting more than 4.5 million people each year. This serious but easily cured disease is three times more common than gonorrhea and six times more common than genital herpes. It's caused by a deceptive little organism *(Chlamydia trachomatis)* that is classified as a bacterium, even though it's similar to a virus. You catch the disease during sex with an infected partner (or a baby can become infected as it passes through an infected birth canal). While you become infected right away, symptoms don't often appear, if they appear at all, before one or two weeks have passed. You remain infectious until you've taken the complete course of antibiotics. Those at highest risk are women under age 24, women who have had more than one sexual partner, and women who have had other STDs (especially gonorrhea). Some studies suggest that if you've ever had chlamydia, you are more vulnerable to re-infection.

The most reliable test for women is a culture taken from the cervical cells (it's 90 percent accurate); you'll get results within 24 hours. Experts recommend all young women be tested for chlamydia, including all college and pregnant women. If you're being tested for any STD, you should also be tested for chlamydia—it's that common.

Symptoms include yellowish-black discharge or bleeding (about 20 percent of women notice a discharge) and pain burning, or a frequent urge to urinate.

Even if you don't have any symptoms, you can infect your partner during sex. The disease is treated with a seven-day course of antibiotics or a 1g single dose of azithromycin (penicillin isn't effective against this bacteria). If you are diagnosed, your sexual partner should be treated, even if he doesn't have symptoms.

If you don't treat the infection, you'll be infectious for years and you may develop complications; chlamydia may lead to infection of the fallopian tubes or uterine lining (endometritis), PID or a higher risk of premature birth and low birth weight infants.

You can lower the risk of infection by using condoms, but they don't provide complete protection. The only absolute way to protect against chlamydia is by not having sex or by having sex only with someone who has not had sex with anyone else.

Genital warts

Genital warts are an extremely common sexually transmitted disease; almost two million Americans are treated for these warts each year, mostly women between the ages of 15 and 24. (Older women may have the virus, but their immune systems control the outbreaks.) Those who are most at risk are women who have more than one sex partner and who don't use condoms.

The virus is transmitted during unprotected sex with an infected partner; you're most infectious when visible warts are present in the genital area, but even if the warts disappear, you still carry the virus. These warts are as incurable as AIDS or herpes. The warts may range from pink to gray and are either raised or flat, cause itching, burning, or bleeding around the genital area. You may find warts on the vulva, vagina, or anus, and occasionally they may crop up on the cervix. Infrequently, warts may grow larger and block the entrance to the vagina, anus, urethra, or (after oral sex) throat. Studies have shown that smoking makes the vaginal cells more susceptible to the wart virus.

At least six strains of the warts have been associated with a higher risk of cervical cancer, especially among women with persistent warts and many sex partners, but the association between this type of cancer and the virus is not well understood. While there are eight different types of HPV associated with genital warts, only two (types 16 and 18) have been associated with cervical cancer. The different types of virus can be distinguished only in a research lab. Most women with genital warts are not at higher risk for developing cervical cancer.

Your doctor can diagnose the warts from their appearance either with the naked eye, through a colposcope or from a biopsy; a Pap smear will indicate an "abnormality" which your doctor can investigate.

(In fact, large number of women infected with HPV never have a wart—and an abnormal Pap smear may be the only sign.) No treatment will remove all traces of the virus, but your doctor will try to remove or shrink the warts themselves with a topical solution, or by freezing them or burning them off with a laser. Unfortunately, genital warts often reappear after treatment. As a last resort, your doctor may turn to surgical removal if the warts are very large or cause problems (but even then, 20 percent of the time they grow back). They are so recalcitrant because the virus remains in the body in a quiescent state no matter what is done to remove the wart itself. Doctors don't know exactly why some women have recurrences and others don't. If you do have warts and have the growths removed, 90 percent of the time you will not have another outbreak unless you are re-exposed to another viral type.

Anyone with genital warts (or who has been diagnosed in the past) should always use a condom during sex, since there is no other way to prevent the disease. Scientists at multiple medical centers and labs around the world are investigating the world's first test of a potential vaccine, but it is not yet available. All women with genital warts need a Pap test every 6 to 12 months to detect early signs of cervical cancer.

Genital herpes

Genital herpes is a very common STD. The medical community has always considered genital herpes to be more of an annoyance than a life-threatening infection. Herpes can be transmitted by any skin-to-skin contact, but the virus for genital herpes usually invades the body during sex, where it remains for a lifetime, usually reactivating several times a year with painful sores in the genital area. It's estimated that there are more than 700,000 new cases each year, and that the disease is responsible for more than 500,000 doctor visits each year.

Herpes simplex type II (HSV-II) causes most of the genital herpes cases; herpes simplex virus type I (HSV-I) causes cold sores, usually above the waist. HSV-II can infect any skin or mucous membrane. While it's normally spread by contact with the genital secretions of a person with an open sore, it's possible for someone without obvious lesions to infect his or her partner. Genital herpes also can be acquired by infants as they pass through the birth canal of an infected mother. Neonatal herpes can cause serious damage to the brain and many other organs; even with therapy, more than 20 percent of the affected infants will die, and many survivors will be seriously impaired. Because of this, thousands of women in the United States with active herpes near the time of delivery undergo a Cesarean section. Women with recurrent herpes infection shouldn't be alarmed: The vast majority of affected babies come from mothers with initial or first herpes infections.

About 60 percent of women with herpes never have any symptoms; if they do, the first infection is usually the worst and can take up to three weeks to recover from. After the sores fade away, the virus remains in your body until it reactivates, triggering lesions on the cervix or vulva, the skin between the vagina and the anus, upper thighs, anal area, or buttocks. The sores usually recur within six months of the first attack. The reactivation is often signaled by a prodrome—a tingling or stinging in the area where the virus first entered the body. Scientists at

Watch Out!
To prevent re-infection for any bacterial STD, don't have sex until all antibiotics have been taken and symptoms have disappeared.

Bright Idea
If your sores are painful or itchy, try taking a lukewarm sitz bath; afterward, dry the sores with a hair dryer set on "cool." A small amount of petroleum jelly on the sores can reduce the irritation during urination. During outbreaks, wear loose cotton underwear, not pantyhose or tight pants.

one time thought there might be a link between herpes and cervical cancer, but new studies show that there is probably no correlation.

The antiviral drugs Famvir and Valtrex can reduce the number and severity of attacks, but it's not a cure—it can't kill the virus. Taking the drug at the very first sign of an outbreak (when your skin starts to tingle) may shorten the healing time from five days to one. If you have more than six episodes a year, you may take acyclovir every day to prevent recurrence, but most women don't take the drug daily for more than three years. Very few women report any side effects. At least two companies are in the final stages of testing for a vaccine to prevent the infection, but so far no vaccine has been approved.

Gonorrhea

Gonorrhea is one of the most commonly reported STDs, although the number of infected women has been declining since 1980. Nevertheless, there are still a million cases reported each year, most by women between the ages of 15 and 24; some experts think the number is actually twice as high.

The infection is caused by a bacteria called *Neisseria gonorrhoea,* which thrives in warm, moist places and is transmitted during sex. Women who have unprotected sex with an infected man have an 80 to 90 percent chance of becoming infected. Contrary to myth, it's not possible to get gonorrhea from contaminated toilet seats or public pools.

About one-half of all infected women will notice symptoms, which include vaginal swelling, green-yellow discharge, vaginal bleeding between periods, itching and burning, or pain during urination. Severe infections may affect your whole body, causing nausea and vomiting, fever, and rapid heartbeat.

About 40 percent of women develop PID as a result of infection, causing scars in the fallopian tubes and infertility. Untreated pregnant women may have smaller babies or premature birth; babies born to infected mothers may have gonorrhea conjunctivitis during delivery (untreated infants can be blinded).

Your doctor can diagnose the infection with a bacterial culture from the cervix and surrounding areas; results are usually available within 48 hours. Because gonorrhea and chlamydia often occur together, your doctor will treat the infection with drugs effective against both. While gonorrhea is becoming resistant to some antibiotics, newer drugs have been developed that will cure the infection.

Hepatitis B

Hepatitis B is the most common preventable STD in the United States. It's caused by an extremely infectious virus that is 100 times more contagious than the virus that causes AIDS.

While experts believe there are 300,000 cases a year, only about 15,000 are reported. Approximately 1.25 million Americans are carriers and remain infectious all their lives. Almost 6,000 Americans die each year from acute hepatitis B or from complications of infection. Tragically, while hepatitis B can be prevented by a vaccine (a three-vaccine series), only about 5 percent of those who account for most of the infections (teenagers aged 15 to 19) ever get vaccinated. The vaccine is now recommended for all children in order to prevent 6,000 death a year. However, some critics are concerned about two deaths reported from the use of the vaccine.

The virus is carried in the blood and in saliva, semen, and other body fluids and is transmitted much as the AIDS virus is—it is not spread by casual contact. The virus must get into a person's blood to cause infection, either by sex, blood transfusions, dirty needles, or by sharing toothbrushes, razors, or utensils. It's also possible to pass the infection to your baby during the final three months of pregnancy, during delivery, or while nursing. The virus is very stable and can survive for days on dry surfaces. Still, more than half of all cases are linked to sex with an infected person.

It may take up to six months after exposure before symptoms appear, which may show up only gradually, if they appear at all. Symptoms may include fatigue, joint and muscle aches, mild stomach pain, poor appetite, hives or rash, and mild diarrhea. About half of those infected may develop jaundice. Approximately a third of women have no symptoms; another third experience only mild illness (the chance of becoming a carrier is greater if there aren't severe symptoms). About 25 percent of carriers develop chronic symptoms and are at greatest risk of developing cirrhosis of the liver. The virus can be found in blood and body fluids several weeks before symptoms appear and several months afterward. People who are chronic carriers are always infectious, although they don't appear to be sick. Those who recover are immune for life.

Hepatitis B is diagnosed by blood tests; other tests can differentiate hepatitis B from other types of hepatitis. Chronic active hepatitis B is treated with alpha-interferons, but the treatment itself causes many flulike side effects. There is no treatment for acute hepatitis B beyond bed rest and a high carbohydrate, low fat diet. After recovery, you will need a blood test to see if you have retained an antigen; if you have, it means you are extremely infectious and are at higher risk for developing complications.

About 10 percent of these chronic carriers lose the antigen each year. A high percentage of patients go on to develop chronic hepatitis, leading to persistent poor liver function. Most people recover from the infection completely and aren't at risk for long-term complications.

While hepatitis B is completely preventable with the vaccine, thousands continue to come down with the disease each year. Anyone at risk for the disease (including all medical and nursing personnel) should have the vaccine. As of November 1991, the vaccine was recommended for all infants; boosters are not currently recommended. Those who haven't been vaccinated but who are exposed can receive immune globulin HBIG for 90 percent protection, if they get the treatment within a week of exposure and begin the vaccine series at the same time.

Carriers should follow standard hygienic procedures to make sure their close contacts aren't contaminated. You should not share razors, toothbrushes or any other object that may become contaminated with blood. In addition, household members (especially sexual partners) should be immunized with the hepatitis B vaccine. If you're a carrier, you should tell your health care workers and dentists of your health status.

Syphilis

This once fatal infection, first recorded as a major epidemic after Columbus returned from his trip to America, has tormented people around the world for centuries. Today, penicillin can cure the disease if it's caught in time, and the rate of infection is currently dropping in the United States after a recent epidemic from 1986 to 1990. Still, thousands of Americans contract the infection each year.

Bright Idea
If you don't want to rely on your partner to wear a condom, you can use an over-the-counter female condom (two rings with a latex sheath between them). The closed end of the sheath is inserted into the vagina, and the ring is placed high up around the cervix. The open end of the sheath remains outside the vagina. Used once and thrown away, it can prevent STDs and pregnancy.

It's caused by the *Treponema pallidum* spirochete, which enters the body via broken skin or mucous membranes during sex, by kissing, or by other body contact with an open sore. The rate of infection during a single contact with an infected person is about 30 percent. The initial sore may be easily overlooked so that the infection is not detected until a rash appears during the second stage of the disease. It can be diagnosed from a blood test or an examination of material from the lesion (there is no culture for syphilis).

Penicillin cures the infection 98 percent of the time if diagnosed early, but if it's not treated, the infection can spread to the central nervous system leading to irreversible nerve damage.

HIV and AIDS

Infection with human immunodeficiency virus (HIV) leads to the condition called acquired immune deficiency syndrome (AIDS). Since its discovery in 1984, AIDS has reached epidemic proportions throughout the world, infecting about 13 million people. Although the disease was originally found primarily among homosexual men, it's now transmitted mostly through heterosexual activities.

In the United States, blood and blood products have been tested since 1985 for HIV and are considered safe. In addition, the FDA inspects the more than 3,000 donor centers where blood and blood components are collected. The risk of HIV transmission dropped from 1 in 2,500 units of blood in 1985 to 1 in 440,000 to 640,000 units by the end of 1995.

HIV infects bodily fluids, such as blood, semen, vaginal secretions, amniotic fluid, breast milk, and urine. It can be transmitted by coming in contact with body secretions during sex, or by being exposed to blood or blood products via blood transfusion. The virus can be and has been transmitted by intravenous drug use; by being accidentally pricked with a needle containing traces of infected blood; by contaminated needles used for tatoos, accupuncture, blood drawing, injections, and so on; and from an infected mother to her baby during pregnancy or breastfeeding.

Practicing safe sex

Spread of the disease through heterosexual activity has led to a dramatic increase in HIV infection among women, who today make up almost 13 percent of AIDS cases. In the United States, AIDS is the fourth leading cause of death in black women of reproductive age in New York and New Jersey. Short of an effective vaccine, the best way to stop the spread of HIV is by avoiding sex with infected individuals and by practicing safe sex. Using a rubber (latex) condom during sex is the best protection, save abstinence; latex condoms should always be used for oral, anal, and vaginal sex if there is a chance that either partner is infected.

Condom manufacturers in the United States electronically test all condoms for holes and weak spots; in addition, the FDA requires that manufacturers use a water test to examine samples from each batch of condoms for leakage. Only water-based lubricants should be used with latex condoms, because oil-based lubricants (such as petroleum jelly) weaken natural rubber.

If you're allergic to latex, the FDA has approved several polyurethane condoms, which are comparable to latex as a barrier to both sperm and HIV virus.

Unofficially...
Outside the body, HIV is easily killed by common household disinfectants, such as alcohol, bleach, and peroxide.

Treatment

While at present there is no cure for AIDS, intensive research has produced new medication combinations that can prolong life. Three groups of medicines currently treat AIDS: Antiviral drugs; prophylactic medicines to protect against certain infections; and other drugs to fight infections and cancer.

An enormous number of new antiretroviral drugs for treating HIV infection have been introduced, including nucleoside agents, HIV protease inhibitors, and non-nucleoside reverse transcriptase inhibitors. In addition, tests to evaluate how much of the virus is circulating in a patient's blood make it possible to monitor the effectiveness of these drugs.

This combination of new agents for fighting HIV infection, in conjunction with improved ways to monitor the effectiveness of therapy, has significantly improved the prognosis for today's HIV-infected women. Combination therapy—the use of more than one antiretroviral drug at a time—is often used. By combining drugs, the likelihood that a woman will become resistant is much lower.

Still a possibility: Preventing tuberculosis

Tuberculosis (TB) is an infectious disease that usually attacks the lungs and is spread from person to person through the air. Most people think of TB as no longer a threat to anyone in the United States, but in recent years it's made a startling comeback.

When people with TB in their lungs or throat cough, laugh, sneeze, sing or even talk, the germs may spread into the air; if another person breathes in these germs, she could become infected.

Latent versus active TB

It's important to understand that there is a difference between being infected with TB and having active TB. If you're infected with TB, you have the bacteria in your body, but your immune system protects you from the germs and you're not sick. By comparison, someone with the disease is sick and can spread the infection to others; a person with TB disease needs to see a doctor as soon as possible. Experts believe that about 10 million Americans are infected with TB, but only about 10 percent of these people will develop tuberculosis. The other 90 percent will never get sick or be able to spread the infection to others.

Who's at risk?

It's not easy to become infected with TB. Usually, you have to be close to someone with the disease for a long period of time. It's normally spread between family members, close friends, and people who work or live together.

Some groups of people are at higher risk for active tuberculosis:

- People with HIV infection (the AIDS virus)
- People in close contact with those known to be infectious with TB
- People with weak immune systems
- Foreign-born people from countries with high TB rates
- Some racial or ethnic minorities, including African Americans
- People who work in or are residents of nursing homes, prisons, and some hospitals
- Undernourished people

Watch Out! You may have tuberculosis, yet feel perfectly healthy—or you may only have a cough from time to time. If you think you have been exposed to TB, get a TB skin test.

- Alcoholics
- Intravenous drug users

How do you know it's TB?

If you simply have a latent infection, you won't have any symptoms; if you have active TB, you may have any, all, or none of the following symptoms:

- A nagging cough
- Fatigue
- Weight loss
- Loss of appetite
- Fever
- Coughing up blood
- Night sweats

Diagnosis: When to get a TB skin test

The Mantoux test is the best way to find out if you're infected. A nurse will place a small amount of testing material just below the top layers of skin of your arm; two to three days later, your arm is checked to see if a bump has developed. If the bump is big enough, the test is positive—which means you have a TB infection. To find out if you have active tuberculosis, your doctor may give you several other tests, including a chest X-ray and a test of your sputum.

You should get a tuberculin test if you have symptoms or if you are living in close contact with someone who recently came down with TB. If you fall into one or more of the high-risk categories for TB (see list above) or you've never had a skin test before, you should be tested. TB can be prevented, even if you are at risk.

Can TB be treated?

Luckily, TB patients no longer have to be isolated in asylums. Treatment for TB depends on whether you have the disease or just the infection. If you are infected with TB but don't have TB disease, you may be given preventive therapy to kill germs that aren't doing any damage right now, but could break out later. You'll need to take medicine for between six months and a year. If you have active disease, it can be treated with very effective drugs. After a few weeks, you probably can even return to normal activities and not have to worry about infecting others.

Preventing mononucleosis

Mononucleosis (mono) is an infection caused by the Epstein-Barr virus (EBV), one of the herpes family of viruses. Studies suggest that most women are infected with EBV at some point, but most rarely have any symptoms at all. Once you're infected, the virus persists in your white blood cells in a latent form, which means it's still there but not actively producing any symptoms. This state is believed to last for life.

There's no way to prevent the disease other than avoiding people you know are infected—but since it's quite possible not to know who's infected, this is almost impossible. People with mononucleosis are not required to observe strict isolation procedures, although they should not give blood after a recent infection.

How do you know it's mono?

If you're going to have symptoms, they'll usually develop four to seven weeks after you're exposed to the virus. They include fever, sore throat, headaches, white patches on the back of your throat, swollen glands in your neck, fatigue, and loss of appetite. Generally, you get mononucleosis only once, and it's most common among people 15 to 35

Unofficially...
Cytomegalovirus, another herpes virus, can mimic the symptoms of mononucleosis.

years old. Because the virus is found in saliva and mucus, it's transmitted from one person to another through coughing, sneezing, and kissing.

Diagnosing the problem

Your doctor can diagnose mono from your symptoms and a blood test. One common test used to diagnose mononucleosis is called the Monospot test; sometimes other blood tests are needed if the results of the Monospot test aren't conclusive. An examination of your blood under a microscope may reveal an increased number of white blood cells known as lymphocytes. Other blood tests may show an increase in antibody levels (antibodies react to infectious organisms in the blood and create immunity). There are a number of different antibody tests for EBV that can reveal useful information to doctors.

Complications

Most of the time, mono is more of a nuisance than a serious infection. The main serious concern with mononucleosis is that the spleen will enlarge and occasionally rupture. Call your doctor if you have the signs of a ruptured spleen:

- Hepatitis (inflammation of the liver), which is caused by the virus infecting the organ
- Pain under the left side of chest
- Lightheadedness
- Heart racing or thudding
- Excessive bleeding
- Breathing problems

Other rare complications include inflammation of the heart muscle (myocarditis), meningitis, encephalitis, or Guillain-Barré syndrome.

Treatment tips

Antibiotics such as penicillin are of no help for treating mononucleosis, which is caused by a virus. But your doctor may give you an antibiotic if you have a bacterial infection in addition to having mononucleosis. Although you can't cure mononucleosis itself, you can treat the symptoms—and the good news is that it will go away on its own, eventually. (Symptoms usually last about four weeks.) Here's what to do until then:

- Rest.
- Drink plenty of fluids.
- Gargle with salt water or suck on throat lozenges, hard candy, or flavored frozen desserts (such as Popsicles) for sore throat relief.
- Take acetaminophen (Tylenol) or ibuprofen (Advil, Motrin, Nuprin) to relieve pain and fever.
- To avoid spleen rupture, avoid exercise of any kind until your doctor tells you it's safe.

Preventing Lyme disease

Lyme disease is a recently identified infection first recognized in Lyme, Connecticut. It's caused by the bite from a deer tick carrying the bacterium *Borrelia burgdorferi*. These tiny ticks (about the size of the period at the end of this sentence) don't hop, jump, fly, or descend from trees—you must come in direct contact with them (although they may blow in a strong breeze). The best defense against Lyme disease is to avoid ticks

- While walking in the woods, stay on trails.
- Avoid brushing up against low bushes or tall grass.

Watch Out!
Do not take aspirin for the symptoms of mononucleosis because doing so while infected with mono has been associated with a disease called Reye's syndrome, a serious illness that can be fatal.

Bright Idea
Eliminate tick habitat around your house—ticks need moisture and a place to hide, so if your yard is neat, you're less likely to attract ticks. Remove brush and leaf litter from your yard and garden. Keep woodpiles neat, under cover, off the ground, and in a dry, sunny place.

- Wear light-colored, long-sleeved shirts, and light-colored pants tucked into boots or socks (this lets you see the ticks more easily).
- Use an insect repellent containing no more than 30 percent DEET (N-diethyl-metatoluamide) on bare skin and clothing, but don't apply it to your hands or face.
- Apply the insect repellant Duranon to clothing only—not to skin.

While the disease has been portrayed as frightening, most of the time it is easily treated with antibiotics and doesn't progress to the chronic stage. It probably causes severe, long-term effects in less than 10 percent of untreated patients.

If you live in the "Lyme disease belt" of the northeast coast from Maine to Maryland, it's possible to be vaccinated against *B. burgdorferi*, the bacterium that causes Lyme disease, which can help you build up an immunity to the bacteria from the tick bite. But it's not foolproof—the three-shot vaccine is expensive (about $150 for all the shots, plus doctor fees) and it doesn't provide 100 percent protection. Other experts worry that the shots only protect you against Lyme disease, but not against other diseases carried by ticks, including Rocky Mountain spotted fever (found all over the country), ehrlichiosis, and babesiosis. While these three diseases combined affect fewer people than does Lyme, they are on the rise and cause far more serious symptoms than does Lyme.

Because of these limitations, the vaccination is recommended only for adults who live, work, or play where Lyme disease is prevalent, or who have frequent or prolonged exposure to tick habitat (wooded areas, brush, and tall grass). In any event, it's not recommended for

- Pregnant women.
- Women who have Lyme disease that hasn't responded to treatment.
- Children under age 15.

Just the facts

- The best way to prevent colds is to wash your hands and disinfect household surfaces regularly.
- A flu vaccine can prevent infection in high-risk women.
- Both sexual partners need to be treated for most STDs, regardless of whether both are symptomatic.
- You can be infected with TB, but never get sick or be able to spread the disease.
- Experts don't advise everyone to get a Lyme disease vaccine; only those specifically at risk should be vaccinated.

GET THE SCOOP ON...
Why women are at risk for autoimmune diseases ▪ How to get your symptoms taken seriously ▪ Possible links between autoimmunity and infertility ▪ New treatments for autoimmune disease

Autoimmune Diseases

One out of every eight American women will be diagnosed with an autoimmune disease. Unfortunately, it may take years for many women to be diagnosed, and many will suffer significant damage as a result of the delay. Individually, most autoimmune diseases are not very common, but taken as a whole, they represent the fourth-largest cause of disability among women in the United States. Overall, autoimmune disease is five times more common in women than in men. The various diseases range from the benign to the severe and cost this country about $86 billion every year.

Symptoms also vary widely from one illness to another (and even within the same disease); different diseases affect many different systems in your body, so symptoms are often misleading. Misguided T cells and antibodies contribute to many autoimmune diseases:

- Connective tissues: Lupus erythematosus, rheumatoid arthritis, and systemic sclerosis
- Neuromuscular systems: Multiple sclerosis or myasthenia gravis
- Endocrine system: Graves' disease or insulin-dependent diabetes mellitus type 1
- Gastrointestinal system: Inflammatory bowel disease
- Skin: Psoriasis or vitiligo

The conditions aren't contagious, nor related to cancer or AIDS. Often genetic, the diseases can be debilitating and life threatening, exacting not just a physical but also a mental toll. In most cases, the risk of getting one of these diseases increases as you get older.

What causes autoimmune disease?

An autoimmune disease occurs when a woman's immune system suddenly malfunctions and begins to attack her own tissues. Scientists now understand that it happens, but so far, they're not exactly sure why.

The immune system is designed to protect your body by producing antibodies or T cells in response to invading viruses or bacteria. Normally, the immune system can tell the difference between its own cells and those of an invading microorganism. But sometimes immune cells make a mistake and start attacking the very cells they're supposed to protect. The exact mechanism behind this is not completely understood, but doctors believe that bacteria, viruses, toxins, and some drugs may play a role in setting off an autoimmune process in someone who already has a genetic tendency to develop

Unofficially... The incidence of autoimmune diseases varies in different ethnic groups, but the specific differences depend on the disease. For example, the incidence of insulin-dependent diabetes mellitus is higher in Caucasians, while noninsulin dependent diabetes mellitus occurs more frequently in African Americans, Hispanics, and Native Americans.

such a disorder. Scientists think that the inflammation triggered by these toxic or infectious agents somehow provokes in the body an autoimmune reaction.

In some cases, there seems to be an association with life events. For example, childhood neck irradiation is associated with later development of thyroid disease. Pregnancy may trigger thyroid autoimmunity (postpartum thyroiditis) in susceptible women. The incidence of some autoimmune diseases varies by geographic location, and diet may be another factor in developing them. There also may be a genetic component to some of the diseases.

Is it my hormones?

Because women face a much higher risk of developing autoimmune diseases, many experts believe this means that female hormones must play a role. The development of many autoimmune diseases (and the severity of symptoms) seems to be related to changes in hormone levels.

Hormones are produced by endocrine glands in comparatively large quantities, and secreted into the bloodstream to act at distant sites in the body. For example, estradiol (a type of estrogen) is produced by the ovaries and influences nerve cells, bone, muscle, and metabolism (the regulation of the body's ability to utilize fuel) in general. It is the sex steroid hormones (including estrogen, progesterone, and testosterone) that seem to influence the symptoms and severity of some autoimmune diseases, but how they do this isn't completely understood.

Hormones affect immune cell functions. In general, androgens (such as testosterone) and progesterone are thought to suppress and protect the

> 66
> Despite their devastating human and economic toll, autoimmune diseases are among the least investigated, most difficult to diagnose, [as well as the most] physically and emotionally painful diseases that face Americans today.
> —Susan Wood, Ph.D., newly appointed acting Deputy Assistant U.S. Secretary for Women's Health, Department of Health and Human Services, National Institutes of Health.
> 99

Unofficially...
The first multidisciplinary center dedicated to the study and treatment of women afflicted with autoimmune disorders is the Barbara Volcker Center for Women and Rheumatic Diseases at the Hospital for Special Surgery in New York City.

immune cells, prolactin stimulates the cells, and estrogen can either stimulate or inhibit immune function. Studies of isolated immune cells in cultures, however, show that sex steroids have a variety of effects. In animal models, hormone effects have been shown to be complex with different results, depending on the strain and the specific disease.

Yet there are many aspects of this relationship that aren't completely understood. The symptoms associated with some autoimmune diseases change with natural shifts in estrogen and progesterone, such as those that occur during the menstrual cycle, pregnancy, and at menopause. Some autoimmune disorders strike women in their 20s and 30s when estrogen levels are high; others hit hard right before puberty, or after menopause, when estrogen levels are low. And during pregnancy—when estrogen levels are highest—many women with rheumatoid arthritis go into complete remission. On the other hand, about 60 percent of pregnant women with systemic lupus erythematosus (SLE, or lupus) find that their condition worsens during these nine months. (Still, in women whose lupus is inactive at the time of conception, pregnancy actually seems to protect against a lupus flare.)

In addition, the typical age of onset varies among autoimmune diseases. For example, SLE onset commonly occurs after puberty and during the reproductive years, while rheumatoid arthritis tends to begin later, peaking around the age of menopause and coinciding with declining estrogen levels. The incidence rates of rheumatoid arthritis for men and women become similar around the age of menopause, however, suggesting that aging may be a more critical factor than hormone changes.

Do autoimmune diseases run in families?

Autoimmune diseases also seem to have a genetic component. Some families predisposed to autoimmune diseases carry a common antibody traditionally associated with rheumatic autoimmune diseases, such as SLE. The antibody (called antiphospholipid antibody) belongs to a class of antibodies called auto-antibodies, which are proteins produced by the body that attack themselves, rather than invading germs. Auto-antibodies are commonly found in women with autoimmune disease.

But genetic predisposition alone does not cause autoimmune diseases—other factors need to be present as well in order for these diseases to develop. Different autoimmune illnesses may cluster in families; for example, a grandmother may have rheumatoid arthritis, her daughter, diabetes, and her granddaughter, lupus.

Rather than one overriding gene for autoimmune disease, it may be more likely to find separate or interrelated genes for different disorders. For example, scientists have zeroed in on the location of a gene that predisposes Caucasians, Asians, and African Americans to lupus in a region near the end of the long arm of human chromosome 1. Identifying genes for lupus will provide new insights into why people get the disease, and should help researchers develop new treatments or preventive measures.

More than one gene determines whether a person will get certain autoimmune diseases, such as rheumatoid arthritis, type 1 diabetes and lupus; disease genes interact with one another and with triggers from the environment (such as a virus or sunlight) to produce disease. Identifying each of the multiple genes involved in complex disorders is

Unofficially...
A 1998 Harvard University study reported that 75 percent of lab mice injected with herpes simplex I virus went on to develop an autoimmune eye disorder.

much harder than finding the genes that cause single-gene disorders, such as Huntington's disease.

Can you catch an autoimmune disease?
While you can't directly "catch" an autoimmune disease, some scientists believe something outside your body (an infection, for example) may trigger the disease. For example, strep throat infections are linked with rheumatic fever (an autoimmune disorder).

Getting a good diagnosis

As a group, autoimmune diseases are among the most poorly understood and recognized of any category of illnesses. Unfortunately, too many women with these diseases are dismissed as hypochondriacs and not properly diagnosed for years because the symptoms can be vague and not specific to a single illness.

The real problem with being properly diagnosed is that these days, most doctors can't spend a great deal of time with you—and yet listening to the patient's description of her symptoms is the only way to diagnose most autoimmune diseases, according to experts. In addition, diagnostic tests for many autoimmune diseases are not standardized. Thus many people who have milder forms of autoimmune diseases may not quite meet the established criteria for a particular disease, and so it could take a long time for the diagnosis to be confirmed.

Autoimmunity has yet to be embraced by the medical community as an "umbrella" category of disease. Doctors haven't focused on autoimmune diseases very much because the conditions cross different medical specialties (such as cardiology or dermatology), which usually focus on diseases within their particular category.

Unofficially... More than 65 percent of women diagnosed with a serious autoimmune disease had been told they were chronic complainers or hypochondriacs prior to being correctly diagnosed, according to a study conducted by the AARDA.

Even when some doctors understand autoimmunity, its victims—mainly women—have suffered from the scattered research approach. Many doctors don't realize the diseases have a genetic component and may cluster in families as different autoimmune diseases. For example, in some families, a mother may have lupus; her daughter, diabetes; her sister, Grave's disease; and her grandmother, rheumatoid arthritis.

Sufferers face problems not only because doctors don't always think of autoimmunity, but also because of who they are—women in their childbearing years. As a rule, this is a time in a woman's life when she seems healthy (at least on the outside) and so, often, women with symptoms of fatigue, weight gain or loss, and listlessness—symptoms of potential autoimmune problems—may not be taken seriously when they consult a doctor. Proper diagnosis is complicated by the fact that fatigue, weight changes, and listlessness are also symptoms of pregnancy, colds, allergies, emotional stress, and a multitude of other disorders. Moreover, a woman's symptoms are likely vague in the beginning, with a tendency to come and go, and she may find it hard to describe them accurately to her physician. Women with autoimmune diseases are often shunted from specialist to specialist, undergoing a battery of tests and procedures before a correct diagnosis is made. This process can sometimes take years.

Tragically, many of the misdiagnosed women suffer significant damage to their organs during the long search for a diagnosis, and end up carrying this health burden with them for the rest of their lives because of the delay.

Experts believe that if women and their doctors were more aware of the genetic predisposition for these conditions, doctors would be more careful about taking a medical history for autoimmune diseases within the family when presented by a patient with confusing symptoms. Early screening of these diseases may not only prevent significant and lifelong health problems, but also actually prevent some autoimmune diseases.

Because diagnoses of most autoimmune diseases are difficult to make and women with these diseases can look very healthy, you must work with your doctor if you want to get a proper diagnosis. Here's how:

- Read as much as you can about autoimmune diseases.
- Know your family history.
- If family members have one or more autoimmune diseases, tell your doctor.
- Sort out and list meaningful symptoms.
- Identify a doctor with good diagnostic skills and a reputation for listening.

Treating autoimmune diseases

There is no cure for autoimmune diseases, but they can be treated if the major deficiencies are corrected. You'll also need to control the activity of the immune system while still maintaining the body's ability to fight disease. The drugs most commonly used to do this are corticosteroids, which also act as immunosuppressants, as well.

Severe disorders can be treated with other, more powerful immunosuppressant drugs, such as methotrexate, cyclophosphamide, and azathioprine.

All of these drugs, however, can damage rapidly dividing tissues (such as bone marrow or a fetus), and so are used cautiously.

Intravenous immunoglobulin therapy is used to treat various autoimmune diseases, reducing circulating immune complexes. Some mild forms of rheumatic autoimmune diseases are treated by relieving the symptoms with nonsteroidal, anti-inflammatory medications.

Connective tissue diseases

Many autoimmune diseases target the connective tissue of the body. Some of the most common autoimmune connective tissue diseases are lupus, rheumatoid arthritis, systemic sclerosis, and Sjogren's disease.

Lupus

When your immune system becomes overactive and produces antibodies that attack healthy tissue in the body, the resulting inflammation, redness, pain, and swelling is diagnosed as lupus. This tendency for the immune system to become overactive may run in families. There's considerable evidence that the development of lupus has a strong genetic basis. For example, studies suggest that a sibling of a person with SLE is 20 times more likely to develop the disorder, compared with the general population.

In some people, lupus becomes active after exposure to sunlight, infections, or certain medications. While it can affect men, 9 out of 10 people who have lupus are women between the ages of 15 and 44. Lupus is three times more common in black women than in Caucasian women.

There are three different forms of lupus:

Watch Out!
Lupus may be hard to diagnose and is often mistaken for other diseases, which is why it's often been called the "great imitator."

- SLE: This most serious form may affect many parts of the body including joints, skin, kidneys, lungs, heart, and the brain.

- Discoid or cutaneous lupus: This type mainly affects the skin.

- Drug-induced lupus: Some prescription medicines trigger this type of lupus, which resembles SLE but is less serious.

The signs of lupus vary and may have periods of exacerbation and remission. Some people have just a few signs of the disease; others have more, but many people with lupus look healthy.

While many people have just one symptom, the following symptoms are more indicative of lupus when they occur together:

- Red rash or color change on the face, often in the shape of a butterfly across the bridge of the nose and the cheeks
- Painful or swollen joints
- Unexplained fever
- Chest pain with each breath
- Unusual loss of hair
- Pale or purple fingers or toes from cold or stress
- Sensitivity to the sun
- Low red or white blood cell count
- Mouth sores
- Unexplained convulsions
- Hallucinations
- Depression
- Repeated miscarriages
- Unexplained kidney problems

Because the signs of lupus often differ from one person to the next, treatment, too, may vary. There is no known cure today for lupus, but in many cases, symptoms of the disease can be relieved. Your doctor may recommend aspirin or similar medication to treat painful, swollen joints and fever. Creams may ease the rash, and stronger medicines may be prescribed for more serious problems. It's a good idea to wear protective clothing and sunscreen when outdoors. The good news is that with the correct medicine and by taking care of themselves, most women with lupus can work, have children and lead full lives.

Rheumatoid arthritis
This disabling disease, which is characterized by inflamed and swollen joints and the appearance of nodules beneath the skin, is found three times more often in women than in men. Rheumatoid arthritis is one of the more difficult of the autoimmune rheumatic diseases to control. The disease begins when immune cells attack and inflame the membrane around joints (most commonly the hands), although it also can affect the heart, lungs, and eyes. Of the estimated 2.1 million Americans with rheumatoid arthritis, approximately 1.5 million (71 percent) are women. The condition generally develops between the ages of 20 and 50, although it may begin at any age.

If uncontrolled, the inflammation may destroy the joints. The severity of rheumatoid arthritis varies from person to person. In some cases, the disease may be mild, while in others, it can be crippling. Its course is unpredictable; it can flare up suddenly, and just as quickly go into remission. Although emotional stress is not a direct cause of rheumatoid arthritis, it can hasten the progression of the disease

Bright Idea
Government scientists hope someday to be able to use a new type of gene therapy (called naked DNA) to treat rheumatoid arthritis—it works by being directly injected into muscle tissue. In rats, the experimental treatment dramatically reduced symptoms in the joints.

and make it worse. Treatment involves rest and exercise; anti-inflammatory drugs can help; more severe cases often require stronger medications, such as corticosteroids or methotrexate.

Arava (leflunomide), the first new drug specifically designed to treat active rheumatoid arthritis in more than a decade, may soon be available if approved by the FDA. It's been recommended for approval for symptom relief and for slowing down structural damage. Scientists suspect Arava works because it interferes with an enzyme involved in the autoimmune process that leads to rheumatoid arthritis. Studies have shown Arava is effective and well tolerated by patients in all stages of disease and that it slows joint deterioration. Since studies have shown that structural joint damage often starts during the first two years after disease onset, early diagnosis and treatment are critical.

Systemic sclerosis (scleroderma)

Scleroderma is an activation of immune cells that produces scar tissue in the skin, internal organs, and small blood vessels. It affects women three times more often than men, but increases to a rate of 15 times higher for women during childbearing years. Like other autoimmune disorders, it appears to be more common among black women.

In most patients, the first symptoms are swelling and puffiness of the fingers or hands, followed by thickened skin a few months later. Other symptoms include skin ulcers on the fingers, joint stiffness in the hands, pain, sore throat, and diarrhea.

The drug D-penicillamine has been shown to decrease skin thickening. Symptoms involving other organs, such as the kidneys, esophagus, intestines, and blood vessels are treated individually.

Sjogren's syndrome (Sjogren's disease)

Sjogren's syndrome (also called Sjogren's disease) is a chronic, inflammatory autoimmune disorder that slowly interferes with the ability to secrete saliva and tears. It can occur alone or with rheumatoid arthritis, scleroderma, or systemic lupus erythematosus. Nine out of ten cases occur in women, most often at or around midlife.

This syndrome is caused by auto-antibodies attacking and destroying the moisture-producing glands in the body (tear ducts, salivary glands and the vagina), which in turn may cause some changes in peripheral nerves and in the trigeminal nerve of the face.

Symptoms include dryness of the eyes and mouth, swollen neck glands, difficulty swallowing or talking, unusual tastes or smells, and thirst. To keep the mouth and eyes moist, drink lots of fluids, use eye drops, and maintain good oral hygiene and eye care.

Neuromuscular diseases

Many autoimmune diseases target the nervous system, causing widespread symptoms throughout the body. Two of the most common autoimmune neuromuscular diseases are multiple sclerosis and myasthenia gravis.

Multiple sclerosis (MS)

MS is a chronic disease of the nervous system that affects mostly young and middle-aged women, damaging the protective sheaths covering nerves in the brain and spinal cord. More than 300,000 Americans now have the disease, which causes a variety of symptoms, including paralysis, eye problems, speech defects, and shaky movements. It's one

Unofficially... Treating rodents orally with copolymer 1 prevents the onset of autoimmune encephalomyelitis, paving the way for the development of the first oral treatment for MS in humans, according to research published in the March 30, 1999 issue of Proceedings of the National Academy of Science.

of the most common neurological disorders affecting young people, first appearing between the ages of 20 and 40. MS is the leading cause of disability among young adults.

While MS is more typically considered to be an autoimmune disease, not an infectious disease, some experts have suspected a slow virus or a bacterium as a potential cause.

Symptoms begin with numbness, weakness, tingling, or paralysis in one or more limbs, impaired vision and eye pain, tremors, lack of coordination or unsteady gait and rapid involuntary eye movement. A history of at least two episodes of a cluster of symptoms is necessary for a diagnosis of MS.

Scientists suspect that one way to treat MS is to block autoimmune cells before they can attack the myelin sheath, for it's in the progressive splitting and swelling of the myelin sheath that the disruption begins. Myelin is a protective sheath that covers literally every nerve in the body. Other treatments include the drug baclofen, which is used to suppress muscle spasticity, and corticosteroids to help reduce inflammation. Interferons also are being used to treat this disease.

MS patients treated with the experimental drug novatrone suffered fewer attacks and were able to delay the disease progression longer than those who took placebo. Even during the third year of follow-up, patients taking novatrone had fewer attacks than those taking placebo.

Myasthenia gravis

This chronic autoimmune disorder is characterized by gradual muscle weakness, often appearing first in the face. It occurs three times more often in women than in men and usually shows up after repetitive use of a muscle, with the weakness fluctuating during the day. Women generally contract this condition between the ages of 20 and 30, while in men it occurs between the ages of 60 and 70.

This disease is caused by a problem in neuromuscular transmission as antibodies form in the muscle membranes, decreasing response to neurotransmitters. Symptoms may involve just the eye muscles, with drooping eyelids and double vision, or may also include facial, swallowing, and speech muscles, causing problems with breathing, talking, chewing, and swallowing.

The condition is diagnosed in part by an injection of the drug edrophonium, which can partially reverse the weakness. If the patient responds to the drug, it's considered to be an indication that the disease is present.

Treatment may include anticholinesterase drugs, plasmapheresis, steroids, and medications designed to suppress the immune system, along with daily rest periods to improve muscle strength. The disease may spontaneously reverse itself, but usually only for short periods.

Endocrine diseases

The endocrine system is responsible for coordinating the body's physiology; autoimmune diseases of this body system affect specific endocrine glands. Hashimoto's thyroiditis (low thyroid function) and Graves' disease (overactive thyroid function), are among the most common endocrine autoimmune diseases.

The disorders develop gradually (it may be several years before vague symptoms begin to appear). Your doctor will diagnose endocrine autoimmunity problems by assessing symptoms and measuring

Watch Out!
Thyroid disease boosts your risk of osteoporosis; if you have a thyroid disease, make sure you get enough calcium, get plenty of exercise, and regular bone-density testing.

hormone levels; antibody tests can confirm the diagnosis. Treatment for endocrine autoimmunity usually consists of hormone replacement or agents to suppress overactive glands.

Hashimoto's thyroiditis

The underlying cause of Hashimoto's thyroiditis is an autoimmune reaction to proteins in the thyroid (the gland that helps set your metabolic rate). As in many autoimmune diseases, there's evidence of a genetic tendency to develop the condition.

The disease, which affects women 50 times more often than men, may occur with other autoimmune diseases, such as pernicious anemia, diabetes, or adrenal insufficiency. Low levels of thyroid hormone cause mental and physical impairment, greater sensitivity to cold, weight gain, coarsening of the skin, and goiter (a swelling of the neck due to an enlarged thyroid gland). The disease process can eventually destroy the thyroid, but typically women have an enlarged thyroid gland with normal or mildly abnormal thyroid function tests. (Just because the gland is enlarged doesn't mean it's not destroyed. And all glands have mechanisms in the pituitary that will compensate for disease to a great extent, which is why women with severe disease may have only slightly abnormal thyroid levels.) It's treated with thyroid hormone replacement therapy.

Graves' disease

Graves' disease is one of the most common autoimmune diseases, affecting 13 million people and targeting women seven times as often as men, usually between the ages of 20 and 30. Patients with Graves' disease (among them, former First Lady Barbara Bush) produce too much thyroid hormone, which leads to bulging eyes and neck. Thyroid hormone plays a major role in metabolism.

Mild forms of the disease can include symptoms such as nervousness, heat intolerance, diarrhea, sweating, insomnia, and weight loss with increased appetite. More serious complications may include irregular heart beat, tachycardia (increased heart beat), tremor and atrial fibrillation, extreme sensitivity to light, swelling in the legs and eyes, and clubbed fingers. The eyes may have a bulging, staring appearance or a surprised expression. In rare situations, there may be cardiovascular collapse and shock or coma.

The condition is treated with radioiodine, antithyroid drug therapy or the surgical removal of the thyroid gland. Graves' disease may transform itself into Hashimoto's over time, since treatments directed at suppressing an over-active thyroid may eventually reduce thyroid function below normal. These individuals may then be treated with thyroxine replacement. Individuals with other autoimmune diseases, such as lupus, rheumatoid arthritis, vitiligo, myasthenia gravis, IDDM, etc., are more likely to also develop thyroid autoimmunity.

Insulin-dependent (type 1) diabetes mellitus (IDDM)

IDDM is a chronic autoimmune endocrine disease that usually begins in childhood or young adulthood and is more common in women. While it's fairly rare (this type of diabetes accounts for less than 5 percent of diabetes cases), it has a much greater impact on a woman's life than the more common adult-onset type of diabetes. Insulin-dependent diabetes is also called type I diabetes, juvenile diabetes, and diabetes mellitus.

Watch Out! Having diabetes doubles your risk for heart disease and increases your risk of stroke.

No one knows exactly why, but it's clear that a diabetic's own immune system turns against itself. The body's T cells begin to attack pancreas islet cells, contributing to diabetes. Most people inherit traits that put them at risk for IDDM, but not everyone who inherits these traits develops the condition; one or more factors in the environment probably trigger the immune system to destroy the insulin-producing cells. In some cases, the trigger may be a viral infection, but in most cases, the trigger for diabetes is unknown.

Whatever the reason, diabetes occurs when the pancreas produces too little insulin, causing severe thirst, increased urination, weight loss, fatigue, nausea, vomiting, and frequent infections. The American Diabetes Association recommends routine screening for everyone at age 45 with one of the following tests:

- Fasting blood glucose: A blood sample is tested for sugar after you have stopped eating for between 10 and 16 hours. A measure of 126 mg/dL indicates diabetes (if confirmed with a repeat test on a different day).

- Nonfasting blood glucose: This blood test can be taken anytime, whether you've eaten or not. A reading above 200 mg/dL would confirm diabetes if the results are the same on a different day (in presence of symptoms).

- Glucose tolerance test: After the first blood sample is drawn, the patient drinks a solution containing 100 mg of glucose, after which blood is drawn every 30 minutes for two hours, and then every hour for four hours. This reveals how your body processes sugar. A level above

200 mg/dL may mean you have diabetes; if the result is confirmed by a test on a second day, you have diabetes.

- Urine test: A test of urine to detect ketones, a byproduct produced in diabetes (and also in starvation and dehydration). Ketones aren't used to diagnose diabetes but can help guide insulin therapy.

Diabetes type I is treated with aggressive control of exercise, diet, and insulin; oral medications are often used in adult-onset diabetes.

Bright Idea
A healthy diabetes diet has 50 to 60 percent of its calories from complex carbohydrates (breads, fruits, and vegetables); 12 to 20 percent from protein, and no more than 30 percent from fats, according to the American Diabetic Association.

Inflammatory bowel disease

Inflammatory bowel disease (IBD) includes two autoimmune disorders of the small intestine—Crohn's disease and ulcerative colitis. These nonspecific inflammatory diseases of the bowel are strongly suspected of having an underlying autoimmune factor in some cases.

The conditions seem to run in families, and family members of a person with IBD have an increased risk of developing the problem. Stress may aggravate the condition, but it's not considered a cause.

The diseases are treated with antidiarrheal pills or bulk formers for mild cases. For more serious cases, anti-inflammatory drugs are effective. Corticosteroids are reserved for acute flare-ups. In some instances, surgery may be required to remove obstructions or to repair a perforation of the colon.

Crohn's disease

Symptoms of Crohn's disease include persistent diarrhea, abdominal pain, fever, and general fatigue. In both Crohn's and ulcerative colitis, there is a risk of significant weight loss and malnutrition.

Ulcerative colitis

Symptoms of ulcerative colitis involve bloody diarrhea, pain, urgent bowel movements, joint pains, and skin lesions. Because of the chronic inflammation of the wall of the colon, it may become thickened and develop scar tissue. The patient may develop polyplike structures as a result of the extended chronic inflammatory response. Moreover, patients with ulcerative colitis also have an increased risk of developing colon cancer.

Autoimmune skin diseases

The skin is one of the first places that symptoms of an autoimmune disease show up. In many of the diseases discussed above, the skin isn't seriously involved, but in others, the skin is the primary site of the disease.

Psoriasis

Psoriasis is one of the most common autoimmune skin diseases, caused by a malfunction in the life cycle of skin cells. The process of skin cell production, which normally takes about a month, is accelerated to several days, resulting in a buildup of thick scales. Psoriasis, which may have a genetic component, waxes and wanes (often in response to sun exposure). It's considered mild if 10 percent or less of the body is affected; psoriasis in more than 30 percent of the body is considered severe.

In mild cases, limited sun exposure can be enough to clear up the problem. Topical medications include steroids, emollients, vitamin D, or coal tar and are used for mild to moderate cases, either alone or with ultraviolet light. For more severe cases, topical treatments are combined with chemotherapy, ultraviolet A light, and oral medications such as Tegison.

Vitiligo

Vitiligo has only recently been identified as an autoimmune skin disease. It occurs when the body produces antibodies directed against the pigment-producing cells (melanocytes), hence destroying them and causing the skin to lighten. Vitiligo is 10 to 15 times more common in patients with other autoimmune diseases and is also associated with thyroid disorders. It has a tendency to run in families and may follow unusual trauma, especially to the head. The disease may also be referred to as leukoderma.

Makeup can disguise the disease, and in mild cases, no further treatment is needed. Phototherapy may induce repigmentation in more than half the cases, but many treatments are needed. Corticosteroid creams also may help. If the skin depigmentation is extensive, topical chemicals may be used to remove pigment from remaining areas of involved skin.

Other autoimmune diseases

Scientists are currently studying a wide range of other illnesses that may prove to be autoimmune diseases.

Chronic fatigue syndrome

Chronic fatigue syndrome (CFS), also called chronic Epstein-Barr, is an inflammatory illness causing exhausting fatigue that is suspected (but not proved) to have an autoimmune component. The Epstein-Barr virus has been implicated as a possible cause for this syndrome. The exhaustion comes on suddenly, and may be relentless or relapsing, causing a debilitating tiredness and weakness that can last for months.

Bright Idea
Women with CFS should try to maintain a healthy lifestyle, with a good diet, plenty of rest, and exercise.

CFS usually includes symptoms in addition to fatigue that may resemble viral illness, such as headache, sore throat, low grade fever, tender lymph glands, muscle and joint aches, and concentration problems. Symptoms do not get worse with time. Because chronic fatigue and these other symptoms are common to many other illnesses (especially those that are autoimmune) doctors must first rule out other diseases, including lupus, MS, Lyme disease, AIDS, antiphospholipid syndrome, thyroid disease, rheumatoid arthritis, fibromyositis, and depression.

The syndrome affects twice as many women as men from all ages, races, and income levels. It was first reported among well-educated women in their 30s, but it is found among all ages and socioeconomic groups. Although the illness sometimes breaks out in groups, the vast majority of people who work and live closely with persons who have CFS don't get sick. It's not considered to be easily contagious, although some experts believe a common virus may be involved in the development of CFS, in combination with a genetic predisposition to acquire the illness.

While there is no effective treatment for CFS, some doctors report slight success with antiviral drugs, antidepressants, and drugs that boost the immune system.

Sarcoidosis

Sarcoidosis is a chronic autoimmune disease that may affect many body systems. It is characterized by small round spots (tubercles) of dead tissue, which is why it is sometimes misdiagnosed as tuberculosis.

Not all cases of sarcoidosis are alike. Some patients have few (if any) symptoms, while others experience many problems. Although sarcoidosis may go away spontaneously without treatment, most people will have it all their lives. There is no cure at this time, but sarcoidosis can be controlled with medications.

Sarcoidosis occurs predominantly between the ages of 20 and 40. There are about 25,000 cases in the United States, most of which are in the southeastern part of the country. The disease varies in severity, may affect any part of the body, and is most common among people of northern European ancestry and African Americans.

Sarcoidosis is now suspected of being an autoimmune disease triggered by an agent, such as a slow virus or possibly a variety of other toxic agents. Genetic predisposition may also be an important factor in its development.

Vasculitis syndromes

This broad group of diseases is characterized by an inflammation of the blood vessel system, believed to be triggered by an autoimmune response. Vasculitis may occur alone, in combination with an allergic reaction, or with other autoimmune diseases; it may be confined to one organ or involve several organ systems.

As chronic inflammation narrows the inside of the blood vessel, it obstructs the flow of blood to the tissue. The lack of blood may damage the tissues, form clots, or weaken or rupture the vessel wall.

Arteries and veins of all sizes and in all parts of the body may be affected. Vasculitis may occur in one area or all over the body, including in major organs such as the lungs, kidneys, heart, and brain. It may develop as an autoimmune disease itself or as a complication of many other autoimmune diseases.

Some forms of vasculitis may be caused by allergy or hypersensitivity to medications (such as sulfa drugs or penicillin), toxins, or other inhaled irritants. Other forms of the condition may be triggered by infection, parasites, or viral infections.

Hematologic autoimmune diseases

Blood also can be affected by an autoimmune disorder. In autoimmune hemolytic anemia, red blood cells are prematurely destroyed by antibodies. Other autoimmune diseases of the blood include autoimmune thrombocytopenic purpura and autoimmune neutropenia. Autoimmune thrombocytopenic purpura, which occurs in a chronic state three times more often among women, is a disease associated with a low platelet count. It occurs when too many platelets are destroyed and too few are produced. Patients tend to bruise easily and have nosebleeds, heavy periods, and bleeding gums—hence the name "purpura," meaning "purplish patches." About 20 percent of those afflicted recover spontaneously; the rest have remissions and recurrences. Autoimmune neutropenia is a disease associated with a low white cell count leading to fever, malaise, mouth ulcers, and often have repeated non-life-threatening infections of the skin, mouth, and upper respiratory tract.

Autoimmunity and infertility

As many as 50 to 60 percent of unexplained cases of infertility may in fact be caused by autoimmune problems. But because infertile women aren't routinely screened for autoimmune diseases, doctors do not have systematic data on the association of autoimmune disease with reproductive failure. Autoimmunity is also a major cause of miscarriages.

Tips for managing autoimmune disease

If you follow a few basic suggestions, you'll be better equipped to manage your autoimmune disorder:

- Ask questions: Understand your illness and the treatment plan. Ask questions about your particular condition, especially what changes and symptoms you can expect.

- Comply with treatment: If you're not sure of the treatment, don't be afraid to ask questions or get a second—or third—opinion. Ask questions about the side effects of medications and medical tests and the impact or benefit they'll have on your condition.

- Report symptoms: Let your doctor know if you have a new symptom. Don't worry that your doctor will think you're a chronic complainer—it's much better to discuss what's going on and how symptoms might be treated than to worry about what your doctor will think.

- Don't be intimidated: Your doctor is your partner in fighting your disease. Be honest about how you feel; you only hurt yourself if you lie to your doctor.

- Be a partner: Play a role in your treatment plan. Once satisfied that the plan is right for you, follow it.

- Pace yourself: Fatigue is common in autoimmune diseases. Learn how to pace yourself so you can control your illness. Listen to your body and stop before you feel tired. Regulating your activities can help you sustain a relatively normal and consistent energy level.

- Follow your diet: If your autoimmune disease requires a special diet, follow it. Understanding

Bright Idea
Learn to spread out your work load—you will be able to accomplish as much, if not more, while feeling better. Resting only when you're sick and then trying madly to catch up can make it harder to manage the disease and wind up boosting your need for medication.

the need for your diet will put you more in control and allow you to better manage your disease.

- Understand your emotions: You can expect to have a variety of emotional responses ranging from anger, denial, bargaining, depression, and acceptance. You may feel isolated or afraid about the future. Be open with friends and family, and don't blame everything that goes wrong on your illness.

- Use "I" messages: If you're not feeling well, say "I'm not feeling well and I could really use some help." Avoid "You" messages, which are usually interpreted defensively.

- Take time to adjust: Nobody adapts overnight to a chronic condition. Realize that you might experience feelings of worthlessness, depression, and self-pity, and that it is normal to experience these feelings.

- Get support: Join a group for women with chronic illness. Mental health counseling may help if you find you can't cope.

- It's not your fault: Understand that you didn't do anything to cause your illness—life's just not always fair. Bad things do happen to almost everyone.

What's new on the research horizon?

Autoimmune diseases run the gamut from mild to disabling to potentially life threatening. Nearly all affect women at far greater rates than men. The question before the scientific community is, why?

We've come a long way in the diagnosis and treatment of autoimmune disease, but more work is needed, especially in the areas of discovering the causes and developing more effective treatments and prevention strategies. Unfortunately, these diseases are significantly understudied when you consider how many people suffer from them and the number of new cases diagnosed each year. Despite the fact that more people have some form of autoimmune disease than have AIDS, the National Institutes of Health doesn't maintain an autoimmune disease study group—by comparison, there are seven such study groups for AIDS.

Nevertheless, there have been some exciting breakthroughs in research focusing on new treatments for autoimmune diseases. Scientists are currently studying drugs that act more specifically on the immune system, perhaps by blocking a particular hypersensitivity reaction. Other new treatments on the horizon include genetically engineered molecules, bone marrow transplants, and immunosuppressive therapies.

Unofficially...
Over the past seven years, several new biotechnology companies have begun to develop new treatments for autoimmune diseases, including AutoImmune, Inc., LaJolla Pharmaceutical, Anergen, and BioGen.

Just the facts

- One out of every eight women has some form of autoimmune disease.
- Autoimmune diseases can be hard to diagnose because many of the symptoms are varied and vague, and many patients appear to be healthy.
- Some autoimmune diseases seem to have a genetic component, making the possibility of developing one more likely if there is a family history of any.
- Autoimmune diseases appear to be linked to hormones, genetics, and environmental triggers, although the exact causes are not known.

PART V

The Ticking Clock: Women and Aging

GET THE SCOOP ON...
Your aging skin ▪ The ins and outs of laser resurfacing ▪ The pros and cons of fruit acids ▪ Removing unwanted hair ▪ The safety of hair dyes ▪ Your memory: Use it or lose it

What to Expect as You Age

As you age, do you think you're getting better or are you just getting older—and fast? Knowing what to expect can help prepare for changes that crop up with each passing year. These changes include alterations in your skin—it's drier, and more prone to wrinkles, discoloration, and funny red patches. Your hair—it may be much thinner, falling out, or turning gray (or even white). Many women do lose their hair, although not in the same way as men, and the products that can boost thinning hair for men don't work for women. Then there's your memory—are you really losing your mind, or does it just seem that way?

Younger-looking skin: The eternal quest

It seems like yesterday we were all broiling on the beach, pouring pure olive oil on unprotected skin in the pursuit of the perfect tan. Today, we're older, wiser, and a good deal more wrinkly. (Wrinkles are caused by reduced collagen production and loss of elasticity of the skin.) In fact, American women fork over more than $3.7 billion a year in their quest for better-looking skin. On the theory that if a small amount is good, more must be better, many women slather on all sorts of these revolutionary skin care products and makeup in all kinds of combinations.

"The bottom line is that people will do whatever is within their means to look the best they can," explained Jeffrey S. Dover, M.D., an associate professor of dermatology at Harvard Medical School and director of the Cosmetic Surgery and Laser Center at Beth Israel Deaconess Medical Center in Boston. "There are a bunch of effective products now on the market that were not available even five years ago that can help them do that."

Laser resurfacing

As we age, most women begin to show signs of routine aging—skin starts to sag and turn a sallow color, as sun-induced brown discoloration and wrinkling begin. In the past, a woman wanting to erase the signs of aging from her skin had only two choices: chemical peels or dermabrasion.

Unfortunately, neither chemical peels nor dermabrasion (a procedure in which a spinning wheel or brush removes layers of skin) could be controlled as well as doctors would like. Today there's a third option: Laser resurfacing, one of the newest techniques for removing medium-to-fine wrinkles using a special pulsed or scanned laser. With these laser treatments, up to 50 percent of a woman's wrinkles and discolorations can fade away. Women get the best results with wrinkles and scars that are sharply defined and shallow.

The pulsed CO_2 laser works by emitting a very brief pulse of high-intensity light that's fast enough to limit heat damage to the skin, yet strong enough to vaporize tissue cleanly. Since the heat penetrates the skin no deeper than one-half the thickness of a human hair, it can remove the wrinkled skin layer by layer without scarring. New lasers developed since the early 1990s pulse or scan rapidly, lingering on cells for less than 1/10,000 of a second. By vaporizing thinner layers than were previously possible, doctors can remove layers of skin with little damage to surrounding tissue. The procedure can be done on an outpatient basis and takes only about 30 minutes to an hour.

Both the discolorations and wrinkling of aging respond very well to the laser's vaporizing action in the hands of a skilled doctor. The laser also is useful for scars from acne or injury, precancerous spots, and some benign growths.

How it works

If you want to understand skin resurfacing, think of what happens when your city's road crew comes around to resurface a road. First, the outer layer of the pavement is broken up and removed, replaced by a new, smooth surface. Laser skin resurfacing works on the same principle. As lasers remove the sun-damaged outer layers of skin, natural regeneration produces smooth, fresh tissue. Health care professionals theorize that shrinkage of underlying collagen tissue may help explain why the new skin appears tighter.

Although laser resurfacing has been available for just a few years (at first, in only a few locations), there has been no shortage of patients, despite the cost (which ranges from $1,000 to $5,000, depending on the extent of treatment—and it's not usually covered by insurance). The experiences of these

Unofficially...
Another version of the laser (the scanned CO_2 laser) doesn't produce a pulse of laser light, but utilizes mirrors to rapidly scan the laser spot in a spiral. While experts don't yet have enough information to make direct comparisons between the two versions, both appear to achieve impressive results.

women are forming the basis for refining laser use, together with the few short-term studies that have been completed and the larger ones under way.

The pros and cons

As more data are collected, health care providers are learning more about the side effects of skin resurfacing. Lasers used for some other procedures leave few telltale signs of surgery and the affected area heals quickly—but that's not the case with lasers used in skin resurfacing. For days after the surgery, women should be prepared to look terrible—as if they've had steel wool rubbed vigorously on their faces. There is oozing, swelling, and redness. The first phase of recovery generally takes from 10 to 14 days, depending on the extent of the treatment and the patient's overall health. During this time, you should take off from work and stay at home to rest.

Also during that time, you'll need to repeatedly soak your skin and apply salves to the treated area to ease burning discomfort and speed healing. To prevent infection, you'll need to take an antibiotic and an antiviral drug, both before the surgery and for a week afterward. Redness tends to last about three months. People who tan easily also seem vulnerable to excessive pigmentation, which usually goes away with retinoic acid and hydroquinone cream within a few weeks or months. Some women also experience lightening of the skin. Scarring is uncommon, but as with all surgical procedures, it is possible.

Because the procedure is relatively new, there aren't many long-term follow-up studies, and the next generation of lasers is already in development. But for now, health care providers say they are seeing extremely good results in the hands of the right practitioners, with faster healing time and fewer complications than previous skin-rejuvenating procedures.

Finding the best doctor

The most important thing you can do if you're thinking about having laser resurfacing is to find a good, experienced doctor to do the procedure. After ads and news stories first trumpeted good early results with laser resurfacing, thousands of consumers began demanding the treatments. This sent floods of doctors to weekend courses in how to use the devices. With this hurry-up push to learn the technique quickly came frightening tales of discoloration and scarring, and of doctors ill-equipped to deal with side effects.

Remember—any doctor can attend laser courses in resurfacing, not just dermatologists and plastic surgeons. Although these doctors may quickly learn the basics of the procedure, a doctor who is not board certified in a specialty relating to skin and cosmetic surgery may not be the best person to perform the procedure or to help you if side effects develop.

Questions to ask

Before you choose a doctor to work on your face, there's a number of things you need to find out first:

- How many cases of skin resurfacing has the doctor done?

- Ask to see before-and-after pictures of patients the doctor has treated, ideally with the "after" picture at least six months beyond the surgery.

- Ask for phone numbers of at least three patients the doctor has treated—and call them.

Bright Idea
For a list of dermatologists qualified to perform laser resurfacing, call the toll-free hot line maintained by the American Society for Dermatologic Surgery at 800/441-2737.

- Find out where the doctor learned to use the laser. It's best if a doctor who is new to the procedure has spent time observing an experienced doctor, treating several patients under that doctor's supervision.

Although you may feel awkward asking these questions, remember that you are putting your face in this person's hands. If a doctor balks at any one of these questions, that's a red flag. Leave and find another doctor. Remember, resurfacing isn't magic; it takes skill and even a sense of artistry to manipulate the laser across the face. Although the process takes only an hour or two in a doctor's office, it's still surgery and requires at least several weeks for healing.

Collagen treatments

Collagen treatment is a temporary way to reduce wrinkles, lines, and scars and to improve soft tissue contours. Because collagen is broken down by the body, repeated injections may be necessary to maintain a more youthful appearance. Found naturally in the body as an important building block of the skin, a highly purified form of injectable collagen was first introduced in 1981. This collagen is derived from cows and is marketed under the trade names Zyderm and Zyplast.

Other types of collagen include Autologen, an injectable form of collagen derived from the patient's own skin, and Dermalogen, a human collagen product designed to provide a matrix to support growth of the patient's own collagen.

Tiny drops of thick collagen are injected via a fine needle underneath the skin to replace collagen lost by the body. During this injection, some patients may feel some stinging. The entire procedure may take between 2 and 10 minutes; you will recover in up to three hours. After treatment, there may be some redness lasting up to 10 days; a few patients also experience bruising, temporary stinging, burning feelings, faint redness, swelling, or fullness. Others have no reaction at all.

One of the least painful ways to temporarily erase wrinkles, collagen injection results last only between 3 and 18 months (averaging about six months). The price varies depending on the part of the country where the procedure is done.

As with all cosmetic surgery, there are risks and potential complications, a thorough discussion of which is an essential part of the consultation process.

Unofficially...
Applying collagen directly to the skin has no proven benefit other than as a moisturizer; it must be injected in order to work.

Botox injections

Botox is a purified form of the toxin that causes botulism, which has been studied as a possible wrinkle remover. When injected locally into a muscle, Botox produces a reversible paralysis of that muscle. In studies, when the substance was injected into the faces of subjects interested in smoothing their skin, it appeared to temporarily paralyze the muscles beneath frown lines and crow's feet. This prevents them from contracting fully, giving a smoother, less furrowed face, the effects of which last between three and six months.

The U.S. Food and Drug Administration (FDA) has approved Botox for use in treating certain eye conditions and disorders of the facial nerve in patients aged 12 and above, but it has not approved its use in wrinkle treatments. Botox as a wrinkle treatment is considered to be an "off label" use in treating expression lines of the face and neck. (It's

> [Using Botox as a wrinkle remedy is] an egregious example of promoting a potentially toxic biologic for cosmetic purposes.
> —Food and Drug Administration, Federal Register notice, Nov. 18, 1994.

used especially to treat wrinkles at the base of the nose, forehead wrinkles, and crow's feet.)

Botox injections are performed in a health care practitioner's office. The substance is injected directly into the muscle via a small needle. Patients usually return to work that day and, in most cases, can participate in a social engagement that evening.

There are risks associated with Botox; however, complications are usually temporary because of the nonpermanent nature of the treatment. The only side effect researchers have reported is a feeling of heaviness in the face of a few patients that lasted for a few weeks. The technique has critics other than the FDA who charge that the slackened muscles can give patients a blank, lifeless look. More seriously, in the hands of inexperienced practitioners, Botox treatments could partly paralyze a person's face.

Dermabrasion

Dermabrasion is used to decrease fine wrinkling or acne scars by using a sort of high-speed sanding. It's the most dramatic resurfacing technique available, and it leaves the skin relatively smooth.

The skin is first numbed with a local anesthetic and with an abrasive wheel, wire brush, or diamond attachment rotating at high speeds, the dermatologist removes layer after layer of skin to reach the smooth skin underneath the wrinkle or scar. The skin heals in about two weeks, although the full effect of the treatment isn't apparent for two months. Pain isn't considered to be a problem, but many women are bothered by the red, raw appearance of the skin that lasts for at least 10 days after the procedure. As with other type of facial peels, dermabrasion may cost several thousand dollars.

Skin peels

Chemical peels typically use trichloroacetic acid, phenol, resorcinol, and salicylic acid to help remove undesirable signs of skin aging, such as discoloration, roughness, and wrinkling. The chemicals cause the skin to shed its outer layer, revealing a fresher-looking layer of skin underneath. Known as chemical exfoliation, the procedure is done in doctors' offices so they can control the process and prevent deep skin burns from the highly acidic solutions.

Chemical peels are often used for more severe cases of adult acne, age spots, and wrinkles. Used less often now (in favor of laser resurfacing), the technique is somewhat less popular because it's basically a controlled second-degree burn using a caustic chemical. It may seem no more harmful than getting a facial, but, in fact, a chemical peel is surgery, using potent chemicals that actually dissolve the top layer of skin, erasing irregular pigmentation and fine cheek wrinkles and tiny lines above the upper lip.

After the peel, a thick crust develops and lasts for about a week, but the purple-red skin color may take six months to fade away. It is a painful, emotionally difficult process to endure, but after the skin heals, the result is pinker, tighter, smoother, and relatively wrinkle- and blemish-free skin, which may remain younger looking for 15 years or more.

The procedure isn't for everybody; women with dark or olive skin may end up with a blotchy appearance and those with poor liver, heart, or kidney function could be affected by the solution that strips away the upper layers of the skin and is absorbed into the blood.

Unofficially...
A surface (or freshening) peel is more like a superficial facial, leaving the skin glowing for a week or two, but not going deep enough to erase wrinkles.

No matter what sort of peel you're interested in, you should make sure your doctor is a board-certified dermatologist who has the ability and experience to perform the technique, since it takes a great deal of expertise to apply a good chemical peel. You should ask whether the procedure makes up a large portion of the person's practice. Ask how many peels the doctor does in a week, and how he or she learned to do the procedure. The cost of a peel ranges from $200 to $3,000 depending on how much and how deeply the skin is treated, and the area of the country where the doctor practices.

When the chemical peel isn't for you...

If you're interested in a facial peel but the thought of caustic chemicals makes you hesitate, you may be interested in the newest products on the market that do basically the same thing in a milder way. These are alpha-, beta- and poly-hydroxy acids, vitamin A derivatives, and vitamin C. These new products really do produce some biological activity in the skin. Each work at a different level of the skin in a different way. For that reason, they are often used together in a treatment plan (but not at the same time).

Vitamin A derivatives

The strongest and potentially most irritating of all the new skin care products designed to improve the appearance of the skin are the vitamin A derivatives Retin-A (tretinoin) and Renova (tretinoin emollient cream), the first FDA-approved skin cream to reduce the appearance of wrinkles.

Retin-A and Renova, available by prescription only, reduce the appearance of wrinkles, mottled dark spots, and rough facial skin. They can eliminate wrinkles, repair sun-damaged skin, or restore skin to its healthier younger structure. (They work wonders in the treatment of acne as well.) The most effective of all the new skin care products, they work by boosting cell turnover. As a result, they can be irritating: Skin can swell, turn red, peel, itch, and burn, especially in the beginning.

Because Retin-A is so drying and irritating to the skin, dermatologists don't recommend combining it with any other topical anti-acne product, skin soaps, cleansers, preparations or cosmetics, or with etretinate. Women who do so risk severe skin irritation. By applying Retin-A (or its milder cousin, Renova) at night and then going to bed without adding anything else to the skin, women can get the benefit of the tretinoin without the risk of added irritation.

The safety of daily Renova use for longer than 48 weeks has not been established, and it should not be used by women who are pregnant or trying to become pregnant. Renova use has not been studied in people 50 and older or in people with moderately or darkly pigmented skin.

Vitamin A-like products

Some products are related to the vitamin-A derivatives, but they aren't the same thing at all. The most popular of these nonprescription items contain "retinol palmitate," a cousin of retinoic acid. Retinol palmitate is not as effective as retinoic acid in helping aged skin, although experts believe it probably does affect the skin to some degree.

Because these products are available without prescription, cost less than Retin-A, and aren't as irritating, they are popular with the public.

Keep in mind that, while the labels may say that a particular cream "contains vitamin A," the active

Bright Idea
While some dermatologists don't recommend it, you could use a moisturizer after Retin-A if your skin is very dry, according to Kathy Fields, M.D., instructor of dermatology at University of California, San Francisco. The Retin-A will probably be slightly less potent but you can still get the benefits.

ingredient is retinol palmitate—not Retin-A. If your cosmetician or hairdresser tells you that retinol palmitate is "a non-prescription Retin-A," that's not true. It's a close cousin, but it's much less effective.

Do-it-yourself peels: Fruit acids

You've probably seen the ads on TV and in magazines—the new "wonder ingredient" in modern cosmetics that is said to take years off your looks. But do they really work—and are they safe?

To some degree, these new fruit acids (called alpha-, beta-, and poly-hydroxy acids) really seem to have an effect on the skin. A recent, large double-blind study has shown that an eight percent alpha-hydroxy acid (AHA) product applied to the skin reversed skin aging in 74 women aged 40 to 70. Daily AHA use clearly improved their skin with limited but measurable anti-aging effects. After six months, the women had an improvement in skin quality and thickness.

AHA is a generic term that refers to any one of several organic "fruit acid" chemicals that serve as a sort of mild chemical peel, loosening dead skin cells so as to expose newer, fresher skin. In six to eight weeks, skin treated with AHA appears softer and smoother, while age spots and freckles seem to fade. The acids can be applied to the skin as an ointment, cream, or lotion. The extent of exfoliation depends on the type and concentration of the AHA, its pH level (acidity), and other ingredients in the product. Most cosmetics sold to consumers contain AHAs at levels up to 10 percent.

AHA cosmetics are derived from the "chemical peels" that dermatologists and plastic surgeons have used for years. Cosmetic manufacturers began to market similar but milder versions of these chemical peels containing AHAs for salon and at-home use around 1989. They quickly caught on, and by 1992, mass marketing had begun. Today, almost every cosmetic company has AHA products. There used to be only three product lines; now there are 20 or more.

AHAs are commonly found in human skin and plants. While synthetic varieties are available, most skin products use AHAs from plant sources. Commonly used AHAs include malic (apples), ascorbic (various fruits), glycolic (sugar cane), gluconolactone (plants), lactic (milk) and tartatic (red wine) acids. Marine sources of AHAs, including certain varieties of seaweed, are also used for skin care products. The AHAs used most often in cosmetics are glycolic acid and lactic acid. Increasingly, manufacturers are using poly-AHAs, which have larger molecules and ingredients such as salicylic acid, because these products may produce less skin irritation.

Less irritating than the tretinoin products, the alpha- and beta-hydroxy acids in lower concentrations help to prevent or reverse signs of sun damage and aging, but they work differently than either Retin-A or retinol palmitate. While the acids aren't as good as Retin-A at removing wrinkles, AHAs can still help prevent and treat fine wrinkles, according to some dermatologists.

Beta-hydroxy acids (BHAs) are a close cousin to the AHAs and have been used to treat acne and warts for many years. Face creams containing BHAs are usually sold over the counter in a two-percent solution, which is strong enough to remove the skin's outer layers. BHAs are stronger than AHAs, penetrating the skin more deeply.

Scientists don't understand exactly how the acids interact with the skin, but the products seem to improve the skin's appearance by speeding up the

Bright Idea
How can you tell if your AHA product will work? If you put a product containing AHA on the skin and it doesn't sting a little, it probably has too low of a pH and it won't be effective.

natural process of shedding dead skin cells. If you use them often enough, they can soften tiny lines around your eyes and mouth, smooth dry skin, and fade dark spots caused by the sun or hormonal changes. You'll get faster results in your dermatologist's office (since doctors can use the stronger products).

In beauty shops, you can find concentrations up to 40 percent; your dermatologist can use an AHA up to a concentration of 70 percent. Some experts recommend starting at home with a 4-percent AHA product, switching to a stronger 8-percent product once your skin has gotten used to the acid. Some companies have introduced a four-step method that gradually acclimates your skin to the higher acid level. Keep in mind, however, that some experts don't think any of these over-the-counter products are really strong enough to do much more than soften the skin.

It's important to note the pH of cosmetic formulations containing AHAs. For example, a moisturizer containing 5 percent lactic acid will affect skin differently depending on the pH of the formulation. That is, a 5-percent lactic acid moisturizer at pH 6.0 (slightly acidic) is nonirritating, while at pH 1.0 (100,000 times more acidic), it is very irritating. Most cosmetic AHA formulations are adjusted between pH 3 and 4, both of which have been clinically shown to be effective.

In general, cosmetic concentration AHAs can improve the look of your skin if you use them every day. You should see some improvement in less than a month and see clear benefits after six months of daily use. Fruit-acid peels are sometimes used by "estheticians" (beauty school graduates who specialize in skin care) for exfoliating acne-damaged skin and darkened sun spots. Estheticians are also using AHAs to reverse premature aging. Unlike the use of cosmetic concentration AHAs, these stronger formulations are used for brief periods of time and are then thoroughly removed so as not to cause a chemical burn.

AHAs versus Retin-A

Retin-A (tretinoin) is a chemical derivative of vitamin A that has been shown to reverse photo-aging, including age spots. It has two major drawbacks, however: It can be very irritating and can damage skin that is later exposed to sunlight. Retin-A is available by prescription and your dermatologist may prescribe its use for certain conditions, such as adult acne. AHAs are not known to cause photosensitive skin reactions.

Of all the different fruit acids, some doctors think lactic acid has particular benefits. "I happen to think lactic acid is tremendously underused and the most effective of all these new products," according to Harvard dermatologist Jeffrey Dover, M.D. In one study in which Dr. Dover participated, patients used 12 percent lactic acid in the morning with Retin-A at night. "I have never seen such a dramatic improvement in my life," he commented. "I could pick out just by sight which women were using the lactic acid-Retin A combination; their skin had a particular glow."

Risks of AHAs

AHAs have been used extensively for skin care by dermatologists and estheticians for more than 30 years for treating dry skin. AHAs are generally considered to be safer to use than other chemicals typically chosen for chemical peels. But there are concerns about AHAs in home-care cosmetic products. Cosmetics that contain AHAs are widely used despite many unanswered questions about their

Watch Out!
Cosmetics manufacturers aren't required to submit safety data to the FDA before marketing products, although they bear the responsibility for manufacturing safe products.

safety. Legally, these products are considered to be cosmetics, not drugs, and therefore not regulated by the FDA.

While not as harsh as Retin A, the hydroxy acids can still redden or blister the skin. Lactic acid in particular is very irritating at its 12 percent prescription strength. Indeed, since 1989, the FDA has received more than 100 reports of adverse reactions in people using AHA products, ranging from severe redness, swelling (especially in the area of the eyes), burning, blistering, bleeding, rash, itching, and skin discoloration. The FDA believes reactions from AHAs are probably even more widespread, guessing there may be as many as 10,000 adverse reactions in people using AHA-containing products.

The FDA is concerned about AHAs because, unlike traditional cosmetics, AHAs seem capable of penetrating the skin barrier and affecting or changing the body structure—which would legally make them "drugs." In reviewing the limited data on AHAs, the FDA concluded in a 1996 report that certain formulations of AHA products can affect the skin more like chemical peels—that is, boosting cell turnover rate and decreasing the thickness of the outer skin. The effect depends on the product's pH level, the AHA concentration, and the cream containing the AHA, as well as how the product is used.

Because they are relatively new (they've been widely available only since about 1992), their long-term effects are unknown. In the spring of 1997, the National Toxicology Program of the National Institute of Environmental Science began a study of AHA safety.

Some people who had reported adverse reactions cited increased sun sensitivity. In addition, one industry-sponsored study found that participants whose skin was exposed to 4-percent glycolic acid twice daily for 12 weeks developed minimal skin redness with 13 percent less ultraviolet (UV) radiation exposure than normal. Three participants developed minimal redness with 50 percent less UV exposure than normal. Another study found that people using the AHA product in the sun had twice the cell damage in areas where the AHA had been applied than those who were treated with the non-AHA product.

Considering the questionable safety status, the FDA and dermatologists advise consumers who use AHA products to follow these precautions:

- Protect your skin: Use a sunscreen product with an SPF of at least 15. Wear a hat with a brim of at least four inches. Cover up with lightweight, loose-fitting, long-sleeved shirts and pants.

- Read labels: Check for a list of ingredients to see which AHA or other chemical acids are in the product, the name and address of the manufacturer or distributor, and AHA concentration and pH level. (The first is mandatory; the second and third are optional.)

- Test the product on your skin: Do a skin-sensitivity test on a patch of skin if you're using an AHA product for the first time, or are using a different brand or a product with a different concentration or pH than you're used to.

- Reactions: Stop using the product immediately if you experience adverse reactions, including sharp stinging, redness, itching, burning, pain, bleeding, or change in sun sensitivity. Even mild irritation is a sign that the product is causing

Bright Idea
Consumers can call or write the manufacturer to get information about a product's AHA concentration and pH level if the label doesn't contain that information.

damage. Despite what the manufacturer may indicate on the product label, cosmetics shouldn't sting or cause irritation.

- See a doctor: If you have an adverse reaction, see a dermatologist, who can tell you whether an adverse reaction is from the product or is an indication of an underlying disease. Dermatologists also can recommend appropriate skin care products, and they will report your case, keeping your name confidential, to the FDA's adverse reaction monitoring program.

Bright Idea
To report an adverse reaction to a cosmetic, call your local FDA office or the FDA's Office of Consumer Affairs at 800/532-4440. Have the label and any other packaging information nearby and give the name of the product, the name and address of the manufacturer or distributor, and any identifiable product code numbers.

Do your cosmetics have AHAs?

To find out if a cosmetic contains an AHA, look on the list of ingredients. All cosmetics must, by law, have this information on their outer packaging. Of the following, the most-often used in cosmetics are glycolic acid and lactic acid. AHA ingredients may be listed as

- Alpha-hydroxy and botanical complex.
- Alpha-hydroxycaprylic acid.
- Alpha-hydroxyethanoic acid plus ammonium alpha-hydroxyethanoate.
- Alpha-hydroxyoctanoic acid.
- Alpha-hydroxypropionic acid.
- Glycolic acid.
- Glycolic acid plus ammonium glycolate.
- Glycomer in cross-linked fatty acids alpha nutrium.
- Hydroxycaprylic acid.
- Lactic acid.
- L-alpha hydroxy acid.

- Mixed fruit acid.
- Sugar cane extract.
- Tri-alpha hydroxy fruit acids.
- Triple fruit acid.

BHA ingredients include

- Salicylic acid.
- Beta hydroxybutanoic acid.
- Tropic acid.
- Trethocanic acid.

Alpha- and beta-hydroxy acids, in combination, are listed as

- Malic acid.
- Citric acid.

Vitamin C: Just a fad?

Vitamin C is a powerful antioxidant that is important in building collagen and in wound healing; theoretically, delivering vitamin C to the skin ought to improve its appearance. Until recently, however, it was almost impossible to formulate a product that would enable vitamin C to penetrate the outer layer of skin cells. You could put tons of it in a product, but none of it would get into a person's skin—until Sheldon Pinnell, M.D., a dermatology professor at Duke University, came up with a way to get high concentrations of vitamin C into the skin, a process for which both he and his university hold the patent.

Since this time, many other vitamin C-containing products have popped up on drug shelves with no proof that any of them actually deliver vitamin C into the skin. It's not enough to have vitamin C in a skin care product; it must be formulated in such a way that it can penetrate the skin, or it won't do any

Unofficially...
While vitamin C is important for building collagen and wound healing, there is no proof that swallowing lots of vitamin C tablets alters the outward appearance of the skin.

more good than if you tried to lower a fever by crushing an aspirin tablet on your cheek.

Should you combine skin products?

In the days when nonprescription beauty products contained nothing more exotic than undigested whale spit and some lanolin, it didn't matter so much what you combined—but today's "cosmeceuticals" pack a lot more wallop, so you need to be more careful. Still, most dermatologists agree that because Retin-A products and the glycolic acids work in slightly different ways, it makes sense to use them both—but not at the same time. If used properly, using two different preparations is probably better than either one alone.

Dermatologists recommend using AHAs in the morning and Retin-A at night. It's a popular treatment regimen; in fact, in the Ortho Pharmaceutical Corporation study of dermatologists, 69 percent of the participants combine AHAs with some form of tretinoin (Retin-A or Renova). (Someone with more sensitive skin may not tolerate this double whammy, but the only way to tell is to try it.) In fact, one recent survey of 200 female dermatologists conducted by Ortho found that 65 percent of the women surveyed reported that they combined skin care products. Yet, while some combinations are helpful, others may dilute each other's effectiveness or cause irritation.

Try Retin-A first before adding other new skin care products to allow your skin to become adjusted to the irritation. Most women start at a low dose of Retin-A and eventually work up to 0.1 percent cream. Once the skin is tolerating the Retin-A, you can add an AHA in the morning. Try combining your products this way:

Bright Idea
If you can't tolerate the swelling, stinging, and redness that accompany high-strength lactic acid, try a bit of lactic acid diluted with your favorite moisturizer. Lactic acid is a tremendous moisturizer that actually draws water from the upper level of skin into the lower level.

1. Wash in the morning with an AHA cleanser.
2. Wait 30 minutes after using the AHA and then apply a vitamin C product on clean, dry skin.
3. Follow this with a moisturizer or makeup.

Because vitamin C must be formulated precisely to get into the skin, it won't be absorbed if it's used together with Retin-A or an AHA or BHA. The buffering of these products is different, and a different buffering can interfere with the effect of the compounds. On the other hand, vitamin C can be used at the same time with moisturizers, sunscreens or makeup, because these products aren't buffered.

Coping with dry skin

One of the big problems with aging is that the skin dries out and becomes leathery and wrinkly (especially if you smoke or spend time in the sun). Your skin gets dry as you age because the outer layer of skin is losing too much water as a result of a drop in moisture-locking skin oil that keeps your skin supple. Environmental conditions such as indoor heat, swimming pool chlorine, cold windy weather, and lots of hand washing can aggravate the problem.

Moisturizers can help because they reduce water loss from the skin and draw moisture from the inner layer of skin up into the outer layer. Just about all lotions and creams contain ingredients to do this—but which kind? The drugstore aisles are filled with lotions and creams for hands, face, and eyelids. The department store cosmetic counters hawk multi-product "skin care systems" promising to restore your ailing epidermis. Fortunately, finding an effective moisturizer is not nearly as complicated as you might think.

Moneysaver
You don't need separate lotions for different parts of the body and you need not spend a lot of money for a good moisturizer, says Dr. Nelson Lee Novick, an associate clinical professor of dermatology at Mount Sinai Hospital-NYU Medical Center in New York. That's marketing, not medicine.

Compounds that reduce water loss by creating a barrier include

- Petrolatum.
- Mineral oil.
- Lanolin.
- Silicone derivatives.

Substances that attract moisture to the top skin layer (called humectants) include

- Glycerin.
- Propylene glycol.
- AHAs.
- Urea.
- Lactic acid.

Dry skin benefits from the use of AHAs more than any other skin type, most likely due to the acids' exfoliation of dead skin cells and stimulation of new cell production. AHAs have been used on dry skin by dermatologists for decades but it is only more recently that their positive effects on anti-aging have been observed. It is very important that dry skin is cared for on a daily basis, care which should include an AHA cream or lotion formulation.

While many products contain these basic active ingredients, you won't find the concentrations of the barrier substances and humectants on the label. So even though any moisturizer can be effective, it's a good idea to do some trial-and-error testing.

Moreover, some products contain a lot of extras, such as fragrances and botanicals, which can cause irritation or allergic reactions in some women. If you have sensitive skin, try moisturizers with only a few ingredients and no lanolin (a common allergen).

Moneysaver
Don't spend lots of money for products containing collagen, elastin, eggs, milk, royal jelly (from bees), placental extracts, or vitamin E—they can't be absorbed by the skin. They don't do much but boost your risk of irritation or allergy.

A few "safe" humectants to look for are urea and lactic acid, both of which are produced naturally by the skin. As we've seen above, AHA moisturizers are also a good choice because they not only peel off dry flakes, but improve the health of the upper skin layer. If you're looking for one lotion for your entire body, oil-free moisturizers (usually containing dimethicone) will work on legs and elbows and not make your face break out.

To get the most out of your moisturizer, apply it just after bathing so you can trap more moisture in your skin. When drying off with a towel, pat your skin so that you leave a trace of water and then put on the lotion.

Bright Idea
To ease skin dryness, boost the humidity in your home and office with a humidifier (or place a pan of water on a radiator or stove during winter). The ideal humidity for skin is about 35 percent.

Here's what else you can do to prevent dry skin:

- Take shorter and less frequent showers or baths.
- Use warm (not hot) water.
- Use soap only on the feet, under the arms and in the groin and buttocks areas.
- Wear gloves in cold weather or while your hands are in dishwater.
- Avoid the sun or wear a hat and use a sunscreen or a moisturizer containing sunscreen.

If your dry skin doesn't get better with over-the-counter moisturizers, see a dermatologist. Sometimes flaky skin is actually caused by seborrheic dermatitis, a condition worsened by creams and lotions.

Plastic or cosmetic surgery

Sometimes the wrinkles and other facial symptoms of age require not just topical treatment, but surgical intervention. Facelifts, eyelid, and eyebrow lifts can usually be performed as "day surgery" so that you can go home the same day. Many surgeons prefer to use "twilight" anesthesia (or twilight sleep)—local anesthesia with intravenous sedation whenever possible.

With all these procedures, you can expect some scarring, but plastic surgeons are trained to close incisions in a way as to make the scars as inconspicuous as possible. Some scars eventually become faintly visible fine lines. Scars from these procedures are, in most cases, quite acceptable, since they are usually placed within normal creases and folds whenever possible. As with all surgery, the type of procedure and your personal healing ability play a large role in the development of any scars.

Also, as with all surgery, complications are possible, but they are usually infrequent and minor when performed by a competent plastic surgeon. All patients experience some bruising and swelling for several days after cosmetic surgery, depending on the extent of the procedure. As with all elective surgery, you should carefully consider risks and potential complications before having the procedure.

Finding a plastic surgeon

Any doctor can call him or herself a "cosmetic" (or plastic) surgeon after obtaining a license to practice medicine. You should carefully evaluate the credentials of your cosmetic surgeon:

- Ask the doctor about board certification, training, qualifications, and the hospital where he or she has admitting privileges.
- Check for certification by the American Board of Plastic Surgery (you can find a listing of all board-certified specialists in the "Official ABMS

Directory of Board-Certified Medical Specialists" in your library.

- Check for membership in the American Society for Plastic and Reconstructive Surgeons and the American Society for Aesthetic Plastic Surgery.

- Ask to see "before-and-after" photos of other patients who've had the same type of surgery you're considering.

- Discuss the doctor's fees and costs, which will probably not be covered by your health insurance.

Face-lifts

A face-lift is a surgical procedure designed to rejuvenate the face by removing excess fat and skin and by tightening the muscles of the face and neck. However it doesn't stop the aging process—it just makes you look a bit younger. How much younger you look, and the rate at which facial aging occurs after surgery, depends on your age and lifestyle. However, years after surgery, most patients look better than if they had never undergone surgery. Many women never have a second face-lift, while others have additional surgery at a later time.

A face-lift is usually performed on an outpatient basis with a local anesthetic. Loose skin is separated from underlying muscle and pulled upward and backward all around the face, going back two to four inches from the side of the face. When the skin is lifted away, it's pulled up and draped over the face. The excess skin that overlaps the incision line is removed and the skin is sewn again at the incision line. Cotton and gauze are placed over the face and eyes and the whole face is wrapped in an elastic bandage. Pads are kept in place for up to 48 hours and then removed; after less than a week, the entire bandage is removed.

You should expect bruising and some discomfort (usually controlled with painkillers); within a few weeks, however, your face should begin to show improvement. Stitches are removed three days after surgery and the scars are usually hidden by natural crease lines and hair. You may be back to work within two weeks, although your bruises may still be apparent for three weeks.

After you've had a face-lift, you must clean your face twice a day with mild soap and avoid creams, which could pull the newly sewn tissue. While most patients are able to return to work in two to three weeks, if you're expecting to attend a major social engagement, you might want to allow more time between the surgery and the event.

Face-lifts should be individualized for each patient. Younger women (under 55) usually don't need as extensive a correction and can sometimes be treated with a more limited procedure, with shorter scars and a quicker recovery time. Many women have combination surgery when they have a face-lift, adding eyelid surgery, neck liposuction, fat transfers, lip augmentation, brow lifts, and limited laser skin resurfacing, depending on the type of aging problems.

Face-lift results should last for up to 10 years; it costs an average of $4,000, depending on the location of the hospital. You can have several face-lifts in your lifetime. Although some people believe that repeated operations result in a masklike appearance of the face, that look really means the skin was tightened too much during surgery.

Eyelid-lifts

An eyelid-lift (blephoroplasty) is an operation on the upper or the lower eyelids, and is designed to remove excess skin and fat. It's one of the most common operations performed by plastic surgeons. In the upper eyelid, a lift is designed primarily to improve the aged, tired appearance caused by the extra fold of skin that moves over the eyelid as you age. A lower eyelid-lift tightens the skin and muscle and removes the excess fat or "bag." Recently, doctors have realized the importance of more conservative fat removal to prevent a sunken or unnatural appearance after surgery. In some operations, doctors focus on repositioning rather than removing fat.

An eyelid lift won't remove the wrinkles around the eyes (crow's feet) or correct droopy eyebrows; these conditions are usually best treated by other means. Dark circles under the eyes may improve if they are related to large bags, but an eyelid-lift won't lighten the dark pigmentation of lower eyelid skin.

Watch Out!
If you have certain conditions (thyroid disease, high blood pressure, or dry eyes), you have a higher risk of suffering from complications after an eyelid-lift.

Brow-lifts

A brow-lift is an operation designed to rejuvenate the upper one-third of the face, improving droopy eyebrows, forehead wrinkles, and vertical "frown" lines, or horizontal creases at the base of the nose. Most brow-lifts are outpatient "day" surgery, performed under local anesthesia and intravenous sedation.

Hair—Too much or too little?

Your hair is made of keratin, the same protein that makes up your nails and the outer layer of your skin. It's actually dead tissue produced by your hair follicles (the bulblike structures beneath your skin that each hold a single hair).

Most women naturally lose some hair as they get older, but age, changing hormones, and genes (hair loss can be hereditary) make some women lose more hair than others. Female-pattern baldness begins when the hairs that grow in to replace those that fall out are progressively finer and shorter. They can eventually become almost transparent. This type of hair loss is usually far less noticeable than it is in men, since it occurs throughout the head and not just on the top, as in men. Most women first experience hair thinning and loss where they part their hair, at the top of the head, but they don't have a receding hairline. About half the women who lose their hair have female pattern baldness. It's usually permanent.

Treating hair loss

There's not a great deal you can do to prevent hair loss. If you're worried about hair loss, you'll need to treat your hair gently. Avoid

- Hair dyes, tints, or bleaches.
- Don't rub your wet hair hard with a towel.
- Don't use a brush on wet hair.
- Don't brush your hair 100 strokes a night; it can damage hair.
- Protect your hair from the sun; wear a hat or stay in the shade.

A medication called minoxidil (Rogaine) is now available without a prescription and it may help stop hair loss in some people. The effectiveness varies from one woman to the next, however, and you need to keep using it to retain your hair.

Unfortunately, the hair regrowing drug Propecia works well in men, but is not effective for women who are suffering hair loss; in fact, a study by the manufacturer found that women on the drug actually lost 8 percent of their hair.

Hair transplants are an option for some men, but they have produced less satisfactory results for women. But a new method, called micrograft hair transplantation, which transplants single hairs, has been successful in some women.

Gray hair

As you age, your hair appears to turn "gray," which is actually a combination of pigmented and nonpigmented hair. Most women with gray hair aren't entirely gray, but have a mix of white hair among those of normal color. As you age, your body produces less melanin; new hair contains less pigment and, eventually, the shaft grows in without any color. The only color left in the hair is the color of the keratin itself, which is yellowish gray. Eventually, more and more hair continues to grow in the same way until your entire head is filled with gray hair.

Most women begin to develop a few gray hairs at about age 30, becoming progressively grayer over the next 20 years as more and more of their hair grows in lacking pigment. By age 60 to 70, the hair often turns completely white, which means that all of the hairs on the head have lost their pigment granules. Hair that turns gray prematurely (while the woman is in her 20s) is usually the result of genetic factors, since the tendency seems to run in families. Severe stress, mental illness, and trauma also are associated with premature gray hair, although scientists don't know why.

Once you start to go gray, you can't reverse the process; however, hair dye specifically designed for use on gray hair can be used to retain hair color. Some gray hair that has a yellow tinge can be

Unofficially...
Throughout history, some famous people have turned gray overnight: Sir Thomas More in the 16th century and Queen Marie-Antoinette in the 18th century were both said to have suddenly gone gray when they got the news they were to be executed.

worsened by tobacco smoke, dry powder shampoos, setting lotions, and especially dandruff shampoos containing resorcinol. The easiest way to get rid of this tinge is to treat the hair with a bluing rinse. Don't use setting lotions or hair sprays, which have a tendency to turn gray hair yellow.

Hair dye: Does it cause cancer?

Researchers aren't quite sure whether hair dye causes cancer, but findings seem to be leaning toward dyes being safe. Still, many reports are inconclusive. The FDA says some studies raise questions about the safety of hair dyes, but, at this point, there's no basis to say that hair dyes pose a definitive risk of cancer. In the final analysis, you'll need to consider the lack of demonstrated safety when choosing to use hair dyes.

A recent study looking at the use of permanent hair dyes and cancer did not find an association between such use and cancers of the blood or lymph systems. The study, by a team of researchers from Brigham and Women's Hospital in Boston, involved more than 99,000 women.

The new study's findings differ from the results of at least eight earlier studies that indicated that women and men who dye their hair frequently may be at increased risk for cancers of the blood and lymph systems. The early studies showed an association between hair dye use and increased risks for multiple myeloma (cancer of cells in the bone marrow), non-Hodgkin's lymphoma (cancer of the lymph system) and leukemia (cancer of blood-forming cells) in both sexes, and ovarian cancer in women. Almost all the early studies indicated that increased risk might be restricted to long-term or frequent hair dye users, particularly users of dark hair dyes.

Research has shown that some of the substances in hair dyes are readily absorbed through the skin and scalp during application. Several studies of cosmetologists and other persons who apply hair dyes to others as part of their work have shown them to be at increased risk of non-Hodgkin's lymphoma, multiple myeloma, and leukemia.

Hair removal

As women age and their hormone levels change, many women notice unwanted hair sprouting on the face and chest. A growing number spend millions of dollars each year on products and services that promise smooth, silky skin free of "unsightly" and "excessive" body hair. There are a variety of home-use hair removal products available over-the-counter, including shaving creams, foams and gels, waxes, chemical depilatories, and electrolysis devices. Professionals at beauty and skin care salons and in dermatologists' offices provide waxing, electrolysis, and now laser treatments to remove hair. (The FDA cleared the first laser for this use on April 3, 1995.)

You need to consider the cost, safety, effectiveness, and ease of use of the various methods, as well as the area and amount of hair growth to be treated when choosing a method and deciding whether to go to a professional.

Depilatories act like a chemical razor blade and are available in gel, cream, lotion, aerosol, and roll-on forms. They contain a highly alkaline chemical (usually calcium thioglycolate) that dissolves the hair. It's very important to carefully follow the use directions for depilatories and to do a preliminary skin test, both for allergic reaction and sensitivity. Hair and skin are similar in composition, so chemicals that destroy the hair can also cause serious skin irritations—possibly even chemical burns—if left on too long. Some depilatories are for use only on the legs, for example, while others are safe for more sensitive areas, such as the bikini line, underarms, and face. You shouldn't use depilatories for the eyebrows or other areas around the eyes, or on inflamed or broken skin. To minimize the chance of skin irritation, they should not be applied more often than recommended on the product label.

While depilatories remove hair at the skin's surface, epilatories, such as waxes, pluck hairs from below the surface. Waxing may be more painful than using a depilatory, but the results are longer lasting. Because the hair is plucked at the root, new growth is not visible for several weeks after treatment. Waxing is mostly done to shape the eyebrows and remove hair on the chin and upper lip, although some women also have their legs, underarms and bikini line waxed. Epilatory waxes are available for use by professionals or over-the-counter for home-use. They contain combinations of waxes, such as paraffin and beeswax, oils, or fats, and a resin that makes the wax adhere to the skin.

The needle epilator used in electrolysis introduces a very fine wire close to the hair shaft under the skin and into the hair follicle. An electric current travels down the wire and destroys the hair root at the bottom of the follicle. The loosened hair is then removed with tweezers. Every hair is treated individually. Because this technique destroys the hair follicle, it is considered a permanent hair removal method. The hair root may persist, however, if the needle misses the mark or if insufficient electricity is delivered to destroy it. Successful electrolysis usually requires considerable time and money.

Watch Out! Over-the-counter waxes should not be used by women with diabetes and circulatory problems, who are particularly susceptible to infection. Waxes also should not be used over varicose veins; moles or warts; or on eyelashes; inside the nose or ears; on the nipples or genital areas; or on irritated, chapped, sunburned, or cut skin.

The major risks of electrolysis are electrical shock, which can occur if the needle is not properly insulated, infection from an unsterile needle or other infection control problem, and scarring. There are no uniform standards governing the practice of electrology. Only 31 states require electrologists to be licensed, and among those, the licensing requirements vary.

Home-use electrolysis devices work the same way as do those for professional use and carry the same health risks, although the voltages and currents for the home-use devices are not very high. The success of electrolysis self-treatment depends largely on the condition of the hair and skin, the equipment and the level of skill developed.

One of the newest techniques in the hair-removal arsenal is the laser, designed to be a non-invasive way to remove unwanted facial and body hair. It's an in-office procedure without the need for anesthesia. After the procedure, you can immediately go back to sedentary activities. Most women experience only a slight stinging—or nothing at all—as the laser pulses are applied.

The laser targets the pigment within the hair follicle (melanin), thus disabling the follicle. It's designed to selectively target the follicle without damaging the surrounding skin. It only treats hairs in their actively growing phase; the number of active follicles will vary with each area of the body. Follicles that are in a dormant phase aren't affected.

Additional treatments are needed as hairs that were dormant become active and begin to grow. The number of sessions will vary with each woman and by body area.

Unlike traditional methods, such as shaving, plucking, and waxing, laser hair removal is intended

Bright Idea
For a list of licensed and certified electrologists, contact the International Guild of Professional Electrologists, 202 Boulevard St., Suite B, High Point, NC 27262; 800/830-3247.

to provide long-lasting or permanent hair reduction. The FDA has approved the diode laser for hair removal; currently, however, no laser has achieved FDA clearance for permanent hair removal.

Laser hair removal differs from electrolysis in that each hair must be individually treated with an electric current. Electrolysis carries the risk of electric shock, infection, and scarring, and the process can take months or even years to complete. On the other hand, the laser noninvasively treats an area with many hairs at one time. For example, it typically takes about 30 seconds to treat the upper lip. The lip and chin are the most common areas targeted for laser hair removal, followed by the bikini line, legs, and armpits, but it's possible to treat most areas of the body.

If you're planning to try laser hair removal, you shouldn't wax or bleach the targeted hair for about six weeks prior to treatment. It's more effective if you avoid sun tanning prior to laser hair removal. As with any medical procedure, there are potential risks, although, with laser hair removal they are minimal.

Memory loss

Women must cope with a variety of physical changes as they age and modern technology has many ways to camouflage those changes. Memory loss, however, is often more disconcerting and unexpected. It is a particular problem among women as they approach menopause.

Contrary to what most people think, however, your memory doesn't automatically self-destruct as you age. You do have some control over when and how much memory you lose as you get older. In fact, judgment, memory accuracy, and general knowledge may increase with each passing birthday.

Some specific parts of memory may decline with age, but you can expect your overall memory to remain strong at least through your 70s. In fact, research has shown that the average 70-year-old performs as well on many memory tests as 30 percent of 20-year-olds. Even more interesting, many older people in their 60s and 70s scored much better in verbal intelligence than did younger people. Still, a mild memory impairment related to age is common, albeit not inevitable.

A simple memory test
Test your working memory. Read a line of numbers, look away and repeat it. See how far down on this list you can go.

QUIZ 17.1: MEMORY TEST

3 9 5 8
2 0 3 5 1
5 9 3 2 8 6
9 3 8 1 4 3 0
3 9 4 3 8 3 8 2
0 4 2 8 4 7 0 3 2
8 3 7 9 8 2 9 3 4 2
3 8 4 7 3 8 7 2 3 4 0

Most women can remember up to seven digits. If you remembered nine or more, you're doing much better than average!

Menopause-related "fuzzy thinking"
Don't ignore memory problems—if you notice a dramatic downturn in memory, discuss it with your health care provider. You're the best one to notice a problem. Memory problems affect almost all of

us as we age, but it becomes especially annoying as a woman enters menopause. Many women report an abrupt "fuzzy thinking" problem, which may be related to the drop in estrogen hormones that, in turn, appear to be related to healthy memory function.

Some studies have shown that estrogen replacement improves symptoms of forgetfulness, short-term memory loss, anxiety, and concentration problems. Recent studies at the National Institute of Aging show that memory for words and images tend to be better in women on estrogen replacement therapy (ERT) than those of the same age who aren't taking the hormone. In another study, ERT altered brain activity patterns that affect memory in postmenopausal women. In fact, brain activity in certain areas of estrogen-treated women were more like patterns normally seen in younger women. Other studies have shown a possible decreased risk for Alzheimer's disease in those on estrogen replacement.

Scientists concluded that ERT significantly alters brain patterns in postmenopausal women, which should predict improvement in memory, although they caution they didn't observe such changes during their study. Studies have also shown that regular exercise improves short-term memory.

Is it Alzheimer's?

Many women start worrying that they have Alzheimer's disease when they begin to forget keys or the location of the car in a parking garage. Most of the time, it's simply memory loss linked to failure to pay attention.

There are ways to tell the difference between the normal breakdown of memory that comes with age and that which accompanies Alzheimer's disease.

While both do begin with forgetfulness, Alzheimer's soon progresses to a far more profound memory loss than simply not being able to find your keys. If you misplace your glasses, that's forgetfulness. If you can't remember that you wear glasses, that could be a sign of Alzheimer's.

There are other differences between simple forgetfulness and dementia. Age-related memory loss may leave your memory unchanged for years, whereas Alzheimer's gets progressively worse, interfering more and more severely with the normal activities of daily life. Alzheimer's also affects more than memory—it interferes with the ability to use words, compute figures, solve problems, and use reasoning and judgment. It also may cause mood and personality changes.

Other causes

As you age, memory function begins to slow, affecting different types of memory in different ways. Many of the reasons for this age-related memory loss are reversible: Depression, medications (especially benzodiazepines used to treat anxiety), poor diet, thyroid deficiency or substance abuse are all common causes of reversible memory loss. Memory problems also may be caused by a number of problems within the brain itself. If you can treat these problems, or switch medications, you may completely alleviate the memory problem.

You may not learn or remember quite as rapidly as you age, but you will remember nearly as well. After about age 30, most people reach a plateau that is usually maintained until about age 60. After that, there are small declines depending on ability and gender. It's not until a person reaches his or her 80s that any sort of serious mental slowdown occurs in most people. Indeed, the memory for general vocabulary and knowledge about the world often stays sharp through your 70s, but memory for names (especially those you don't use a lot) begins to decline after age 35. The ability to recognize faces and find your car has already begun to wane by the time you leave your 20s.

Preventing memory problems

It's really fairly simple: The healthier life you live, the better your memory should be. Since memory is part of how you think, it follows that anything that interferes with brain function is going to affect how well you store information in memory and how quickly you can retrieve it again.

Remember, your body and your mind (and hence, your memory) are influenced by a wide range of lifestyle choices, including diet, medications, stress, exercise, smoking, and relaxation.

Stress affects mood, and mood affects your ability to remember. In fact, anxiety and depression are the two major causes of memory problems at any age. When you're deeply depressed or stressed, you turn inward and stop recording information the way you normally would. Did you ever hear bad news in your health care provider's office? If you did, you may recall that after the bad news, you forgot everything else the practitioner said.

Stress and anxiety can take over and prevent you from remembering much of anything. Even minor stress can interfere with memory. If you stand still and try to think where you left your keys, chances are you'll have a hard time remembering where they are because the physical sensation of stress is interfering with your concentration. The harder you try to remember, the more likely you are to go blank.

Watch Out! Caffeine may keep you up at night, but that's not all it can do—it can also interfere with memory. One study of college students showed that drinking coffee lowered their ability to remember a list of words.

Experts aren't sure how diet affects memory, but they know that essential nutrients are important for enhancing chemical processes. Imbalances in diet can cause memory problems. Your ability to remember is affected by deficiencies in iron, other minerals, vitamins, and protein. Without sufficient levels of thiamine, folic acid, zinc, and vitamin B12, the brain can't function properly and experiences memory and concentration problems.

Water helps maintain memory systems, especially in older people. Lack of water in the body has a direct, profound effect on memory. Dehydration can quickly lead to confusion and other thinking problems.

Getting adequate rest is also important. In order to function with peak memory skills, it's essential to get enough sleep so you can rest your brain. During certain periods of deep sleep that occur every hour and a half, the brain disconnects from the senses and processes, reviews, consolidates, and stores memory. Interfering with this critical time of sleep will seriously affect memory.

Drugs, like alcohol and nicotine, also interfere with memory. Studies have found that even a few drinks four times a week can interfere with your ability to remember; the issue is much more serious for alcoholics, who may have serious short-term memory problems.

Smoking cuts down on the amount of oxygen in the brain and studies have found that smokers consistently score lower on memory tests than nonsmokers, especially if they smoke more than a pack a day.

Some prescription and over-the-counter drugs affect memory, particularly when taken by older people, especially benzodiazepines (including Valium and Ativan). In addition, muscle relaxants,

Unofficially...
Studies at UCLA found that people over age 40 experience the most memory problems after drinking, but even those between 20 and 30 experience some memory loss. Women are more susceptible to the toxic effects of alcohol, especially in relation to short-term memory.

tranquilizers, sleeping pills, and anti-anxiety drugs can produce confusion and memory loss. As a general rule, any drug that warns you not to drive when you take it may impair your ability to remember. If you're having memory problems while taking medications, check with your doctor or pharmacist to see if the medication may be contributing to the problem.

There are ways for you to avoid medication-related memory problems:

- Fill all prescriptions at the same pharmacy so your pharmacist can recognize potentially troublesome interactions.

- Bring a list of all your medicines to your health care provider's office, including vitamins and supplements.

- Follow your health care provider's prescription; if you miss a dose, never double the next one without permission.

- Don't combine alcohol and drugs (not even over-the-counter medications)—and especially not drugs that affect the central nervous system, including tranquilizers, sedatives, and barbiturates.

Unofficially... Italian researchers found that monounsaturated fats (found in olive, canola, sunflower, and soybean oils; walnuts; pork; chicken; beef; turkey; eggs; and herring) may help slow the mental decline that comes with normal aging.

You can improve memory

Fortunately, it's possible to improve your memory, even if you're older. Studies of nursing-home populations showed that patients were able to make significant improvements in memory through the use of rewards and brain challenges.

Experts suspect that age-related memory problems may be caused by differences in the ability to store information. Those with the best ability to remember at any age tend to give new information lots of details and images. When they are introduced to a new person, for example, they might notice the physical appearance of the person and link that in some way to the person's name. As you get older, it's harder to organize this information effectively. For these reasons, older people have the most problems when trying unfamiliar tasks that require rapid processing, such as learning how to program a VCR or operate a computer.

Stimulating the brain is one of the best ways to stop brain cells from shrinking with age. It can even lead to an increase in brain size and memory improvement. Living in an enriched environment, with plenty of colors, sounds, sights, and smells, is good for both mind and memory. This may be one reason why your socioeconomic status can affect your memory and mental decline; if you have the money to buy lots of "toys," you'll have a more stimulating environment. Take adult education courses, learn to play chess or a musical instrument. Keep music playing, have plenty of pictures around, take trips, and meet new people.

Just the facts

- Laser resurfacing is one of the newest ways to erase wrinkles on your face with less risk than with older forms of cosmetic surgery—but make sure your cosmetic surgeon has plenty of experience with this procedure.
- Fruit acids (AHAs) do appear to have some effect on the skin but they can cause side effects; the strongest acids work the best, but they are only available at your health care provider's office.

- Women, as well as men, can have an age-related hair loss.
- Laser hair removal is the newest technique in hair reduction.
- The best way to keep your memory sharp is to live and work in a stimulating environment and keep learning new things.

Chapter 18

GET THE SCOOP ON...
How to tell if you're entering menopause ▪ The difference between PMS and menopause ▪ The pros and cons of hormone replacement therapy ▪ The "anti-estrogens" (raloxifene) ▪ HRT: Pill, patch, ring, injection? ▪ Cenestin: Newest natural estrogen

Menopause

Between 1995 and 2010, the number of women over age 50 entering menopause in the United States will grow from 37 million to 52 million. As women age, they face increasing risks for diseases such as heart disease, breast cancer, and osteoporosis related to their declining levels of estrogen). Indeed, hormones influence almost every bodily system and can be associated with a wide range of disorders, including Alzheimer's disease and even skin changes. The risks for developing these problems can be minimized by making healthy lifestyle choices.

Ovulation

Each month starting in your teenage years, your body releases one of the more than 400,000 eggs stored in your ovaries—as well as the layers of cells that cover the eggs, which are the primary producers of the hormones estrogen and progesterone. A woman's monthly cycle begins when the pituitary gland in your brain secretes follicle-stimulating hormone (FSH), which causes the ovaries to produce estradiol (the body's natural estrogen). This triggers the release of an egg from a follicle in one of the ovaries—also known as "ovulation"—which will probably occur more than 500 times in your life if you never get pregnant or use birth control pills.

The estradiol also triggers your uterine lining to thicken in anticipation of receiving a fertilized egg. Once ovulation has occurred, the follicle produces progesterone; if the egg isn't fertilized, progesterone levels drop and the uterine lining sheds and menstrual bleeding begins.

As you age, your store of eggs gradually diminishes and the estrogen-secreting layer of cells becomes less responsive to the signals from the brain. Some months you won't ovulate at all, which means you don't produce any estrogen or progesterone. The result: You skip a period. Some women in this situation have longer periods with heavy flow (if you still have enough estrogen to thicken the uterine wall, you may experience heavy bleeding when progesterone is finally produced). Others find they have shorter cycles and hardly any bleeding. Some have a combination of the two, and others will begin to miss periods completely. During this time, you also will experience a decrease in your ability to become pregnant.

Eight out of every one hundred women stop menstruating before age 40. At the other end of the spectrum, 5 out of every 100 continue to have periods until they are almost 60. In any case, by the time you reach your late 30s or 40s, your ovaries are beginning to shut down, producing less estrogen and progesterone and releasing eggs less often.

The gradual decline of estrogen causes a wide variety of changes in tissues that respond to estrogen: Your vagina, vulva, uterus, bladder, urethra, breasts, bones, heart, blood vessels, brain, skin, hair, and mucous membranes may all begin to change. You may notice that you get more colds and flu, since almost all tissues in your body have estrogen receptors; when the level drops, they may not function as well. Over the long run, the lack of estrogen can make you more vulnerable to osteoporosis (which can begin in your 40s) and heart disease.

As the levels of hormones in your body decrease, you will begin to experience the symptoms of perimenopause, that is, the time right before menopause. In fact, some women find that the very worst symptoms of the entire menopausal transition occur during the perimenopausal phase.

When will you enter menopause?

Unfortunately, there's no easy way to predict when you will enter the menopause years, but you can get a general idea based on your family history, body type, and lifestyle. There's no link between the age when you started menstruating and the age when you'll stop; instead, you'll probably enter menopause at about the same age as your mother—the average age is 51.

Of course, it's also true that the hormonal situation for many women today may be quite different than the experience of their ancestors. Because women in the past married fairly soon after puberty and spent much of their lives either pregnant or nursing, they had many fewer periods than we have today. This means that their lifetime exposure to estrogen was actually far lower than ours. How this

Unofficially... Early onset of menopause can be triggered not just by age but also by smoking, hysterectomy with the removal of ovaries, damaged reproductive organs, being underweight, or by having a severely restricted diet.

difference in long-term exposure to hormones will affect when modern women enter menopause isn't fully understood.

On average, menopause begins at age 51. Your menopause may be earlier than average (that is, before age 51) if you

- Are thin and small boned.
- Have never had children.
- Smoke.
- Live at a high altitude.
- Have eaten poorly throughout your life.
- Have a higher standard of living.
- Have had a hysterectomy (even if your ovaries aren't removed, a woman whose uterus has been removed enters menopause a few months earlier than otherwise).
- Have shorter-than-average cycles (less than 25 days).
- Have had several abortions.

Your menopause may be later than average if you

- Are heavy or big-boned.
- Have had several children (each child you've had will delay the onset of menopause by about five months).
- Don't smoke.
- Live at sea level.
- Have had diabetes, cancer of the breast or uterus, or uterine fibroid tumors.
- Have a lower standard of living.
- Had your first child after age 40.
- Have taken birth control pills for many years.

Is it me or is it hot in here?

Menopause doesn't start abruptly one day; it's a gradual shift in the production of hormones. Therefore, the onset of symptoms may not be obvious, either. The most common symptom of menopause is a change in your menstrual cycle, but there are a variety of other symptoms, too, such as

- Hot flashes.
- Insomnia.
- Mood swings.
- Memory or concentration problems.
- Vaginal dryness.
- Breast changes.
- Headaches.
- Heart palpitations.
- Loss of libido.
- Urinary problems.
- Excessive facial hair.
- Depression.

Menstrual period changes

Although there is a wide variation in the length of menstrual cycles from woman to woman, as you enter menopause your own cycles will become more irregular. Your periods may come farther apart or lighter. Some women notice their periods change month to month. This is the most common symptom of menopause. If your periods come closer together or they get heavier, this is abnormal and must be evaluated by your health care provider to rule out endometrial cancer.

Shorter cycles can be an indication that you aren't ovulating anymore. Ovulation usually occurs in the middle of a menstrual cycle; as the amount of estrogen in your body drops, the number of days before you reach the midpoint of your cycle will decrease. At the same time, as the amount of progesterone drops, the number of days after the cycle midpoint varies. Low levels of both hormones will have a strong affect on your cycle.

Missed periods aren't uncommon because there are some months when you don't ovulate, which means you won't produce progesterone and you won't shed your uterine lining. You can tell the difference between a missed period and a pregnancy by the presence of other symptoms. A missed period that occurs along with dryness of the vagina and hot flashes is most likely related to menopause. A missed period together with nausea, fatigue, and breast tenderness may be pregnancy. Still, if you are still a reproductive-aged woman who misses periods, you need to rule out pregnancy. See your health care provider to be sure.

Almost a quarter of all hysterectomies in the United States are performed in an effort to control prolonged abnormal bleeding. If the only reason you're having problems with bleeding is due to menopausal hormone changes, hormone replacement therapy (HRT) may make a hysterectomy unnecessary. Keep in mind that this abnormal bleeding will stop once menopause is complete. Before agreeing to a hysterectomy, get a second or third opinion.

If your bleeding is related to fibroids, your health care provider may recommend removal if there is painful pressure on the rectum or bladder.

Watch Out!
If you notice heavy bleeding, long intervals of spotting, you should talk to your health care provider. These symptoms—especially heavy bleeding—may be due to more serious problems such as polyps, fibroids, or even cancer.

Fibroid growth can be measured by an ultrasound scan; an endometrial biopsy can check for the possibility of cancer, although it's still possible to miss a small malignancy.

Hot flashes

The second most common symptom of menopause is hot flashes. According to a 1991 Gallup survey, 87 percent of menopausal women report they have experienced hot flashes, and more than half say they also experience night sweats. About half of women, according to another study, experience hot flashes while they are still menstruating regularly.

While some women may notice only an occasional hot flash that prompts them to remove a sweater or briefly fan themselves, other women wake in the middle of the night, drenched in sweat, with soaking sheets. Others find it difficult to function because they are so uncomfortable. Your face may suddenly feel flushed or blotchy; sweat may roll off your body and your skin may feel hot to the touch. Most of the time, the feeling of heat begins at just about your waist, spreading quickly to the chest, back, neck, face, and scalp. The sensations of searing heat may last anywhere from a few seconds to an hour, either once or twice a day or as often as 40 or 50 times daily.

While hot flashes usually occur only for about a year—it's one of the most transitory of all the menopause symptoms—some women struggle with them for up to five years. Most of the time they occur when you're sitting still or when you're asleep, but they can also be triggered by exercise, eating spicy food, or drinking something hot. The precise cause of hot flashes isn't completely understood, but

Bright Idea
If you're bleeding heavily and irregularly, you should be checked for signs of anemia. If you have low levels of hemoglobin, eat more iron-rich foods and take iron supplements. Heavy or irregular bleeding also can be caused by a dysfunctional thyroid gland. Have your thyroid checked for abnormally low or high levels of the thyroid hormone.

experts think they are related to changes in the hypothalamus, which regulates body temperature, as your hormone levels decline. When your hypothalamus gets confused and senses the body is hotter than it really is, your skin gets cold and clammy; your blood vessels dilate and your heart rate speeds up. Skin temperature may rise by up to 8°F and you begin to sweat. You start experiencing a hot flash. Some women notice feelings of tingling, throbbing, or dizziness as they feel the first flush of heat. In addition, more than 68 percent of women also experience night sweats. Some women are more affected by hot flashes than others because their level of estrogen doesn't drop slowly and evenly, but instead fluctuates wildly. As the body tries to repeatedly adjust, the hot flashes become stronger and more frequent.

Doctors believe estrogen plays a role in hot flashes, since they begin as estrogen levels drop. Studies have shown that the more abruptly your estrogen levels fall, the more severe the hot flashes will be. This is why women who have had their ovaries removed experience much more severe hot flashes than those whose ovaries are intact. This is also why thin women have stronger hot flashes; fat cells produce estrogen even after menopause is complete.

One reason why scientists are certain that estrogen is linked to hot flashes is that when a woman starts estrogen replacement, hot flashes stop. The exact interaction between estrogen and the brain is unclear, however, since once you have been menopausal for some time, your estrogen levels remain low yet you don't continue to have hot flashes. Hot flashes have also been reported during pregnancy, when estrogen levels are high. For this reason, experts suspect hot flashes are more likely the result of estrogen withdrawal, and not low estrogen levels.

It's probably true that estrogen doesn't act alone; other hormones and various brain chemicals may also be involved. Progesterone, for example, appears to rise during the second half of your cycle, raising your body temperature and making you feel warmer. And several types of neurotransmitters are intimately related to the functioning of your hypothalamus.

If you can't sleep...
About 2 in 10 women experience "menopause insomnia," the inability to fall asleep during menopause. Experts believe the sleep problems are due to falling levels of estrogen. Insomnia during this time may be caused by the same vasomotor symptoms that cause hot flashes.

Night sweating is another problem, which often follows hot flashes. When you're in bed, you'll feel especially hot because your body underneath the covers is warmer at night and because, if you're asleep, you won't be able to do anything to head off the hot flash. Hot flashes and night sweats can cause chronic sleep deprivation, which can make you even more irritable, moody, depressed, or forgetful.

Irritability and mood swings
You're standing at the checkout counter and the cashier tells you she's all out of Milk Duds. You burst into tears. No, you're not losing your mind or becoming emotionally unbalanced—mood swings and irritability are classic signs of menopause.

At least three out of every five women report they have experienced anxiety, irritability, or nervousness during menopause, and nearly 58 percent say they have experienced mood swings or some depression. As your hormones fluctuate, it's perfectly normal to feel tense and irritable and to cry easily.

Estrogen and progesterone effect chemicals in the brain that control sleep, pain perception, and a wide variety of emotions, diminishing your ability to cope with the problems you normally handle with ease.

Thinking and memory problems

Some of the most disturbing symptoms of menopause are the mental problems that can occur, including disorientation, concentration problems, and memory loss. The problems with mental acuity may well be linked to the dropping estrogen level, according to researchers.

The brain, like the uterus and breasts, contains estrogen receptors (sites where hormones can affect cells). The more abrupt your estrogen withdrawal, the more pronounced the symptoms. This is why women recovering from surgery or chemotherapy may experience memory problems.

Of course, some problems with memory and concentration are an inevitable part of aging for both men and women. But there is a difference between the age-related problem of retrieving information you have stored in your memory bank, and menopause-related forgetfulness. If your short-term memory is dramatically worse—not only can't you remember where you parked your car, but you have no recollection of even driving into the parking garage—your symptoms may be linked to estrogen withdrawal. Memory and concentration may be made worse if you also have problems in getting to sleep at night. If you often forget where you put your keys, that's probably normal. If you're holding

Unofficially... In one study at Rockefeller University, researchers found that lower estrogen levels in lab animals may reduce the number of connections between brain cells, leading to problems of concentration and memory.

your keys and don't know what they're for, that's probably not normal.

Vaginal dryness

You may notice vaginal dryness during menopause, which can be severe enough to make intercourse uncomfortable. It may not be something that you discuss with your friends or even your partner, but it is very common. As you enter menopause, estrogen levels fall and your vaginal walls become drier and thinner. This dryness is your body's response to the declining level of estrogen; the vaginal secretions also become less acidic. This opens the way for more vaginal infections. Eventually, the vagina itself may become shorter and narrower. If untreated, the vagina can actually atrophy. This lack of lubrication can make sex uncomfortable—and even painful. In severe cases, the vaginal walls can actually tear and bleed.

Breast changes

It's quite common to experience breast tenderness or fullness during the menstrual cycle and pregnancy; this also occurs during menopause. Breast tissue is very sensitive to estrogen and progesterone, even in amounts produced during a normal cycle. Women undergoing HRT may also experience breast tenderness. This should diminish or become tolerable in a few weeks after beginning therapy; if it doesn't, you should check with your doctor.

Watch Out!
Report any lumps or thickening you may find in your breast at any time to your health care provider, who may recommend a mammogram, depending on your family history.

Headaches

Fluctuating levels of estrogen can cause headaches, especially if you were prone to premenstrual migraines before menopause. In addition, if you are on HRT, you may experience intense headaches at first in response to the initial boost in hormones.

Bright Idea
If you are on HRT and you know you tend to get headaches anyway, you can choose the patch instead of a pill; patches provide a more constant absorption of hormone, which can lessen the incidence of headaches.

Heart palpitations

The rapid, out-of-control sensation of heart palpitations are a fairly common symptom of menopause, caused by a vasomotor response in the brain. It's important to realize they can also be caused by a variety of other factors, including too much caffeine or nicotine—or a heart condition. You need to discuss any heart palpitations with your health care provider.

Loss of sexual interest

Declining levels of estrogen can have a direct affect on your libido. Lower estrogen levels also can make your genitals less sensitive and make sex painful because of dry vaginal tissues. Of course, it's also possible that your loss of interest in sex is related to something else—either exhaustion from lack of sleep, depression, or premenstrual syndrome (PMS).

Urinary changes

Many women report changes in urination beginning with menopause. You may find yourself facing stress incontinence—the inability to hold in your urine during moments of stress, such as when you sneeze, laugh, or run. Or you may feel as if you need to go to the bathroom all the time. Other women complain that the urge to urinate is so strong they can barely restrain it until they reach a bathroom. When you do urinate, you may find it has become painful.

Losing urine control during times of stress occurs because the muscles around the bladder and urethra begin to loosen. As the vaginal wall weakens as a result of estrogen depletion, it can no longer support the bladder, which can drop out of place. Without the support of the vaginal wall and other muscles, even the tiniest pressure of a sneeze or a cough can lead to a small loss of urine.

Women who have had hysterectomies sometimes experience incontinence because the missing uterus has left the bladder and urethra without support, and occasionally the surgery itself can damage urinary tract tissues.

Moreover, lower estrogen levels can lead to changes in the urethra, much like those that occur in the vagina, setting off or worsening incontinence problems. Urinary infections, which can cause that urge to urinate, frequency of urination, or pain, are also due to a drop in estrogen. The urethra has estrogen receptors and, without the hormone, it can atrophy in the same way as the vagina. As the urethral walls become thinner and weaker, they are more prone to developing infections.

You may experience more urinary tract infections because the urethra and bladder tissue become thinner and less elastic. This makes these tissues more vulnerable to infection. Because repeated infections may endanger your kidneys or bladder, you should contact your health care provider at the first sign of a urinary tract infection.

Facial hair

As you enter menopause, you may notice the appearance of darker hair on your face. As the level of estrogen drops, male hormones are no longer balanced by estrogen. As a result, hair may begin to grow in response to these hormones. You may notice hair appearing in a more typically "masculine" pattern—on the upper lip, chin, and cheeks. If you start HRT, you'll notice this hair growth stopping, although the hair already present on your face won't go away.

Bright Idea
If you're bothered by urinary tract infections, ask your health care provider to look at the vagina or make a wet smear and look at the cells under the microscope. If they seem very thin and less elastic, consider using an estrogen cream.

Unofficially...
In the United States, about 46 percent of women try HRT; in Japan, only about 6 percent use HRT.

Depression

While a mild depression affects many women and may be related to many of the symptoms of menopause, experts no longer believe that depression is directly caused by the onset of menopausal symptoms. In fact, studies have failed to find any link between depression and menopause; women who do become depressed during this time don't appear to have symptoms any different from younger depressed women.

Of course, this doesn't mean you won't ever get depressed as you enter menopause. Menopause can disturb healthy sleep patterns and cause other annoying symptoms that can make you feel depressed, but it's important to note the difference between symptom-related feelings of depression and emotional illness. It's also true that if you're already depressed, you may be more disturbed by menopause symptoms; women who are already depressed are more than twice as likely to see a professional to complain about hot flashes, cold sweats, and irregular periods. If you are feeling depressed, consult a mental health care expert about treatment for depression.

How to cope with menopause symptoms

The easiest way to deal with menopausal symptoms is to take hormone replacement (or estrogen replacement if you no longer have a uterus). However, some women don't want to or can't take hormones; for these women, here are some tips and suggestions on coping with the various menopause symptoms in natural ways.

Hot flashes

You can handle hot flashes by

- Breathing: Do 10 minutes of slow, deep abdominal breathing every morning and night.

- **Exercising:** Studies show that hot flashes are half as common in women who are physically active (for instance, practice aerobic activity) as in those who are sedentary.

- **Not smoking:** Smoking constricts blood vessels, which can intensify a hot flash.

- **Wearing natural fabrics:** Cotton and other non-synthetic fabrics tend to breathe and don't trap perspiration. Cotton sheets and short-sleeved night clothes with v-necks are a good choice if you have night sweats.

- **Eating a good diet:** Avoid sugar, coffee, alcohol, spicy foods, teas, colas, chocolate, salt, and hot soups and drinks.

- **Tracking symptoms:** Keep track of your hot flashes so if you find a pattern, you can more easily manage the symptoms.

- **Drinking:** Keep a thermos of cold juice or water nearby to sip on.

- **Showering:** Take a cold shower or splash cold water on your wrists or face.

- **Getting cool air:** Use an air conditioner in your bedroom and buy a portable fan to carry in your purse.

- **Using herbs:** Ginseng is a root that has been used by Asians for centuries to enhance vitality; it is also a popular remedy for night sweats in doses of 1,000 mg daily. (Ginseng is also a stimulant; overdoses can lead to insomnia and anxiety); black cohosh (Remifemin) can help reduce hot flashes.

- **Taking vitamin E:** Thousands of women report that vitamin E can ease hot flashes, although studies have not yet provided conclusive proof.

Herbalists advise between 800 mg and 1,000 mg daily (far more than the 100 mg recommended by the Food and Drug Administrations [FDA]). Since extremely large doses of vitamin E can cause muscle weakness and fatigue, don't exceed 1,000 mg a day. Although vegetable oil, nuts, whole grains, and wheat germ are the best sources of this vitamin, you'll need supplements to get 1,000 mg every day. Since vitamin E can raise blood pressure, consult your health care provider before taking it.

- Taking vitamins B and C: Take one vitamin B (50 mg tablet) and 500 mg of vitamin C every day.

- Eating soy products: Take supplements or eat more tofu if you're bothered by hot flashes and can't take hormone replacement.

Heavy bleeding

If you're troubled by heavy bleeding, you may be able to control symptoms by making some lifestyle changes:

- Avoid hot baths or showers—remember that heat dilates blood vessels, which can increase your flow during the time the vessels are dilated.

- Don't take aspirin. Remember that aspirin is a "blood thinner," which means that it can increase your blood flow by interfering with the clotting ability of blood platelets.

- Avoid alcohol. When you drink a lot, fewer blood platelets form, which means your blood won't clot as well and you may experience a heavier flow during your periods.

- Exercise.

Insomnia

Here's how to handle insomnia:

- Drink a glass of warm milk, take a hot bath, listen to soft music, or read at bedtime.
- Avoid caffeine, chocolate, and spicy food late at night.
- Exercise—but avoid working out any later than two hours before bedtime or your heightened metabolism may block sleep.
- Go to bed the same time each night.
- Relax: Because insomnia may be related to stress, you may find relief through meditation, yoga, prayer, or a progressive relaxation. (See Chapter 9.)
- Avoid alcohol: While you may have been able to tolerate alcohol in the past, your present insomnia may be alcohol-related. Cut back and see.
- Stop smoking.
- Cut back on some types of antihistamines; they may be related to insomnia, even if you've never had a problem with them in the past.
- Don't eat a big meal right before bed.
- Keep your bedroom cool and dark.
- If all else fails, you may want to try biofeedback or visiting a sleep disorders clinic.

Mood swings and irritability

If you're feeling irritable

- Eat a well-balanced diet high in fruits and vegetables.
- Get plenty of exercise.
- Reduce stress (meditation has been shown to help ease menopausal symptoms).

Bright Idea
Exercising will help ease many symptoms of menopause by affecting the release of FSH and luteinizing hormone (LH).

- Join a support group for menopausal women.
- If symptoms are unbearable, see your health care provider for possible medication.
- Take B vitamins: Take 50 mg or 100 mg of a vitamin B complex daily.
- Take calcium supplements: Increasing your calcium intake to 1,300 mg a day may make you feel calmer.

Memory problems

If you're having trouble with memory problems:

- Make lists and notes for yourself.
- Carry a tiny battery-powered, microchip "note recorder" to keep track of appointments, reminders, and other things you need to remember.
- Pay attention. Many memory lapses occur because we are distracted, stressed, or thinking of something else when we put down our glasses or park our car.
- Get enough sleep if you want to boost your concentration the next day.
- Exercise your brain; take up new hobbies, learn a foreign language or chess, work on your computer skills.
- The herb ginko biloba may help improve short-term memory by improving blood flow to the brain.

Vaginal dryness

To cope with vaginal dryness

- Use estrogen cream on vaginal tissues.
- Before having sex, place a few teaspoons of a water-soluble lubricant (such as K-Y jelly or

Astroglide) on the outside of your vagina, and a little bit on the inside. Water-based lubricants are superior to oil-based because they are less likely to cause infection. You should use a jelly specifically made for use during sex. Astroglide is a light lubricant that doesn't have any medicinal taste or smell; it is applied right before intercourse.

- Try a vaginal moisturizer (such as Replens), which can be applied hours before sex. These moisturizers claim to replenish vaginal moisture when used regularly. To use, insert the applicator into the vagina three or four times a week so that it coats the surface of the vagina and moisturizes the tissues.

- Drink plenty of water; you can also drink fruit or vegetable juices, or herbal teas. (Coffee and alcohol will dehydrate you, so you might want to avoid them.)

- Stimulate the vaginal area to boost blood flow and improve lubrication; have regular sex or masturbate regularly.

- Avoid douches and perfumed toilet paper, bath bubbles, soaps, and oils that can dry or irritate your vagina.

- Don't become anxious, since tension can lead to painful intercourse.

- Avoid antihistamines and other drugs that cause vaginal dryness.

- Engage in longer foreplay so your body has time to release its own lubricants. By the time you reach your mid-50s, you will need longer stimulation to become fully lubricated.

Watch Out!
Don't use petroleum jelly as a lubricant during sex; it can break down the latex of a condom, increasing your vulnerability to sexually transmitted diseases, and, because it's made from petroleum, it can cause irritation.

- Don't wear tight pants or underpants that don't have a cotton lining.

Headaches

If you're getting lots of headaches:

- Avoid anything that triggered headaches before you entered menopause—certain types of food, caffeine, alcohol, or stress.
- Try regular exercise or biofeedback.
- Your health care provider may prescribe pain medication if you are having severe headaches.

Loss of libido

If you're having a problem with your interest in sex:

- Keep having sex. The less often you have sex, the less you may begin to enjoy—or miss—it.
- Take more time to make love.
- Experiment—try new things, as long as they aren't emotionally uncomfortable for you or your partner.
- Take a mini vacation, even if it's just a hotel room in your own town. Get a sitter and go out to dinner, try a Jacuzzi.

Urinary problems

If this is your problem:

- Kegel exercises can help with bladder control, tightening and toning the vaginal area; try to do at least 10 sets of 20 each day: Contract your vaginal muscles as if you were trying to stop yourself from urinating. Hold for a count of five; relax for a count of five; repeat this sequence 20 times. Contract and release in quick succession.
- If you don't want to try Kegels, you may be interested in pelvic training weights, a set of weights

that look like small cones with attached strings, ranging from 20 to 70 grams. You begin by inserting the smallest weight into the vagina, wearing it for 10 to 15 minutes twice a day. Your circumvaginal muscles must hold the weight in the vagina (otherwise, it falls out). When you can hold the weight in place even when coughing, you graduate to the next bigger weight.

- Lose weight; extra weight may put too much stress on the bladder and urethra, causing them to sag and leak.
- Some drugs (such as antihistamines and tranquilizers) can aggravate bladder control problems.
- Some foods (spicy foods, citrus beverages) can irritate the bladder and worsen leakage. Cut back or eliminate caffeine and alcohol for the same reason.
- Exercise to strengthen your abdomen and pelvic muscles.

Watch Out!
Pelvic relaxation that is too severe to respond to Kegels or hormone replacement may require surgical intervention. However, surgery should be a last resort. Be sure to have your doctor assess your bladder function with urodynamic testing by a urogynecologist.

Is it PMS or the beginning of menopause?

Because so many of the symptoms of the beginning of menopause seem to mimic those of PMS, some women find it hard to tell the difference. The seven million women with PMS notice that symptoms usually begin either with the first period or after the first pregnancy. Some doctors believe that an attack of PMS which suddenly appears in your 30s may not be PMS at all, but very early signs of menopause. Certainly some of the symptoms—moodiness, irritability, breast tenderness, headaches—are the same for both problems.

There is no agreement as to whether women with significant PMS that begins in the teenage years will go on to develop problems as menopause approaches. Likewise, there doesn't appear to be a correlation between severity of PMS and severity of menopause symptoms.

If you suspect you have PMS and not the beginning of menopause, it helps to keep a diary of symptoms. Note the date when symptoms begin, and any changes in symptoms. PMS symptoms tend to be cyclical; menopause symptoms are not. Keeping a diary will help to chart when these symptoms and what, if anything, appears to set them off.

Experts have begun to realize that menopause isn't so much an abrupt health event, but a gradual process of aging that occurs as your body begins to shift gears as the reproductive years pass away. Symptoms can appear up to 10 or 15 years before menopause begins; other women go through the early stages of perimenopause in just a month.

Some lucky women—about 20 percent—have such an easy time they don't notice early menopause at all, and are completely unaware of the gradual decrease in hormones as their body is gearing down. Another 5 to 10 percent have minor problems (maybe a few irregular periods or a couple of hot flashes). But between 10 and 35 percent of women experience severe, long-lasting symptoms, including irregular periods, hot flashes, insomnia, mood swings, and breast tenderness. For these women, the symptoms are much like having a constant bout of PMS, and they can seriously interfere with their daily lives.

The problem is that because many women think of menopause as the month their periods finally stop, they don't often connect these symptoms with hormonal changes. Women may believe they are suffering from PMS, from stress-related irritability, or age-related memory loss. Just as they begin to see their vision worsen because of age-related eye changes, they assume that short-term memory loss must mean the beginning of Alzheimer's disease.

Those women who become concerned enough to see their health care provider may still be told that they're too young to be entering menopause, reflecting the common notion that menopause is an abrupt change. If you're still having periods, some health care providers insist that symptoms must be either due to another cause or are all in your head.

Finding the right health care provider

If you think you're having menopause symptoms, you should seek help from a practitioner trained in the treatment of menopause. There are a wide range of specialists, in addition to internists or family physicians, from whom to choose. You'll want to find someone you can work with, and someone who won't dismiss your complaints and overlook symptoms—someone you can work with as a team. It's important to be able to trust your health care provider and to feel comfortable with that person.

Many women have tended to rely on their gynecologist for all their health care needs. As you age, however, and your health care concerns broaden, you may want to find an internist or family care doctor. If you choose to see a family care physician or internist for your gynecological care, you'll need to be sure this specialist also performs an annual pelvic exam and Pap smear. On the other hand, you may

Bright Idea
To find a menopause clinician or specialist, forward your request to North American Menopause Society, P.O. Box 94527, Cleveland, OH 44101, or fax it to 216/844-8708. You may also register your request with the 900-number program by calling 900/370-6267. Finally, you may submit your request via e-mail to nams@apk.net.

want to choose a gynecologist, nurse practitioner, nutritionist, acupuncturist, herbalist, therapist—or a combination of these.

Consulting an expert

As you enter menopause, you may prefer to locate a health care provider who is an expert in the field of menopause. One way to find such an expert is to contact the North American Menopause Society for its multistate list of NAMS members. This list includes physicians, nurses, psychotherapists, social workers, and others who describe themselves as "menopause clinicians" in their geographic area.

Sometimes you may need specialized care, especially if you're having a hard time regulating your HRT. Some women see a reproductive endocrinologist if they are having a hard time working with their regular health care provider in easing their menopausal symptoms. A reproductive endocrinologist can be of special help to you if your symptoms are severe and aren't responding to traditional treatment, or if you've had breast cancer or have had close family members with the disease and you want someone with the latest information on HRT.

Unless you live in a large urban area or near a medical center, you may have to travel to find a good specialist (who will also be more expensive). But it's possible to have most of your needs taken care of by your regular health care provider while simply relying on the specialist for diagnosis and consultations. Many gynecologists receive extensive training in the management of menopause. And since reproductive endocrinologists don't provide regular, ongoing gynecological care anyway, but will refer you back to your original provider once your situation has stabilized.

Bright Idea
If you want to find a reproductive endocrinologist yourself without a referral from your regular health care provider, you can obtain a list of members from the American Fertility Society. Call 205/978-5000.

You can also ask friends or co-workers for recommendations, or get a recommendation from your current family practitioner. You can also call your local hospital to get a list of names of doctors who are affiliated with the institution. Check out the library resources, including the *Compendium of Certified Medical Specialists* or the *Directory of Medical Specialists*. These sources list physicians' credentials and whether or not they are board certified. (Board-certified doctors have undergone extra training in their field and have passed written exams.)

Now that you have some potential names, schedule an office visit. Talking on the phone to get some basic information is one thing, but you won't know how the doctor actually deals with you as a patient until you are sitting in the office. Be sure to let the doctor know that you're there for an interview, and be prepared to pay the regular office visit cost.

10 questions to ask

1. Is the provider knowledgeable about menopause?

2. What is the person's training in menopause and aging? Has the person recently attended any menopause classes, courses, or workshops?

3. Does your provider give you information about menopause, with ongoing support and/or classes? If not, can he or she refer you to workshops or classes?

4. How much time does the provider spend with you? Is there enough time to adequately explain your lifestyle issues and your family history?

5. Is the provider readily available? Having to wait a month or more for an appointment may be too long.

6. Can you talk openly, as an equal? How does the provider respond to your questions? Does he or she get upset when you question advice or information?
7. Is the provider aware of, or at least open to, alternative therapy or natural methods?
8. Is the provider willing to consult with other professionals on alternative possible treatments?
9. Does the person explain things in a way you can understand?
10. Is the provider willing to review the pros and cons of HRT, including pros and cons of synthetic and natural forms of estrogen?

Hormone tests: Do they work?

Even as your body is trying to cope with a dramatic readjustment and the rebalancing of your reproductive organs, your entry into mid-life means you may be dealing with maturing children, job changes—and problems with your own aging parents. How can you tell whether your symptoms are the result of stress or menopause? A simple test to determine for sure the onset of menopause would be handy—but none exists.

Some doctors will tell you that a simple FSH blood test can determine whether you are going through menopause—but unfortunately, it's not quite that simple. The FSH test is a measure of the level of FSH in your blood, which triggers the release of an egg from your ovaries. FSH rises as you get older and the eggs left in your body lose their ability to function. The brain senses they need more of the hormone to become fertilized, so FSH levels rise. When this happens, it's a sign of the erratic ability of your ovaries to produce estrogen.

The problem is that while it's true that FSH levels do rise as you age, women have varying patterns of FSH levels and menopause symptoms. In one recent study, scientists discovered that it's possible for some women to keep on menstruating with high levels of FSH, even as other women have high levels of FSH and low levels of estrogen. Some women experience wild fluctuations of FSH, with readings typical of postmenopause one moment, which then plummet to pre-menopausal levels the next.

If it's been at least three months since your last period, a test of your FSH level might help determine whether you've finally begun menopause—but even this is no guarantee. It's possible to stop having periods for several months and then abruptly begin bleeding again. In fact, one study found that this is exactly what happened to about 20 percent of women who had apparently stopped having their periods. As a result, most health care providers believe that the FSH test alone can't be used as proof that you've entered menopause. In other words, it's possible that you are indeed beginning early menopause, but that your test won't show it.

An FSH test is a simple blood test done at a particular time, depending on a woman's symptoms. If you're having irregular periods or hot flashes, you should do the test on the second or third day of your cycle. If you have missed your period or have some menopause symptoms, you can do the test any time. If the reading is between 10 and 12, it's a sign of the beginning of ovarian failure. FSH above 25 is a sign that menopause is complete.

Bright Idea
If you want a hormone test, insist that you have a test that checks not just estrogen, but levels of estrogen, progesterone, testosterone, and other hormones. Contrary to popular belief, estrogen isn't the only hormone that changes during perimenopause.

Hormone replacement therapy: Yes or no?

Most experts agree that menopause is not a "disease" that needs to be cured, but a natural transition that has become inappropriately burdened with negative symbolism. But if it's obvious that you're entering menopause and you're struggling with symptoms, it's time to decide what you are or aren't going to do about it.

The goal of HRT is to replace estrogen that's lost at menopause, easing symptoms like hot flashes and safeguarding women against health risks linked to low hormone levels, including heart disease and osteoporosis. But it's also true that HRT causes breakthrough bleeding and sore breasts, and it may trigger other diseases, such as breast cancer.

There are really about 200 different kinds of estrogen, a family of hormones found in humans, animals, and even plants. The three common human estrogens:

- Estradiol
- Estrone
- Estriol

Estradiol is the strongest, created mostly in the ovaries and circulated in the blood. Once thought to affect only sex and reproduction, today scientists know that estrogen influences cells in the brain, the bones, and throughout the cardiovascular system. It's no surprise that a plunge in estrogen as you enter menopause has effects throughout your body!

What kind of HRT?

When you reach menopause, replacing estrogen alone exposes you to the risk of estrogen-related uterine cancer; as a result, unless you've had a hysterectomy, hormone replacement includes progesterone, which protects your uterus from the harmful effects of estrogen.

If you decide to take HRT, the next question is, what kind? Premarin is one of the best-known types of estrogen, purified from the urine of pregnant mares. Widely prescribed in this country in typical doses of 0.625 mg and 1.25 mg, it contains dozens of estrogens. It is the form used in studies that show both benefits and risks of HRT. Some women object to Premarin because they believe that the method of obtaining the mare's urine is inhumane. Other women find taking hormones from a horse to be "unnatural." Many of the recent studies are showing that some of the effects linking hormone replacement to Alzheimer's may arise from horse estrogens and not from estradiol.

The most common human estrogen (17-beta-estradiol) is the only one that has been synthesized in a form potent enough for replacement therapy. Produced from yams, it's marketed under the name Estrace.

While all the patches and creams seem to protect your bones, pills such as Premarin and Estrace seem to be the most effective against heart disease because they are processed by the liver, where cholesterol levels are adjusted. (Skin patches and creams bypass the liver.)

Estrone conjugate is a type of estrogen (Ogen or Ortho EST) derived from the primary type of hormone produced by the ovaries after menopause. It can both ease symptoms and protect against osteoporosis. Estradiol has about 100 times the effect in the body as does Estrone on a dose-for-dose basis. Different doses of different estrogens are required to bring about the same effect on bones. In fact, a dose of one estrogen that protects the wrist from loss of bone may not protect the hip, while a lower dose of a different estrogen may protect the hip but not the wrist.

Plant estrogens are the least studied forms of estrogen. Over-the-counter forms of phytoestrogens (plan estrogen-like compounds such as soy powder or the herb black cohosh) are largely unregulated, so no one knows how much estrogen they contain.

Progestins

Progestin is a family of agents that have progestational effects. There aren't as many different types of progestins as there are estrogens. One brand name progestin, Provera, is the trade name for medroxyprogesterone acetate. Amen and Cycrin are also trade names for medroxy progesterone acetate. Aygestin is a trade name for Norethindrone acetate, another progestin. Most progestins are found in oral contraceptives along with an estrogen that is about six to eight times as potent as premarin.

Progesterone is not well absorbed orally—natural progesterone (in an oral form) is given in doses of 100 to 200 mg per day, depending on dosing schedule. Progestins (synthetic) like Provera are given in doses of 2.5 to 5 mg per day, again depending on dosing schedule. Synthetic progestins like Porvera are not meant to be taken vaginally.

You also can take progestin as a vaginal or rectal suppository twice a day, but these are messy. The latest FDA-approved progestins are actually two versions of natural progesterone—Crinone 4 percent, a vaginal gel, and Prometrium, a pill.

Also newly approved by the FDA is the estrogen ring (Estring). Inserted into the top of the vagina, it gradually releases the hormone for up to three months. It can be easily removed if there is a problem and provides constant levels as long as the ring is in place.

Progestin injections are painful and aren't a good choice for HRT. In May 1999, the FDA approved a combination estrogen/progestin patch called Combipatch; it contains estradiol and the progestin norethindrone acetate.

Alphabet SERMs

Some of the newest types of HRT are the selective estrogen receptor modulators (SERMs) that offer some of the protection against bone loss that estrogen does, perhaps without the increased risk of breast cancer. In fact, one SERM—raloxifene (Evista)—seems to have reduced by more than 50 percent the incidence of breast cancer among women enrolled in ongoing osteoporosis studies, according to at least one recent study.

SERMs modulate specific estrogen receptors, of which there are now known to be at least two (and probably six or more). Raloxifene doesn't stimulate the receptors in the breast and endometrium, so it doesn't have a growth effect on cells there (i.e., it doesn't cause breast cancer). On the other hand, tamoxifen stimulates the receptors in the endometrium, but not the breast.

Like estrogen, raloxifene works by attaching to an estrogen "receptor," much like a key fits into a lock. When the hormone "key" clicks into the receptor "lock" in the breast and uterus, it blocks estrogen at these sites by physically keeping estrogen from binding to the receptor. This is the secret of its cancer-fighting property. (Many tumors in the breast are fueled by estrogen.)

Watch Out! Women with a history of blood clots in their veins should not use raloxifene, estrogen, or tamoxifen without consulting a physician; depending on when, where, and why the clots occurred, you may or may not be advised to avoid these drugs.

At the same time, preliminary results from a study of more than 12,000 women suggest that raloxifene increases bone density by up to 3 percent. It also appears to protect against heart attacks by lowering total cholesterol, LDL ("bad") cholesterol and fibrinogen. In addition, raloxifene does not produce breast tenderness or bloating, as do other hormones. So far, experts don't know if it protects against Alzheimer's disease as Premarin appears to.

Raloxifene is already approved for treating osteoporosis, For women who don't undergo HRT for fear of breast cancer, raloxifene could be a logical. There are a few catches, however. There is no evidence that raloxifene boosts HDL ("good") cholesterol and it doesn't ease hot flashes or other menopausal symptoms (and actually worsens hot flashes in about 40 percent of women). Moreover, there is a significant risk of developing blood clots with raloxifene. Additionally, experts are still discovering new benefits of estrogen replacement and it's not clear if SERMs will be as effective and versatile as estrogen itself.

Still, experts are hoping that the new generation of SERMs may offer many of the benefits of HRT with fewer risks or side effects.

The most serious side effect associated with raloxifene was a 2.5 fold increased risk of blood clots that form in the veins, which may break off and travel to the lungs. Other commonly reported side effects were hot flashes and leg cramps.

Low-dose estrogen

Fortunately, doctors today may have a new option for postmenopausal women who have turned against HRT because of unpleasant side effects. Scientists can reduce headaches, breast tenderness,

Unofficially...
A new seven-year study called "STAR" (Study of Tamoxifen and Raloxifene) will be the first large, direct comparison of both drugs' ability to prevent breast cancer. STAR will enroll 22,000 women at hundreds of centers around the United States.

and other side effects by cutting the estrogen dose in half, and by giving progesterone only twice a year instead of every month. The lower levels of hormones still control menopause symptoms, according to a May 1999 report by California researchers. However, scientists at Kaiser Permanente Medical Care in Oakland still need to find out if taking progesterone only twice a year is safe. The monthly progesterone dose included in traditional HRT protects the uterus from the cancer-causing effects of estrogen.

A little more, a little less...

Even though women know that long-term HRT can help prevent osteoporosis and may help the heart, as many as 80 percent stop filling their prescriptions after three years because of unpleasant side effects.

Most women may discover that it can be hard to find just the right dosage of hormones, and find themselves returning again and again to their health care provider's office. It appears as if this tinkering is critical to getting the most out of your HRT, since it's possible to adjust not just the dose, but the method of administration—pill, patch, injection, and so on. The goal is to find the lowest possible dose that will control your symptoms and protect you from heart disease and osteoporosis. Even in the best of cases, most women should count on between three to five return visits to get the adjustment just right.

Testosterone: Yes or no?

In addition to estrogen and progesterone, your ovaries also produce a small amount of male hormone and continue to do so even as female hormone levels drop. As you enter menopause, the levels of male hormones decrease by as much as 50 percent.

If you're taking estrogen and you're still experiencing problems with poor sleep, mood swings, hot flashes, and especially loss of libido, your testosterone levels may be too low—and adding testosterone may help. Ask your health care provider to test your testosterone levels to see if they are abnormally low. Some women never need testosterone replacement, but others find it can help many of their menopausal symptoms. Testosterone can improve your libido and decrease anxiety and depression. (Adding testosterone especially helps women who have had hysterectomies.) Testosterone also eases breast tenderness and helps prevent bone loss.

You can take testosterone in the form of Estratest, which combines estrogen and testosterone and is taken each day, or you can alternate with estrogen every other day.

Of course, no treatment is perfect, and testosterone has its side effects. Some women experience mild acne, loss of hair on the head, and some facial hair growth. However, since testosterone levels in Estratest are very low, more typically, most women don't appear to have extremely masculine changes.

Watch Out!
Long-term use of testosterone supplements in women have not been studied, so doctors don't know what good or bad effects it may have after 20 or 30 years.

Testosterone shouldn't be given to women who could become pregnant while using it, depressed women, or women on antidepressants, or to those whose testosterone levels are normal. In addition, testosterone won't help women whose lack of interest in sex is related to serious history of abuse, body image, or other psychological issues.

Unfortunately, some health care providers are not open to the idea of testosterone supplementation for some menopausal women, believing that somehow testosterone is only a "men's hormone."

There also may be a lingering sexist belief that a man with lagging sexual desire needs to be helped immediately, but a declining interest in sex among menopausal women is not too serious, often dismissed with advice to "just use a lubricant."

In fact, one study found that between 40 and 60 percent of women in the United States lose interest in sex during menopause. If you've always had a normal attitude and interest in sex and suddenly your libido plummets as you approach menopause, see your health care provider for a testosterone test. Loss of desire is not something you should just have to accept.

Birth control pills as HRT

There is another choice for women struggling with perimenopause symptoms who are still having at least occasional periods and who don't want to choose HRT, but whose symptoms don't go away just by making lifestyle changes in diet, exercise, and so on. For some of you, low-dose birth control pills can solve many of these problems.

Oral contraceptives with low estrogen doses can produce regular, predictable cycles and can regulate the erratic release of estrogen. By reining in this burst of estrogen, the pill can ease hot flashes, vaginal dryness, and insomnia. (A side benefit: It can protect against unexpected pregnancy, which can occur during perimenopause.)

However, the Pill is not prescribed as often as it might be because of ingrained concerns about a possible link between stroke in older women and oral contraceptives. While an analysis of the effect of birth control pills on the risk of breast cancer found no increased risk among women aged 24 to 39, there was a risk for both younger and older women who took the Pill. Women aged 46 to 54 had

Watch Out!
Viagra, the medication that restores the ability for many men to have an erection, does not affect libido in men or women.

double the risk of breast cancer; once they stopped using the Pill, the additional risk disappeared after three years. In addition, women over 45 who smoke and take the Pill have a significantly elevated risk of stroke and heart attack.

There may be other reasons why some women don't want to take the Pill. Some women just don't get relief with the Pill and others can't tolerate the side effects—bloating, moodiness, and weight gain.

HRT: What method should you use?

Just as there are different kinds of hormones, there are different ways to take them. Today you can choose from pills, patches, creams, vaginal rings and injections.

Hormone pills

Hormone pills are portable, neat, and easy to take, and it's easy to manipulate dosages. Oral hormones must pass through the liver, however, which can increase the liver's production of clotting factors. This puts you at risk for blood clots, although the risk is fairly low unless you have a history of blood clots. Other possible side effects are high blood pressure, nausea, and bloating. Slipping a pill under your tongue instead of swallowing it may help ease at least some of these symptoms. If you get nauseated from the hormone pill, try taking it at bedtime. On the plus side, it gives you a significant protection against heart attack.

Skin patch

One of the most popular new ways to administer hormones is with the skin patch (transdermal patch), which provides a constant supply of estrogen while bypassing the liver. The transparent dollar-sized patch must be changed every three to four days. You can wear it on your abdomen or buttocks, where it delivers estrogen through the skin in a slow, even dose—just as your ovaries would if they were still functioning at peak efficiency.

The patch is handy—you don't have to worry about taking a pill and it is helpful for women with liver disease. It's also easy to change dosages. Unfortunately, some women are allergic to the adhesive on the patch. And while you can swim and bathe with the patch, it may not stay on for marathon tub soaks.

If you live in a hot, humid climate, you may have trouble keeping the patch on your skin; paper tape can help hold the patch in place. If the patch bothers your skin, remove it and try putting it on a new spot on your abdomen or buttocks. Some women, however, show continued sensitivity to the adhesive. If this happens to you, you may need to find another form of HRT.

If you notice that your symptoms continue even if you are using the higher dose patch, ask your doctor to check your estradiol blood levels. Some women have problems absorbing the estradiol from the patch. (The same holds true for oral estrogen—some women do not absorb oral estrogen well and do better with a patch.)

Vaginal cream

If you suffer from vaginal dryness, you may want to consider a hormone cream, which you can insert into your vagina. This form of HRT is used mostly for problems of the vaginal area or the urinary tract. It can take a long time to heal a dry, atrophied vagina. Women with this problem who are taking other forms of hormones may want to add vaginal cream to relubricate the vagina.

Bright Idea
The patch is available in the United States in 0.05 mg and 0.1 mg dosages, and in a lower dose of 0.025 mg (FemPatch). If you want to start out with lower dose (to ease initial side effects), try placing a bandage under the 0.05 mg patch to reduce the amount of estradiol that enters the bloodstream.

Bright Idea
Now you can wear a patch and swim, shower, and dive without worrying about it coming off. The smallest-ever approved patch, by Noven Pharmaceuticals, is a nearly transparent tiny sticker containing 17-beta-estradiol in four dosing strengths (0.0375, 0.05, 0.075 and 0.10 mg per day).

While some of the hormones are absorbed into the bloodstream from the vagina, the levels aren't high enough to protect you against heart disease and osteoporosis. Dosage is usually a quarter of an applicator each day for four weeks, followed by an occasional dose every couple of days per week afterward. After a few months, the oral or patch forms of estrogen should be enough to thicken the vagina.

While women like the speed of response when using the cream, it can be difficult to apply and can cause unpleasant breast tenderness. Moreover, you shouldn't use the cream right before sex (your partner could absorb the cream through the penis).

Injections

If you hate taking pills or remembering to change a patch and find creams messy, you may want to consider once-a-month estradiol injections. The problem with these (besides the shot, which some women find unpleasant) is that you can't adjust the dosage once you've gotten the injection, even if you develop side effects. Also, the level of hormone is high at the start, and then rapidly falls and stays low for the rest of the month.

Vaginal rings

The estrogen ring Estring was approved by the FDA in April 1996. Once inserted into the top of the vagina, it gradually releases the hormone for up to three months. It can be easily removed if there is a problem, and provides constant levels as long as the ring is in place.

On the drawing board...

Crystalline 17b-estradiol pellets have not yet been approved by the FDA, but are used in Europe. The pellets can be surgically implanted under the skin so the estrogen is absorbed directly into the blood. The pellets can remain in place for up to six months. The good news about this method is that you don't need to think about your hormones for six months. The bad news is that the pellets can be hard to remove if you are having side effects or other problems. Some women also have developed a tolerance to the high levels of estradiol in the pellets and need more frequent insertion or higher doses.

Pros and cons of HRT

The decision to have HRT is very personal. You need to weigh the risks and benefits with your health care provider, and discuss new alternatives such as raloxifene, which can ease symptoms but doesn't seem to boost breast cancer risk.

You may also want to consider natural estrogens derived from soy and wild yam. Natural alternatives also include lifestyle changes: quitting smoking; cutting back on alcohol; eating a low-fat diet rich in fruits, vegetables, and whole grains; and exercising. Instead of taking hormones, some women try to avoid stress, hot weather, warm rooms, hot drinks, caffeine, and spicy foods. Each woman has a unique collection of health issues and concerns, and her therapy needs to be tailored to her own requirements.

As a general rule, if you have a high risk of breast cancer in your family, you should be at least a bit concerned about taking estrogen supplements. On the other hand, for women at high risk for osteoporosis with no family history of breast cancer, the benefits of estrogen might outweigh the risks.

Beyond that very basic statement, leading experts often come to opposite conclusions about the risks and benefits of HRT. In fact, two of the largest recent

Unofficially...
Up to 20 percent of women who try HRT stop within nine months because of various side effects.

studies published in the *Journal of the American Medical Association* came to opposite conclusions about whether giving replacement estrogen to menopausal women increased the risk of breast cancer.

However, a third study of 37,000 women, released on June 8, 1999, found that taking hormones after menopause does not increase the risk of breast cancer, except for some uncommon forms of the disease that are slow growing and highly treatable. Women who took hormones and those who didn't had no difference in their risk of getting the fast growing, life threatening tumors that make up 90 percent of all cases of breast cancer.

This was the first hormone study to categorize cases of breast cancer according to whether they were slow growing or fast growing. Researchers say it may help to explain the conflicting data in other studies, and why hormone takers survive breast cancer more often than those who don't take hormones. One possible explanation is that the women on hormones develop more favorable tumor types, according to Melody Cobleigh, Director of the Comprehensive Breast Center at Rush-Presbyterian-St. Luke's Medical Center in Chicago (she was not involved in the study).

Years ago, when a woman's life span was not so long, taking hormones didn't present such a problem. But since today you may well survive into your mid-80s, beginning hormones in early menopause and taking them for the rest of your life, as some health care providers recommend, means you would be taking hormones for a third of your life. Some experts recommend taking hormones just for the few years when symptoms are difficult, gradually tapering off after menopause is complete.

Still others suggest that it might make better sense to prescribe hormone replacement for women in their 60s who are at imminent risk of developing osteoporosis or heart disease, rather than prescribing it for all healthy women in their 40s on the chance that a few of them might develop these problems.

Some doctors believe that all women, except those with certain cancers, should be taking hormones as they approach menopause because of the low chance of getting breast cancer and the benefits of protection against heart disease, osteoporosis, and uterine cancer. Critics of HRT say that the benefits of taking hormones to ease menopause symptoms are not worth the risk (however small) that the hormones might trigger cancer. They argue that menopause isn't a disease, and not all women should automatically be given hormones to "cure" themselves of what is actually a very natural process of aging.

Unofficially...
Only 1 out of 25 women in the United States will get osteoporosis. Also, more women will die of heart disease than will ever get breast cancer.

HRT risk and heart attacks

While HRT traditionally has been thought to help prevent heart problems in menopausal women, it can cause problems in women who already have heart disease when they begin HRT. Duke University researchers warn that health care providers should think twice about prescribing HRT for women who have heart disease. A Duke study released in 1999 is the second in a year that finds an association between the new use of hormones in women who have previous heart disease and the occurrence of a second "cardiac event" (such as a heart attack or angina). This was not the case among women using such hormones before they developed heart disease.

However, the increase in a second cardiovascular event only seems to be a problem in the first year after HRT is begun. After that, it is protective.

This suggests that the message that hormone therapy is good for the hearts of all postmenopausal women must be considered further. While HRT has benefits and may still help protect the hearts of women without heart disease, women who have heart disease should probably not start hormone replacement, experts say. But experts also say there is no reason to suggest women stop using hormones if they develop heart disease after treatment begins.

A 1998 study reported that women with heart disease should not start HRT because it appeared to boost the risk of a heart attack, especially in the first year of treatment in postmenopausal women with heart disease. The California researchers concluded that there was no overall cardiac benefit to hormone use in these women during the four years of the trial, and that the risk of heart attacks seemed to increase soon after starting hormones. The result was unexpected in light of the growing consensus that hormones helped hearts.

What the experts agree on

Most doctors would agree that short-term use of estrogen is a sensible choice for those women with annoying symptoms, such as hot flashes or night sweats, who don't have a history of breast cancer.

Is HRT right for you?

HRT seems a bit like a two-edged sword. On the one hand, HRT can protect your bones (whether it protects the heart is still controversial), but at the same time it might be causing breast or uterine cancer. How do you decide whether HRT is right for you?

> 66
> I think it's important for women who choose estrogen therapy for relief of hot flashes or night sweats not to feel that this is a bad choice... No studies have found that short-term use of estrogen is dangerous and it can certainly improve your quality of life.
> —Susan Love, M.D., in *Dr. Susan Love's Hormone Book*
> 99

The answer is by keeping up with the latest medical findings, locating a health care provider who will discuss the controversies in an open-minded way, and weighing the risk factors against your lifestyle and your own family history.

Not every woman wants to take HRT. In fact, only 15 to 20 percent of the 37 million postmenopausal women in the United States undergo HRT, and only 70 to 80 percent of women with prescriptions ever fill them.

You're a good candidate
HRT might make a good choice for you if you

- Need to prevent osteoporosis.
- Have had your ovaries removed.
- Have a family history of heart disease.
- Have significant symptoms.

Women at risk
You may not want to take HRT if you have a history of the following conditions, because the therapy puts you at slightly higher risk for serious side effects. You need to discuss HRT with your doctor if you are postmenopausal and have

- Clots or stroke (history of).
- Deep vein thrombosis.
- Diabetes.
- Endometriosis.
- Fibroids.
- Gallstones.
- High blood pressure.
- Kidney or liver disease.
- Obesity.

- Migraines.
- Pulmonary blockage.
- Sickle cell anemia.
- Varicose veins.

You're a bad risk

You would be a poor candidate for HRT if you

- Have ever been diagnosed with breast or endometrial cancer (however, women treated for both breast and endometrial cancers may take HRT if an analysis of potential benefits outweighs potential risks).
- Have had liver disease.
- Have blood clots or phlebitis.
- Are a heavy smoker and have high triglyceride levels.

Some women with liver disease can take HRT, but they may want to consider the patch so the hormones will bypass processing by the liver.

Who should absolutely avoid HRT

You should definitely never go on HRT if you

- Have undiagnosed vaginal bleeding.
- Have a current, acute blood clot.
- Current, untreated breast or endometrial cancer.
- Acute liver disease.

What to ask your health care provider

Ask the following questions of a health care provider who is interested in prescribing hormone replacement to ease your menopause symptoms:

- Which hormones are you recommending for me and why?
- What are the hormones supposed to do?

- What are the short and long-term side effects of this hormone treatment?
- How soon should the hormone therapy be started?
- How long will I be taking the hormones?
- In what form and how often will the treatment be given?
- Will I be given the hormone therapy along with other forms of treatment?

Side effects of HRT

Taking hormones to replace the ones that you have lost can successfully eliminate hot flashes, vaginal dryness, urinary incontinence, insomnia, moodiness, memory, heavy irregular periods and poor concentration. It sounds like a wonder drug, and some women do think of it as a sort of "youth pill."

Unfortunately, there are side effects that can include bloating, breakthrough bleeding, headaches and nausea. Of course, the dosage and the method of HRT can influence the side effect profile. If your therapy includes progesterone, you may also experience fluid retention, breast tenderness, moodiness, and headaches. About one in four women say they gain weight while undergoing HRT, and many insist the hormone makes them hungrier. However, estrogen itself will not increase your weight.

HRT dosage regimens

There are a variety of ways to schedule your HRT and the method you choose may depend in large part on whether or not you want to deal with a regular period. Women who take estrogen alone won't have a period, but adding progestin will bring on bleeding if you take it cyclically (not continuously). Women who had unpleasant symptoms when taking birth control pills years ago may assume that they aren't good candidates for HRT, but it's important to realize that the amount of estrogen needed to suppress ovulation is much higher than the amount required to ease menopause symptoms.

When your ovaries were producing estradiol before menopause, your blood levels usually fluctuated between 40 pg/ml to 400 pg/ml during your cycle. A blood level of 50 to 65 pg/ml is usually enough to ease symptoms and protect your heart and bones. If all you want is to stop your hot flashes during the beginning of menopause, you can take HRT for a few years and then gradually wean yourself off the hormones. If you're troubled with vaginal dryness or atrophy, you may need a longer treatment regimen, but still you should not need treatment for more than about four years.

Continuous estrogen and cyclic progestin

Since estrogen alone has been linked to the development of endometrial (uterine) cancer, women whose uteruses are intact need to add progestin (a synthetic form of progesterone) to their HRT programs. This combination eliminates the added risk of endometrial cancer.

Natural progesterone can also be used. There are now two FDA-approved natural progesterones available for postmenopausal HRT—Crinone 8 percent (a vaginal gel) and Prometrium (an oral pill). Side effects seem to be less with the natural progesterone.

Most experts recommend this dosage regimen for women with severe menopausal symptoms. With this method, you take estrogen every day and add progestin for only part of the month. Because you're taking progestin, you may have a period, although the periods eventually become light.

Your menopausal symptoms won't reappear because of the estrogen, but you'll still have a period because of the progestin.

Cyclic estrogen and progestin
In this treatment plan, you take estrogen on days 1 through 25, adding progestin on days 14 through 25. On the 26th day, you don't take either hormone and you will then have a period. The periods eventually become light, but you will bleed. The problem with this method is that your menopausal symptoms may return during the five or six days you're not taking estrogen.

Continuous estrogen and progestin
For women who want to avoid having a period, take both hormones every day (although the progestin is taken in a lower dose). If you take the hormones all month long, you take lower doses of progestin together with estrogen every single day. Since there are no days you don't take hormones, you don't bleed.

Because there may be breakthrough bleeding at any time with this method, many women prefer the cyclical method so they will know when to expect bleeding. About 80 percent of women who keep taking hormones continuously, however, will stop bleeding completely after about a year; 20 percent will continue to have bleeding.

Continuous estrogen
If your uterus has been removed, you can take estrogen alone each day (usually as a skin patch or in a pill), since you are at no risk of getting uterine cancer.

Cyclic estrogen

Once a popular method of taking estrogen alone, it's not used often today because this method can trigger menopausal symptoms in the days when you aren't taking estrogen. Very few women take cyclic estrogen today.

Continuous progestin

If you can't take estrogen, you may want to try just progestin to relieve hot flashes. This hormone won't protect you from heart disease, but it may help you retain bone mass. It is of no use against dry vaginal tissue or urinary problems.

Knowing when to stop

Watch Out! Remember that if you stop taking replacement hormones, the protective benefits of the treatment will also stop.

Many health care providers recommend HRT for menopausal women only for a few years. When you stop, you may notice that some or all of your symptoms return—but it's also possible that you won't notice any symptoms at all because you've passed through the transition time.

Many other physicians recommend that HRT be continued indefinitely, especially to maintain protection against bone loss. The reduction in deaths from hip fracture alone is enough to make it worthwhile to keep taking estrogen, according to many doctors.

Natural hormone replacement

There are three classes of plant-derived estrogens: isoflavones, lignans, and coumestans. Most plants contain phytoestrogens to some degree, but those that are most like human estrogen are the isoflavone-containing legumes such as soy products, lentils, and kidney and lima beans. Lignans are found in bread and cereal grains, fruit, and vegetables. Coumestans are found in seed sprouts and fodder crops. These plant estrogens supplement the effects of human estrogen when levels are low, and they interfere with human estrogen when levels are high. Their ability to adapt is why they appeal to women in early menopause, whose hormones fluctuate wildly.

Other natural plant-derived estrogens contained in herbs include dong quai and ginseng, traditional Chinese remedies for a variety of gynecological problems; black cohosh, and vitex (chasteberry), a Mediterranean plant traditionally used to relieve menopausal symptoms.

What concerns some critics of natural hormones is that many people think that "natural" estrogen means they are harmless. In large doses, according to anecdotal reports, phytoestrogens can promote the abnormal growth of cells in the uterine lining. Unopposed estrogen can lead to endometrial cancer, which is why women on conventional estrogen replacement therapy (ERT) usually take progestin along with their estrogen. It's important to remember that any substance taken in too high a dose can be toxic. Be very cautious about using too much of any product or using it too often; it's very hard to control the dosage of a skin cream, and too much natural progesterone—just like its synthetic cousin—can cause fluid buildup, irritability, and weight gain.

University of Pittsburgh researchers have found that some natural estrogen products, such as American ginseng and black cohosh, do indeed produced estrogen-like effects in animals. Their findings confirm that these plants can relieve menopausal symptoms, especially hot flashes. The effects after long-term use are not clear, however. If you've decided you don't want to take estrogen because of a family history of breast cancer, for example, you should avoid these natural products, too.

Proponents of plant estrogens argue that some phytoestrogens appear to act as antigrowth factors in the uterus and breast. The results of smaller preliminary trials suggest that the estrogenic compounds that soy contains (genistein and diadzein) can relieve the severity of hot flashes and lower cholesterol. But no one yet has proven that soy can provide all the benefits of estrogen replacement without its negative effects.

It is true that people in other countries who eat foods high in plant estrogens (especially soy products) experience a lower risk of heart disease and breast cancer; in fact, while up to 80 percent of menopausal American women complain of hot flashes, night sweats, and vaginal dryness, only 15 percent of Japanese women have similar complaints. And women in Indonesia, India, and Taiwan likewise have lower rates of heart disease, breast cancer, and hip fractures. All things being equal, the soy-based diet seems to be making the difference—and soy is very high in plant estrogens. However, the low consumption of fats and animal products, the very active lifestyles, and the lower rate of smoking in these other cultures may also play a role.

Unfortunately, experts are unsure about the dosage of phytoestrogens a woman should consume. In one study at Bowman-Gray Medical School in North Carolina, women were able to ease symptoms by drinking a soy beverage with 20 mg of isoflavones. You could mimic that amount by eating a large amount of fruits and vegetables, whole grains, and four ounces of tofu four times a week. It's important to eat tofu every day if you want to enjoy the protective benefits of plant estrogens.

Unfortunately, no one knows how soy interacts with estrogen supplements in birth control pills or

Unofficially...
Blood levels of phytoestrogens are 10 to 40 times higher in Japanese women than in American women. There isn't even a word for "hot flash" in Japanese.

in hormone replacement. And the isoflavone content of soy differs depending on the variety of the soybean and how it's used. In general, soy sauce and soy oils are low in isoflavones, and roasted soy nuts, tempeh, and tofu are high (about 40 mg per ½ cup).

If you want to add soy products to your diet, add them slowly—otherwise, they may cause gas. Japanese women eat between 30 and 50 mg of isoflavones a day (although many Asians routinely consume up to 100 mg a day with no ill effects).

The following soy foods are not good sources of isoflavones:

- Soy sauce
- Soybean oil
- Miso
- Soy food made from soy protein concentrate (such as many veggie burgers)
- Combination foods with soy and other ingredients (such as tofu yogurt)

Bright Idea
Wild Mexican yam (available in creams, pills, and suppositories) contains a natural substance similar to progesterone that many women have been recommending for the treatment of vaginal dryness, hot flashes, and a host of other perimenopause symptoms.

TABLE 18.1: ISOFLAVONE LEVELS

Food	Serving	Isoflavones (mg)
Soy nuts (roasted)	½ cup	60
Tempeh	½ cup	35
Tofu (low fat/regular)	½ cup	35
Soy milk (regular)	1 cup	30
Soy milk (low fat)	1 cup	25
Soy butter (roasted)	2 tbsp	17

The following foods are rich in plant estrogens:

- Apples
- Asparagus
- Barley
- Beans

- Carrots
- Cherries
- Corn
- Fennel
- Garlic
- Legumes
- Licorice
- Oat bran
- Olive oil
- Onions
- Peas
- Pears
- Peppers (green)
- Rice bran
- Seaweed (dried)
- Squash
- Stone fruits (peaches, apricots, etc.)
- Sunflower seeds
- Wheat germ

Bioflavonoids

Bioflavonoids have a mild estrogen effect and are used to treat vaginal dryness, bladder problems, water retention, and hot flashes. You can find the most bioflavonoids in the inner peel of citrus fruits; you can also find them in vitamin C supplements.

Cenestin

In March 1999, the FDA approved the marketing of Cenestin tablets, a new plant-derived, synthetic conjugated estrogen product designed to treat hot flashes, night sweats, and other menopause symptoms. Synthesized from soy and yam plants, it's available in two strengths (0.625 mg and 0.9 mg). Currently, Cenestin is approved only for short-term use and no long-term studies have been completed.

In the past 56 years, the only other complex mixture of conjugated estrogens product that women could choose has been derived from pregnant mares' urine (Premarin). Cenestin was shown to be safe and effective in controlled studies of 120 women. Most often reported side effects were headache and insomnia. However, no studies have shown whether Cenestin reduces the incidence of osteoporosis, heart attack, and Alzheimer's the way that Premarin does.

The risk of developing cancer of the uterus increases with the dosage and duration of any estrogen replacement therapy used without opposing progesterone. Therefore, it's important to figure out the lowest effective dose, and to use it no longer than necessary.

Watch Out!
Like all estrogen drug products, Cenestin should not be taken by women with known or suspected pregnancy, breast cancer, heart disease or estrogen-dependent cancer, undiagnosed abnormal genital bleeding, or blood clotting problems.

Just the facts

- Menopause is a gradual process of aging, and symptoms can appear up to 15 years before menopause begins.
- Your onset of menopause is more closely linked to when your mother entered menopause than whether you began your menstrual period early or late.
- You should not have HRT if you already have heart disease; otherwise, HRT can help protect you from getting heart disease.
- One of the most recent studies found that taking hormones after menopause doesn't

increase the risk of breast cancer except for some uncommon forms of the disease that are slow growing and highly treatable.
- Plant estrogens can affect the body in ways similar to other estrogens.

Resource Directory

Acupuncture

National Commission for the Certification of Acupuncturists
1424 16th St. NW
Washington, DC 20036
202/232-1404

Aging

Resources for Mid-Life and Older Women
226 E. 70th St., Suite 1C
New York, NY 10021
212/439-1913
A nonprofit social service agency for women in mid-life and older that offers quick information and medical/psychological referrals. Also offers referrals to agencies providing services in areas such as personal financial management, legal rights, employment, and so on.

Women's Action Alliance
370 Lexington Ave., Room 603
New York, NY 10017
212/532-8330
Provides referrals for women in midlife.

Transitions for Health
621 S.W. Alder, Suite 900
Portland, OR 97205
800/888-6814
Has a free mail-order catalog of natural health care products for women in midlife.

OWL (Older Women's League)
730 11th St. NW, Suite 300
Washington, DC 20001
202/783-6686
A politically active group that lobbies for equal opportunities for midlife women, with local chapters nationwide that provide referrals to support groups. Publishes a bimonthly newspaper, *The Owl Observer.*

National Aging Information Center
U.S. Administration on Aging
330 Independence Ave. SW; Room 4656
Washington, DC 20201
202/619-7501
www.aoa.dhhs.gov/naic
Central source for a wide variety of program- and policy-related materials, demographic, and other statistical data on the health, economic, and social status of older Americans. NAIC develops special reports on key aging issues for publication and dissemination to the aging community, produces statistical reports and data tables, and compiles an annual compendium of Title IV products.

American Geriatrics Society
770 Lexington Ave. Suite 300
New York, NY 10021
212/308-1414

American Society on Aging
833 Market St. Suite 512
San Francisco, CA 94103
415/882-2910

AIDS

CDC National AIDS Clearinghouse
800/458-5231, 800/243-7012 (TTY)
www.cdcnpin.org

CDC Clinical Trials Information Service
800/874-2572
Provides current information on federally and privately sponsored clinical trials for AIDS patients and others with HIV infection, and on the drugs used in those trials.

Immune Deficiency Foundation
301/461-3127

National AIDS Hotline
800/342-AIDS (English)
800/344-AIDS (Spanish)
800/AIDS-TTY (deaf)

Project Inform HIV/AIDS Treatment Hotline
800/822-7422 (10 a.m. through 4 p.m. Monday through Saturday Pacific time)
415/558-9051 (California only)
Provides treatment information and referral for HIV-infected individuals and information on clinical trials. No diagnosis.

National Gay Task Force Crisis Line (for AIDS)
800/221-7044
212/529-1604 (when calling from within NY or from AK, and HI)

Women and AIDS Resource Network
Suite 513
30 Third Ave.
Brooklyn, NY 11217
718/596-6007

National Association of People with AIDS
Suite 700
1413 K St. NW
Washington, DC 20005
202/898-0414

Alcoholism/Substance Abuse

National Clearinghouse for Alcohol and Drug Information
P.O. Box 2345
Rockville, MD 20847
800/729-6686; 301/468-2600
800/487-4889 (TTY/TDD); 301/230-2867 (TTY/TDD)
www.health.org

Sponsored by the Center for Substance Abuse Prevention, Substance Abuse, and Mental Health Services Administration. Gathers and disseminates information on alcohol and other drug-related subjects, including tobacco. Distributes publications. Services include subject searches and provision of statistics and other information. Operates the Regional Alcohol and Drug Awareness Resource Network, a nationwide linkage of alcohol and other drug information centers. Maintains a library open to the public, 8 a.m to 6 p.m., Monday through Friday. Toll-free number offers 24-hour voice mail service.

National Institute of Alcohol Abuse and Alcoholism
600 Executive Blvd.
Willco Bldg.
Bethesda, MD 20892
301/443-3860
www.niaaa.gov
NIAAA supports and conducts biomedical research on the causes, consequences, treatment, and prevention of alcoholism and alcohol-related problems.

National Institute on Drug Abuse
www.nida.nih.gov
NIDA brings the power of science to bear on drug abuse and addiction.

The National Drug Information, Treatment, and Referral Line
800/662-HELP; 800/66-AYUDA (Spanish)
The free hot line operates Monday through Friday from 9 a.m. to 3 a.m. and Saturday and Sunday from noon to 3 a.m. for confidential answers to women seeking help and referrals to local drug treatment programs for themselves or for someone they care about.

Substance Abuse and Mental Health Services Administration
www.samhsa.gov
This site provides access to the home pages of the Center for Substance Abuse Treatment (CSAT), the Center for Substance Abuse Prevention (CSAP), and the Center for Mental Health Services (CMHS).

Substance and Alcohol Abuse Treatment Program
www.health.org/daatpp.htm

Alcoholics Anonymous
475 Riverside Dr.
New York, NY 10163
212/870-3400
For local meetings or information, check your Yellow Pages.

Al-Anon/Alateen
Al-Anon Family Group Headquarters, Inc.
1600 Corporate Landing Pkwy
Virginia Beach, VA 23454
800/344-2666
www.Al-Anon-Alateen.org

National Association for Children of Alcoholics
11426 Rockville Pike, Suite 100
Rockville, MD 20852
301/468-0985

Alternative Medicine

National Center for Complementary and Alternative Medicine (NCCAM) Clearinghouse
P.O. Box 8218
Silver Spring, MD 20907
888/644-6226 (Voice–Toll-free); 888/644-6226 (Voice–TTY/TDY)
800/531-1794 (Fax-back)
www.altmed.od.nih.gov/nccam/clearinghouse
Develops and disseminates fact sheets, information packages, and publications to enhance public understanding about complementary and alternative medicine research supported by the National Institutes of Health (NIH). NCCAM public information is currently free of charge; however, due to printing and duplication costs, only a limited number of copies can be requested. Information specialists can answer inquiries in English or Spanish. After

normal business hours, callers have the option of receiving fact sheets and other information by fax.

Alzheimer's Disease

Alzheimer's Disease Education and Referral Center
P.O. Box 8250
Silver Spring, MD 20907
800/438-4380
301/495-3311
www.alzheimers.org
Sponsored by the National Institute on Aging. Provides information and publications on Alzheimer's disease to health and service professionals, patients and their families, caregivers, and the public.

Alzheimer's Association, Inc.
919 North Michigan Ave.
Suite 1000
Chicago, IL 60611
800/272-3900; 312/355-8700

Anorexia/Bulimia
See also Eating Disorders.

American Anorexia/Bulimia Association, Inc.
165 West 46th St., Suite 1108
New York, NY 10036
212/575-6200
www.members.aol.com/amanbu
E-mail: AmAnBu@aol.com
A nonprofit organization dedicated to preventing eating disorders through research and advocacy, and to providing resources for women with eating disorders and their families. Offers referrals for doctors and treatment centers.

Anorexia Nervosa and Related Eating Disorders, Inc. (ANRED)
www.anred.com
514/344-1144

National Association of Anorexia Nervosa and Associated Disorders
P.O. Box 7
Highland Park, IL 60035
847/831-3438
E-mail: anad20@aol.com
ANAD is a national self-help organization dedicated to alleviating eating disorders; it provides counseling and doctor/treatment center referrals. ANAD sponsors self-help groups with chapters in 46 states and 15 foreign countries.

National Eating Disorders Organization (NEDO)
6655 South Yale Ave.
Tulsa, OK 74136
918/481-4044
www.laureate.com
An excellent resource for finding treatment programs, NEDO can provide information on treatment options and what to look for in a good program, both locally and nationally. NEDO also offers education and prevention information.

Anxiety/Stress

Anxiety Disorders Association of America
11900 Parklawn Dr., #100
Rockville, MD 20852
301/ 231-9350
www.adaa.org

American Institute of Stress
124 Park Ave.
Yonkers, NY 10703
914/963-1200; 800/24-RELAX

International Stress Management Association
10455 Pomerado Rd.
San Diego, CA 92131
619/693-4698

Arthritis

National Arthritis and Musculoskeletal and Skin Diseases Information Clearinghouse
1 AMS Circle
Bethesda, MD 20892
301/495-4484; 301/565-2966 (TTY)
301/881-2731 (Fax-back, 24-hour service)
www.nih.gov/niams
Designed to help patients and health professionals identify educational materials concerning arthritis and musculoskeletal and skin diseases. Distributes publications and maintains a file on the Combined Health Information Database (CHID) that indexes publications and audiovisuals. Personal information requests from patients are referred to appropriate organizations for additional information.

Arthritis Foundation
P.O. Box 19000
Atlanta, GA 30326
800/283-7800
www.arthritis.org

Autoimmunity

American Autoimmune Related Diseases Association, Inc.
15475 Gratiot Avenue
Detroit, MI 48205
313/371-8600; 800/598-4668
www.aarda.org

National Institute of Arthritis and Musculoskeletal and Skin Diseases
www.aamc.org/research/adhocgp/niams.htm

National Organization for Rare Diseases
www.NORD-RDB.com

Chronic Fatigue and Immune Dysfunction Syndrome Association of America
P.O. Box 220398
Charlotte, NC 28222
800/442-3437

National Chronic Fatigue Syndrome Association
Suite 222
3521 Broadway
Kansas City, MO 64111
816/931-4777

Cancer

The American Cancer Society
1599 Clifton Rd. NE
Atlanta, GA 30329
800/ACS-2345
www.cancer.org

American Institute for Cancer Research
1759 R St. NW
Washington, DC 20009
800/843-8114
www.aicr.org

National Cancer Institute
31 Center Dr., NSC 2580
Bldg. 31, Room 10A07
Bethesda, MD20892

National Alliance of Breast Cancer Organizations
1180 Avenue of the Americas, 2nd floor
New York, NY 10036
212/719-0154

Cancer Information Service
Office of Cancer Communications
National Cancer Institute
31 Center Drive, MSC 2580
Building 31, Room 10A07
Bethesda, MD 20892-2580
800/4-CANCER; 800/332-8615 (TTY); 301/496-5583
www.cis.nci.nih.gov
Provides information about cancer and cancer-related resources to patients, the public, and health professionals. Inquiries are handled by trained information specialists. Spanish-speaking staff members are available. Distributes free publications from the National Cancer Institute. Operates 9 a.m. to 7 p.m., Eastern time.

Child Abuse

National Clearinghouse on Child Abuse and Neglect Information
330 C Street SW
Washington, DC 20447
800/FYI-3366; 703/385-7565
www.calib.com/nccanch
Serves as a national resource for the acquisition and dissemination of child abuse and neglect materials and distributes a catalog of free publications upon

request. Maintains bibliographic databases of documents, audiovisuals, and national organizations. Services include searches of databases and annotated bibliographies on frequently requested topics.

Chronic Fatigue Syndrome

Chronic Fatigue and Immune Dysfunction Syndrome Association of America
P.O. Box 220398
Charlotte, NC 28222
800/442-3437

Colitis
See Irritable Bowel Syndrome.

Contraception

Emergency Contraception Hotline
800/584-9911

Crohn's Disease
See Irritable Bowel Syndrome.

Depression

National Depressive and Manic Depressive Association
730 North Franklin, Suite 501
Chicago, IL 60601
800/826-3632
www.ndmda.org

Depression After Delivery
P.O. Box 1282
Morrisville, PA 19067
800/944-4773; 215/295-3994
www.pleiades-net.com/org/DAD.1.htm

Diabetes

American Diabetes Association
P.O. Box 25757
1660 Duke St.
Alexandria, VA 22314
800/342-2383
www.diabetes.org

National Diabetes Information Clearinghouse
1 Information Way
Bethesda, MD 20892
301/654-3327
www.niddk.nih.gov/health/diabetes/ndic.htm
The National Diabetes Information Clearinghouse (NDIC) is an information and referral service of the National Institute of Diabetes and Digestive and Kidney Diseases, one of the institutes of the NIH. The clearinghouse responds to written inquiries, develops and distributes publications about diabetes, and provides referrals to diabetes organizations, including support groups. The NDIC maintains a database of patient and professional education materials from which literature searches are generated.

Diet/Nutrition

American Dietetic Association
216 West Jackson Blvd.
Chicago, IL 60605
312/899-0040
www.eatright.org

Drug Abuse

Center for Substance Abuse National Drug Hotline
800/662-4357

Narcotics Anonymous
P.O. Box 9999
Van Nuy, CA 91409
818/780-3951

National Institute on Drug Abuse
800/662-HELP

Eating Disorders
See also Anorexia/Bulimia.

Eating Disorders Awareness and Prevention
603 Stewart St., Suite 803
Seattle, WA 98101
206/382-3587
www.members.aol.com/edapine

National Eating Disorders Organization
6655 South Yale Ave.
Tulsa, OK 74136
918/481-4044
www.laureate.com

Exercise and Women's Health

Aerobics and Fitness Association of America
15250 Ventura Blvd.
Suite 200
Sherman Oaks, CA 91403
800/446-2322
www.afaa.com
www.aerobics.com/100000.asp

American Council on Exercise
5820 Oberlin Dr. Suite 102
San Diego, CA 92121
619/535-8227
www.acefitness.org

American Running and Fitness Association
4405 East West Highway, Suite 405
Bethesda, MD 20814
301/ 913-9517

Melpomene Institute for Women's Health Research
1010 University Ave.
St. Paul., MN 55104
612/642-1951
Since 1981, the institute has focused on the link between physical activity and women's health. Annual membership includes the *Melpomene Journal* three times a year.

National Coalition for Promoting Phusical Activity
P.O. Box 1440
Indianapolis IN 46206
317/637-9200

President's Council on Physical Fitness and Sports
200 Independence Ave. SW
Hubert H. Humphrey Building, Room 738-H
Washington, DC 20201
202/690-9000
www.whitehouse.gov/WH/PCPFS/html/fitnet.html
Conducts a public service advertising program, prepares educational materials, and works to promote the development of physical fitness leadership, facilities, and programs. Helps schools, clubs, recreation agencies, employers, and federal agencies design

and implement programs. Offers a variety of testing, recognition, and incentive programs for individuals, institutions, and organizations. Materials on exercise and physical fitness for all ages are available.

Family Planning

Natural Family Planning (Couple-to-Couple League)
www.itek.net/~mission/cathlc/ccl

Emergency Contraception Hotline
800/584-9911

Genetic Diseases

Alliance of Genetic Support Groups
35 Wisconsin Circle, Suite 440
Chevy Chase, MD 20815
800/336-GENE

National Society of Genetic Counselors
233 Canterbury Dr.
Wallingford, PA 19086
610/872-7608
www.members.aol.com/nsgcweb/nstchome.htm

Headache

National Headache Foundation
5252 North Western Ave.
Chicago, IL 60625
800/843-2256
www.headaches.org

Heart Disease

American Heart Association
7320 Greenville Ave.
Dallas, TX 75231
214/373-6300

Provides the latest information about heart disease, perimenopause, and hormone replacement therapy (HRT). Check your phone book for the nearest local chapter.

National Heart, Lung, and Blood Institute (NHLBI) Information Center
P.O. Box 30105
Bethesda, MD 20824
301/251-1222
www.nhlbi.nih.gov/nhlbi/infcntr/infocent.htm
NHLBI serves as a source of information and materials on risk factors for cardiovascular disease. Services include dissemination of public education materials, program and scientific information for health professionals, and materials on work-site health, as well as responses to information requests. Materials on cardiovascular health are available to consumers and professionals.

The American Medical Women's Association Education Project on Coronary Heart Disease in Women
801 N. Fairfax St. #400
Alexandria, VA 22314
703/838-0500
www.amwa-doc.org

American Society of Hypertension
515 Madison Ave.
Suite 1515
New York, NY 10022
212/644-0650

National Hypertension Association
324 East 30th St.
New York, NY 10016
212/889-3557

Herpes

The Herpes Zone
www.herpeszone.com

Herpes
www.azstarnet.com

Herpes Home Page
www.racoon.com/herpes

Herpes Resource Center
American Social Health Association
P.O. Box 13827
Research Triangle Park, NC 27709

Hysterectomy

Hysterectomy Educational Resources and Services Foundation (HERS)
422 Bryn Mawr Ave.
Bala Cynwyd, PA 19004
215/667-7757

An organization that provides information and counseling for women considering a hysterectomy, or who have already had one. Publishes a quarterly newsletter, and sponsors conferences around the country.

Infectious Diseases

National Institute of Allergy and Infectious Diseases
Office of Communications
Building 31; Room 7A50
9000 Rockville Pike
Bethesda, MD 20892
301/496-5717
www.niaid.nih.gov

Distributes publications to the public and to doctors, nurses, and researchers.

Infertility

American Reproductive Health Professionals
2401 Pennsylvania Ave. NW, Suite 350
Washington, DC 20037
202/723-7374
Provides a free copy of a brochure on perimenopause.

Planned Parenthood Federation of America, Inc.
810 Seventh Ave.
New York, NY 10019
www.ppfa.org/ppfa/menopub.html
Offers counseling and gynecological care.

Association of Reproductive Health Professionals
2401 Pennsylvania Ave. NW, Suite 350
Washington, DC 20037
202/466-3825

Resolve, Inc. (infertility support)
1310 Broadway
Somerville, MA 02144
617/623-0744

Society for the Prevention of Human Infertility
877 Park Avenue
New York, NY 10021
212/288-3737

Women's Health and Fertility Branch
National Center for Chronic Disease Prevention and Health Promotion
1600 Clifton Rd. NE
Atlanta, GA 30333
404/329-3286

Insurance Problems

Health Insurance Association of America
555 13th St. NW
Washington, DC 20004
202/824-1600
www.hiaa.org

National Medicare Issues Hotline
Health Care Financing Administration
200 Independence Ave. SW
Washington, DC 20201
800/638-6833

Irritable Bowel Syndrome

Crohn's and Colitis Foundation of America
444 Park Avenue South
New York, NY 10016
800/343-3637

National Digestive Diseases Information Clearinghouse
P.O. Box NDDIC
9000 Rockville Pike
Bethesda MD 20892

Lupus

Lupus Foundation of America, Inc.
www.lupus.org/lupus

Lyme Disease

The American Lyme Disease Foundation, Inc.
Mill Pond Offices
293 Route 100, Suite 204
Somers, NY 10589
914/277-6970 or 800/876-LYME
www.w2.com/docs2/d5/lyme.html

Lyme Disease Information Resource
www.sky.net
Senate bills on insurance, new drugs, support guide, discussion, and general health.

Lyme Disease Network
www.lymenet.org
Newsletter, discussion groups, and diagnosis/treatment.

Menopause

American College of Obstetricians and Gynecologists
409 12th St. SW
Washington, DC 20024
202/638-5577
Provides three free pamphlets (send self-addressed, stamped envelope) about estrogen, osteoporosis, and menopause. Also offers a listing of physicians in your area.

American Menopause Foundation, Inc.
Empire State Bldg.
350 Fifth Ave., Suite 2822
New York, NY 10118
212/714-2398
An independent nonprofit foundation interested in research, education, advocacy, and support of women and menopause. They operate a national network of support groups that deal with alternative treatments (among other issues).

Power Surge Reading Room
www.members.aol.com/dearest/news.htm (accessible in part)
An online menopause discussion area with an electronic newsletter. It can be accessed in its entirety

through America Online, with the keyword "Women" followed by the "well-being" icon.

United Soybean Board
P.O. Box 4192000
St. Louis, MO 63141
800/825-5769
For more information about incorporating soybeans into your diet to ease perimenopause symptoms.

North American Menopause Society
P.O. Box 94527
Cleveland, OH 44101
216/844-8748
www.menopause.org
A group that offers a mainstream perspective on menopause treatment, with lists of suggested readings and physicians in your area who specialize in menopause. Answers written requests for information about menopause and publishes a medical journal.

American Association of Retired Persons (AAR) Women's Initiative
601 East St. NW
Washington, DC 20049
800/424-3410
Free fact sheet about hormone replacement therapy.

Wellspring for Women
303/443-0321
Offers phone consultations with licensed nurse practitioners who can answer questions about conventional hormone therapy, herbal remedies, and natural hormones, and put you in touch with doctors who can prescribe them. A 45-minute consultation costs $120.

Mental Health

American Psychiatric Association
1400 K St. NW
Suite 501
Washington, DC 20005
202/682-6220
www.psych.org

American Psychological Association
750 First St. NW
Washington, DC 20002
202/336-5500

National Mental Health Association
1021 Prince St.
Alexandria, VA 22314
800/969-6642

National Institute of Mental Health (NIMH)
Information Resources and Inquiries Branch
5600 Fishers Lane, Room 7Cû02
Rockville, MD 20857
301/443-4513; 301/443-5158 (Mental Health Fax Information System); 800/64-PANIC (Panic Disorder Education Program information); 800/421-4211 (Depression/Awareness, Recognition, and Treatment Program information)
www.nimh.nih.gov
Responds to information requests from the public, clinicians, and the scientific community with a variety of printed materials on such subjects such as children's mental disorders, schizophrenia, depression, bipolar disorder, seasonal affective disorder, anxiety and panic disorders, obsessive-compulsive disorder, eating disorders, learning disabilities, and Alzheimer's disease. Information and publications

on the Depression/Awareness, Recognition, and Treatment Program (D/ART) and on the Panic Disorder Education Program—NIMH-sponsored educational programs on depressive and panic disorders, their symptoms, and treatment—are distributed. Single copies of publications are free of charge. A list of NIMH publications, including several in Spanish, is available upon request.

Nutrition

American Dietetic Association Consumer Nutrition Hotline
800/366-1655

Osteoporosis

The National Osteoporosis Foundation (NOF)
A nonprofit organization and leading resource for people seeking up-to-date, medically sound information on the causes, prevention, detection, and treatment of osteoporosis.
800/223-9994
www.nof.org

Osteoporosis and Related Bone Diseases National Resource Center
1150 17th Street NW, Suite 500
Washington, DC 20036
800/624-BONE; 202/223-0344; 202/466-4315 (TDD)
www.osteo.org
This organization seeks to create awareness of osteoporosis, Paget's disease, and osteogenesis imperfecta, and of the general possibilities for therapy, and is sponsored by the National Institute of Arthritis and Musculoskeletal and Skin Diseases. Provides patients, health professionals, and the public with resources and information on metabolic bone diseases.

Specific populations include the elderly, men, women, and adolescents.

National Institute of Arthritis and Musculoskeletal and Skin Diseases
www.nih.gov/niams
The government research institute affiliated with the NIH charged with investigating osteoporosis.

National Osteoporosis Foundation
1150 17th St. NW, Suite 500
Washington, DC 20036
202/223-2226
800/464-6700 (action line)
Action line can provide you with the bone-mass testing center nearest you. The Foundation also publishes a booklet called "Boning Up," available by mail ($1).

The American Academy of Orthopaedic Surgeons
www.aaos.org/wordhtml/pat_educ/osteo98.htm
This physician group maintains an information section on osteoporosis on their Web site.

OsNET, Inc.
www.osnet.org
This nonprofit, membership-driven network specializes in clinical research for the pharmaceutical industry in osteoporosis and women's health. OsNET has 21 high-quality health care locations in the U.S. to conduct clinical research.

Plastic Surgery

American Academy of Facial Plastic and Reconstructive Surgery
1101 Vermont Ave. NW, Suite 220
Washington, DC 20005
202/842-4500

American Society of Plastic and Reconstructive Surgeons (ASPRS)
444 East Algonquin Rd., Suite 110
Arlington Heights, IL 60005
708/228-9900
Plastic Surgery Information Online
www.plasticsurgery.org
This Web site allows you to find a plastic surgeon by name or geographical location.

Plastic Surgery Network
www.plastic-surgery.net/home.html
This Web site can provide information on procedures and an online free service to help find a plastic surgeon near you.

Pregnancy/Childbirth

American College of Nurse Midwives
1522 K St. NW
Suite 1000
Washington, DC 20005
202/289-0171

Childbirth Organization
www.childbirth.org
This Web site gives you many links to other sites dealing with pregnancy and childbirth.

Association of Women's Health, Obstetric and Neonatal Nurses
700 14th St. NW, Suite 600
Washington DC 20005
202/662-1600

The Babies Planet
www.thelastplanet.com
You'll find excellent information about pregnancy, morning sickness, babies, and so on.

StorkNet
www.storknet.org
This friendly site gives you pregnancy news, a bookstore, message boards, and more.

Sidelines
www.sidelines.org
This site is aimed at women with high-risk pregnancies and their families.

National Center for Education in Maternal and Child Health
2000 15th Street N
Suite 701
Arlington, VA 22201
703/524-7802
www.ncemch.org
Sponsored by the Maternal and Child Health Bureau, Health Resources, and Services Administration. Provides information to health professionals and the public, develops educational and reference materials, and provides technical assistance in program development. Subjects covered are women's health, including pregnancy and childbirth; infant, child, and adolescent health; nutrition; children with special health needs; injury and violence prevention; health and safety in day care; and maternal and child health programs and services. Types of materials include professional literature, curricula, patient education materials, audiovisuals, and information about organizations and programs. Appointment preferred for on-site visits.

National Maternal and Child Health Clearinghouse
2070 Chain Bridge Road, Suite 450
Vienna, VA 22182-2536
703/356-1964
www.circsol.com/mch

Sponsored by the Maternal and Child Health Bureau, Health Resources, and Services Administration. Centralized source of materials and information in the areas of human genetics and maternal and child health. Distributes publications and provides referrals.

International Childbirth Education Association
P.O. Box 20024
Minneapolis, MN 55420
800/624-4934

La Leche League International
P.O. Box 1209
Franklin Park, IL 60131
708/455-7730

Psoriasis

National Psoriasis Foundation
6443 S.W. Beaverton Highway, Suite 210
Portland, OR 97221
503/297-1545

Sex

American Association of Sex Educators, Counselors, and Therapists
P.O. Box 238
Mount Vernon, IA 52314
319/895-8407
www.aasect.org

Council for Sex Information and Education
2272 Colorado Blvd., #1228
Los Angeles, CA 90041

Sexuality Information and Education Council of the United States
130 W. 42nd St., Suite 350
New York, NY 10036
212/819-9770

Sexually Transmitted Diseases (STDs)

CDC National Prevention Information Network (AIDS, HIV, STDs)
P.O. Box 6003
Rockville, MD 20849
800/458-5231
800/243-7012 (TTY)
www.cdcnpin.org

The Centers for Disease Control and Prevention (CDC) National Prevention Information Network (NPIN) develops, identifies, and collects information on the prevention, treatment, and control of HIV/AIDS and other STDs, and makes this information available to health care providers, patients, grassroots community organizations, and organizations working in prevention, research, and support services. NPIN offers a variety of services, including reference and referrals to public and private resources, access to online databases, and publications. NPIN maintains resource centers in Maryland and Georgia and offers a Web site with up-to-date information.

National STD Hotline
800/227-8922

American Social Health Association
P.O. Box 13827
Research Triangle Park, NC 27709
919/361-8400

Skin

American Academy of Dermatology
888/462-3376

Thyroid Disease

The Thyroid Foundation of America
Ruth Sleeper Hall, RSL 350
40 Parkman St.
Boston, MA 02114
800/832-8321

Tuberculosis

CDC National Prevention Information Network (TB)
P.O. Box 6003
Rockville, MD 20849
800/458-5231
800/243-7012 (TTY)
www.cdcnpin.org
The Centers for Disease Control and Prevention (CDC) National Prevention Information Network (NPIN) develops, identifies, and collects information on the prevention, treatment, and control of tuberculosis (TB), and makes this information available to health care providers, patients, grassroots community organizations, and organizations working in prevention, research, and support services. NPIN offers a variety of services, including reference and referrals to public and private resources, access to online databases, and publications. NPIN maintains resource centers in Maryland and Georgia and offers a Web site with up-to-date information.

The People's Plague Online
www.pbs.org/ppol
Educational site on TB.

TB Weekly
www.newsfile.com/1t.htm
News abstracts, research, and journal articles.

TB Resources
www.cpmc.columbia.edu/tbcpp
Columbia-Presbyterian Hospital and the New York City Health Department series of pamphlets.

Urinary Tract Infections

National Kidney and Urologic Diseases Information Clearinghouse
3 Information Way
Bethesda MD 20892
301/ 654-4415

Vaccines

CDC Immunization Information Page
www.cdc.gov
Hypertext file details diseases and treatments.

Vaccines and Diseases News
www.bio.tsukuba.ac.jp
Journal abstracts.

Vaccine Adverse Event Reporting System
P.O. Box 1100
Rockville, MD 20849
800/822-7967
E-mail: vaers@cais.com

Violence

Educational Fund to End Handgun Violence
100 Maryland Ave. SE, #303
Washington, DC 20002

National Safety Council
1121 Spring Lake Dr.
Itasca, IL 60143
630/285-1121
www.nsc.org

International Society for Traumatic Stress Studies
435 North Michigan Ave., Suite 1717
Chicago, IL 60611
312/644-0828

National Coalition Against Domestic Violence
P.O. Box 18749
Denver, CO 80218
303/839-1852

National Coalition Against Sexual Assault
P.O. Box 21378
Washington, DC 20009
202/483-7165

National Crime Prevention Council
1700 K St. NW
Washington DC 20006
202/466-6272

Weight Control

Overeaters Anonymous
505/891-2664
www.overeastersanonymous.org

Shape Up America!
www.shapeup.org
A national campaign to reduce obesity, led by former U.S. Surgeon General C. Everett Koop.

Take Off Pounds Sensibly (TOPS)
800/932-8677
www.tops.org

Weight Control Information Network
1 WIN Way
Bethesda, MD 20892
301/984-7378; 800/WIN-8098
www.niddk.nih.gov/health/nutrit/win.htm

Healthy Weight Network
402 South 14th St.
Hettinger, ND 58639
701/567-2646
www.healthyweightnetwork.com

Network for Size Esteem
P.O. Box 9404
New Haven, CT 06534

Size Acceptance Web Site
www.bayarea.net/~stef/Fatfaqs/size.html

Women's Health (General)

American Medical Women's Association
801 N. Fairfax St.
Suite 400
Alexandria, VA 22314
703/838-0500
www.amwa.org

Boston Women's Health Book Collective
465 Mt. Auburn St.
Watertown, MA 02172
617/625-0271
A nonprofit organization devoted to women's health education, offering health-related materials through its Women's Health Information Center.

CHOICE
Concern for Health Options, Information, Care, and Education
125 South 9th St., Suite 603
Philadelphia, PA 19107
215/985-3355

Federation of Feminist Women's Health Centers
633 E. 11th Ave.
Eugene, OR 97401
503/344-0966

International Center for Research on Women
1717 Massachusetts Ave. NW, Suite 302
Washington DC 20036
202/797-0007

International Women's Health Coalition
24 E. 21st St., Fifth floor
New York, NY 10010
212/979-8500

National Self-Help Clearinghouse
33 W. 42nd St.
New York, NY 10036
212/840-1259
Offers referrals to support groups and a self-help newsletter.

National Women's Health Information Center
U.S. Public Health Service
800/994-WOMAN
www.4woman.gov
Well respected center launched by the U.S. Surgeon General, the Web site contains links to more than 1,000 other women's health Web sites, including more than 300 federal sites, hundreds of

government-screened private organizations, and more than 2,700 federal documents on women's health.

National Women's Health Network
1325 G St. NW
Washington, DC 20005
202/347-1140
A national public interest organization dedicated to women and health that sponsors many educational and research projects. The organization has published a booklet on hormone replacement therapy and offers a newsletter, *The Network News*. Offers a packet of resource material for a $5 fee.

National Women's Health Resource Center
1440 M St. NW, Suite 325
Washington, DC 20037
202/293-6045

Office on Women's Health
Office of the Assistant Secretary for Health
200 Independence Ave. SW
Washington, DC 20201
202/690-7650

Society for the Advancement of Women's Health Research
1920 L St. NW
Washington, DC 20036
202/223-8224

Women's Health America Group
429 Gammon Place
P.O. Box 259641
Madison, WI 53725
800/558-7046
E-mail: wha@womenshealth.com

Women's Health Initiative
Federal Bldg., Room 6A09
7550 Wisconsin Ave.
Bethesda, MD 20892
800/54-WOMEN
www.nih.gov/od/odp/whi

Women's Helpline (now called the NYC Service Fund)
15 W. 18th St., 9th floor
New York, NY 10011
212/989-7230
Provides referrals to midlife women's groups and services.

Further Readings

Covington, Stephanie S., *A Woman's Way Through the 12 Steps* (Hazelden)

Dunnewold, Anne and Sanford, Diane G., *Postpartum Survival Guide* (Hyperion)

Eisenberg, Arlene, *What to Expect When You're Expecting* (Workman Press)

Jacobowitz, Ruth, *150 Most-Asked Questions About Menopause: What Women Really Want to Know* (William Morrow)

Jibrin, Janis, *The Unofficial Guide to Dieting Safely* (Macmillan)

Johnson, Robert V., *Mayo Clinic Complete Book of Pregnancy and Baby's First Year* (Morrow)

Kearney, Brian, *High Tech Conception: A Comprehensive Handbook for Consumers* (Bantam)

Kitzinger, Sheila, *The Complete Book of Pregnancy and Childbirth* (Knopf)

Love, Susan, *Dr. Susan Love's Breast Book* (Perseus Press)

Love, Susan, *Dr. Susan Love's Hormone Book* (Random House)

MacDougall, Jane, *Pregnancy Week-by-Week* (HarperCollins)

Northrup, Christiane, *Women's Bodies, Women's Wisdom: Creating Physical and Emotional Health and Healing* (Bantam Doubleday Dell)

Steinberg, Alan J., *Insider's Guide to HMO's: How to Navigate the Managed Care System and Get the Health Care you Deserve* (Plume)

Statman, Jan Berliner, *The Battered Woman's Survival Guide* (Taylor)

Turkington, Carol A., *The Perimenopause Handbook* (Contemporary Books)

Turkington, Carol A., *Stress Management for Busy People* (McGraw-Hill)

Turkington, Carol A., *Making the Prozac Decision* (Lowell House)

Vedral, Joyce, *American Medical Women's Association Guide to Cancer and Pain Management* (Dell)

Westcott, Patsy and Black, Leyardia, *Alternative Health Care for Women: A Woman's Guide to Self-Help Treatments and Natural Therapies* (HarperCollins)

A

Abdominal recontouring
(tummy tucks), 76–77
Abortion, 168–70
   medical, 169–70
   spontaneous (miscarriage),
      258–59
   surgical, 170
Abruptio placentae, 225–26
Absorptiometry
   DEXA (dual-energy X-ray),
      105–6, 464–66
   dual-photon, 105, 106
Accutane (isotretinoin), 376
Acetaminophen, 221
Acne, 370–79
   adult, 373
   causes of, 371–73
   myths about, 371
   prevention of, 373–74
   rosacea distinguished from,
      378–79
   scars, 378
   treatment for, 374–78
Acupressure, for menstrual
      cramps, 119
Acupuncture
   for depression, 304
   heart disease and, 452–53
   for quitting smoking, 351
   resources, 645
Adapalene (Differin), 375
Addiction. *See* Substance abuse
Addictive personality, 345
Adenomyosis, 118
Aerobic exercise, 54
   for older women, 57
Aerobics and Fitness
   Association of
      America, 658
Afterbirth, 253

Aging, 549–89. *See also*
      Menopause; Older
      women
   hair, 575–82
   memory loss and, 582–89
   resources, 645–47
   skin. *See* Skin (skin
      diseases),
      younger-looking
Agras, Stewart, 65
AHA (alpha-hydroxy acid),
      560–69
AIDS, 508–10
   during pregnancy, 231
   resources, 647–48
   substance abuse and,
      360–61
Air travel, during pregnancy,
      222–23
Al-Anon, 359, 650
Alateen, 359, 650
Alcohol (alcoholic
      beverages), 48
   cancer and, 400
   infertility and, 172
   memory and, 587, 588
   during pregnancy, 218–19
   premenstrual syndrome
      (PMS) and, 128
   stress and, 327
Alcohol abuse (alcoholism),
      351–59
   health risks of, 353–54
   quiz on, 354–57
   resources, 648–50
   treatment for, 357–59
Alcoholics Anonymous,
      359, 650
Alendronate (Fosamax), 474,
      475–76
Alliance of Genetic Support
      Groups, 660

Alpha-fetoprotein (AFP) test, 203–4
Alpha-hydroxy acid (AHA), 560–69
Alternative medicine, resources, 650–51
Alzheimer's Association, 651
Alzheimer's disease, 584–85
  resources, 651
Alzheimer's Disease Education and Referral Center, 651
Amen, 620
Amenorrhea, 116–18
American Academy of Dermatology, 674
American Academy of Facial Plastic and Reconstructive Surgery, 669
American Academy of Orthopaedic Surgeons, 669
American Anorexia/Bulimia Association, 651
American Association of Retired Persons (AARP) Women's Initiative, 666
American Association of Sex Educators, Counselors, and Therapists, 672
American Autoimmune Related Diseases Association, 654
American Cancer Society, 420, 654
American College of Nurse Midwives, 670
American College of Obstetricians and Gynecologists, 665
American Council on Exercise, 659
American Diabetes Association, 657
American Dietetic Association, 657
American Dietetic Association Consumer Nutrition Hotline, 668
American Geriatrics Society, 647
American Heart Association, 660–61
American Institute for Cancer Research, 654
American Institute of Stress, 653
American Lyme Disease Foundation, 664
American Medical Association, 4
American Medical Women's Association, 677
American Medical Women's Association Education Project on Coronary Heart Disease in Women, 661
American Menopause Foundation, 665
American Psychiatric Association, 667
American Psychological Association, 667
American Reproductive Health Professionals, 663
American Running and Fitness Association, 659
American Social Health Association, 673
American Society for Reproductive Medicine (ASRM), 184
American Society of Hypertension, 661
American Society of Plastic and Reconstructive Surgeons (ASPRS), 670
American Society on Aging, 647
Amniocentesis, 205–6
  CVS versus, 206–7
Anesthesia
  for Cesarean birth, 255–56
  during labor, 237–39
Angiography, coronary, 455
Anorexia nervosa, 58–62
  resources, 651–52
Anorexia Nervosa and Related Eating Disorders, Inc. (ANRED), 652

Antacids, during pregnancy, 222
Anti-anxiety drugs, 334
Antidepressants, 292–300
  lithium, 299–300
  MAOIs (monoamine oxidase inhibitors), 297–99
  for premenstrual syndrome (PMS), 129
  questions to ask about, 293–94
  St. John's wort, 302–4
  tricyclic, 295–97
  types of, 292
Anxiety (anxiety disorders), 330–35
  generalized anxiety disorder, 333
  memory and, 586
  panic disorder, 331–32
  phobias, 332–33
  resources, 652–53
  risk factors, 330–31
  treatment for, 334–35
Anxiety Disorders Association of America, 652
Arrhythmia, 441–42
Arthritis
  resources, 653
  rheumatoid, 529–30
Arthritis Foundation, 653
Artificial insemination, 181. *See also* Sperm banks
Artificial sweeteners, during pregnancy, 221
Aspirin, during pregnancy, 221
Aspo/Lamaze, 233
Assistive reproductive technology (ART), 184–87
  frozen embryos, 187
  gamete intrafallopian transfer (GIFT), 186
  in vitro fertilization (IVF), 185–86
  zygote intrafallopian transfer (ZIFT; tubal embryo transfer), 186
Association of Reproductive Health Professionals, 663
Association of Women's Health, Obstetric and Neonatal Nurses, 670
Atherosclerosis, 436–37
Autoimmune diseases, 519–45
  causes of, 520–24
  chronic fatigue syndrome (CFS), 539–40
  connective tissue diseases, 527–31
  diagnosis of, 524–26
  endocrine diseases, 533–37
  hematologic, 542
  infertility and, 542
  inflammatory bowel disease (IBD), 538
  neuromuscular diseases, 531–33
  resources, 654
  sarcoidosis, 540–41
  skin diseases, 538–39
  tips for managing, 543–44
  treatment of, 526–27
  types of, 520
  vasculitis syndromes, 541–42
Autologen, 554
Aygestin, 620
Azelex (azelaic acid), 375

B

Babies (infants). *See also* Newborns
  choosing a doctor for, 80–82
Babies Planet, 670
Bacterial vaginosis, 493–94
Barrier methods of birth control, 152–58
  cervical cap, 156
  condoms, 153–54
  diaphragms, 155–56
  intrauterine devices (IUDs), 158–59
  spermicide, 153
  sponge, 156–58
Basal body temperature method of birth control, 152
Basal cell carcinoma, 383–85

Baths, hot
　for menstrual cramps, 119
　premenstrual syndrome (PMS) and, 128
Battered Women's Justice Project, 341
B-complex vitamins, stress and, 328–29
Behavior therapy, for depression, 288
Benzodiazepines, 334, 587
Beta-carotene, cancer and, 399
Beta-hydroxy acids (BHAs), 561
BHAs (beta-hydroxy acids), 561
Binge eating (bingeing), 64–65
　bulimia nervosa and, 62–64
Bioflavonoids, 642
Biopsies, for breast cancer, 411–14
Birth. *See* Childbirth
Birth care providers, 192
Birth control (contraception), 102–3, 149–70
　abortion, 168–70
　barrier methods of, 152–58
　　cervical cap, 156
　　condoms, 153–54
　　diaphragms, 155–56
　　intrauterine devices (IUDs), 158–59
　　spermicide, 153
　　sponge, 156–58
　Emergency Contraception Hotline, 656
　hormonal methods of, 159–65
　　implants, 162–63
　　injections, 163–65
　　interactions, 165
　　oral contraceptives (birth control pills), 160–62
　methods of, 150
　"morning after" pill, 167
　natural methods of, 151–52
　sterilization, 165–67
Birth defects, 261–62
Birthing centers, 198–99

Birthing classes, 232–33
Birthing rooms, 197
Birth sites, 196–200
Blackheads, 371–72
Bladder, endometriosis and, 137
Bleeding, vaginal, 121–23
　during pregnancy, 226–27
Blood glucose (blood sugar levels)
　diabetes and, 536
　monitoring (testing), 17, 88
Blood pressure
　heart disease and, 452
　high, 447–48
　　smoking and, 346
　taking (monitoring) your, 88, 448
　　at home, 17
Blood tests, for pregnant women, 202
Bloody show, 242
Body dysmorphic disorder (BDD), 45
Body image, negative, 43–45
Bogus "cures," 20
Bone density tests, 104–6, 464–67
Bones. *See* Osteoporosis
Boston Women's Health Book Collective, 677
Botox injections, 555–56
Bradley, 233
Bradycardia, 441
Bras, sports, 53
BRCA1 genes, 403–7, 424
BRCA2 genes, 404, 405, 407, 424
Breaking of waters, 242–43
Breast augmentation, 66–68
Breast cancer, 401, 402–20
　alcohol abuse and, 352
　clinical trials, 414
　family history of, 403–7
　mammograms to detect, 409–11
　needle and tissue biopsies, 411–14
　risk factors, 402–8
　screening for, 408
　surgery for, 415–16

treatment of, 415–16
warning signs of, 408–9
Breast Cancer Information
    Clearinghouse, 420
Breast exams, 88
    frequency of, 101
Breastfeeding
    newborns, 266
    weight and, 49
Breast reduction, 68–70
Breast self-exam, 101
Breast surgery, cosmetic,
    66–70
Breast tenderness, menopause
    and, 601
Breathing
    deep, 316–19
    stress and, 315–19
Breathing exercise, 317–18
Breathing problems, 52
Brow-lifts, 575
Bulimia nervosa, 58, 62–64
    resources, 651–52

C

Caffeine, 48
    depression and, 306
    infertility and, 173
    during pregnancy, 220–21
    stress and, 326–27
Calcitonin (Miacalcin),
    474, 480
Calcium, 48
    foods rich in, 98
    menopause and, 49–50
    for menstrual cramps, 119
    during pregnancy, 215
Calcium intake, osteoporosis
    and, 460–61, 468–69
Calcium supplements, 97,
    108, 128
    osteoporosis and, 469–70
    premenstrual syndrome
        (PMS) and, 128
    for teenagers, 96
Calendar method of birth
    control, 152
Caloric intake, 50
    pregnancy and, 49
Cancer, 397–98
    breast. *See* Breast cancer
    cervical, 427–31

comprehensive cancer
    centers, 35–36
coping with, 431–32
early detection of, 398–99
endometrial, 136–37,
    425–27
hair dyes and, 578–79
lifestyle choices and,
    399–401
ovarian, 420–25
resources, 654–55
Cancer Information Service,
    420, 655
Carbohydrates, 48
Cardiologists, 445–46
Cardiovascular disease (heart
    disease), 433–55
    atherosclerosis, 436–37
    congestive heart failure,
        440–41
    coronary heart disease, 437
    general heart-smart
        strategies, 451–53
    heart rhythm disturbances,
        441–42
    high blood pressure, 447–48
    mitral valve prolapse, 440
    questions to ask your
        cardiologist, 445–46
    resources, 660–61
    risk factors for, 442–45
    smoking and, 346
    stroke, 437–40
    symptoms of, 435–36
    tests, 453–55
CDC Clinical Trials
    Information Service, 647
CDC Immunization
    Information Page, 675
CDC National AIDS
    Clearinghouse, 647
CDC National Prevention
    Information
    Network, 673
CDC National Prevention
    Information Network
    (TB), 674
Celaxa, 295
Cenestin, 642–43
Center for Substance Abuse
    National Drug
    Hotline, 658

Centers for Disease Control and Prevention, 112
Certified nurse midwives (CNMs), 192
Cervadil, 248
Cervical cancer, 427–31
Cervical cap, 103, 156
Cervical cultures, for pregnant women, 202
Cervical mucous method of birth control, 152
Cervical stenosis, 118
Cervix, incompetent, 224
Cesarean birth (C-section), 254–57
  need for, 254–55
  recovery after, 256–57
  vaginal birth after, 257
CFS (chronic fatigue syndrome), 539–40
Checkups, 79–80
Chemical peels, 557–58
Chemotherapy, for breast cancer, 415–17
Chicken pox, during pregnancy, 229
Chicken pox vaccine, 83–85, 87, 111
Child abuse, resources, 655–56
Childbirth, 235–71. *See also* Delivery; Labor; Newborns
  afterbirth, 253
  Cesarean (C-section), 254–57
    need for, 254–55
    recovery after, 256–57
    vaginal birth after, 257
  first week after, 267–70
  hospital preparation, 246–47
  hospital stay after, 266–67
  problems, 257–63
  what to expect at the hospital, 246
  what to take to the hospital, 245–46
Childbirth Organization, 670
Children. *See also* Teenage girls
  vaccines for, 83–87
Chinese restaurants, 47

Chlamydia, 94, 100, 488, 499–500
  during pregnancy, 229–30
CHOICE (Concern for Health Options, Information, Care, and Education), 678
Cholesterol
  diet and, 452
  exercise and, 451
  measuring, 448–50, 452
Chorionic villus sampling (CVS), 202, 206–7
Chronic Fatigue and Immune Dysfunction Syndrome Association of America, 654
Chronic fatigue syndrome (CFS), 539–40
  resources, 656
Citalopram, 295
Clomid, 180
Coffee, infertility and, 173
Cold medicines, during pregnancy, 222
Colds, preventing, 486–88
Collagen treatments, 554–55
Colon cancer, 18, 401
Colostrum, 266
Community Breast Health Project, 420
Community hospitals, 34–36
Complete blood count (CBC), 88
Condoms, 102
  as birth control method, 153–54
  sexually transmitted diseases (STDs) and, 498, 509
Congestive heart failure, 440–41
Contraception. *See* Birth control
Contraceptive implants, 162–63
Contractions, labor, 243–44
  pushing, 251–52
Coronary angiography, 455
Coronary heart disease, 437
Cosmetic surgery. *See* Plastic surgery
Coumestans, 638–39

INDEX

Council for Sex Information and Education, 672
Counseling, for depression, 285–92
Cramps, menstrual (dysmenorrhea), 118–19
C-reactive protein, blood test for, 455
Crohn's and Colitis Foundation of America, 664
Crohn's disease, 537
Crowning, 252
CT scan, ultrafast, 454–55
CVS (chorionic villus sampling), 202, 206–7
Cyclic antidepressants, 296–97
Cyclic hormone replacement therapy, vaginal bleeding and, 122
Cycrin, 620
Cysts, ovarian, 140, 141–43
Cytomegalovirus, during pregnancy, 230
Cytotec (misoprostol), 248

D

Dalkon Shield IUD, 158
Danazol, 138
D-chiro-inositol, 146
Deep breathing, 316–19
Delivery
    depression after, 281–83
    pushing during, 251–52
Densitometry, ultrasound, 465
Depilatories, 579–80
Depression, 275–307
    after childbirth, 269
    after delivery (postpartum), 281–83
    drugs and, 283
    hormones and, 280–81
    incidence among women, 276–77
    menopause and, 604
    quiz on, 276
    resources, 656
    risk factors, 283–84
    treatment for, 285–307. *See also* Antidepressants
        acupuncture, 304
        alternatives, 301–7
        analysis versus talk therapy, 287–88
        coffee, 306
        electroconvulsive treatment (ECT), 300–301
        exercise, 306–7
        finding a therapist, 285–86
        ginkgo biloba, 306
        inappropriate or unethical behavior of therapist, 290–92
        paying for, 288–89
        relaxation, 305
        sexism and, 290
        social support, 304–5
        St. John's wort, 302–4
        vitamin supplements, 305–6
    in winter, 278–80
Depression After Delivery, 656
Dermabrasion, 556
Dermalogen, 554
Dermatologists, finding, 367–70
DEXA (dual energy X-ray absorptiometry), 105–6, 464–66
Diabetes. *See also* Blood glucose (blood sugar levels)
    resources, 657
    screening for, pregnant women, 202
Diabetes mellitus, type 1 (insulin-dependent, or IDDM), 535–37
Diaphragms, 102, 155–56
    sexually transmitted diseases (STDs) and, 498
Diarrhea, during labor, 243
Diet. *See also* Nutrition
    heart disease and, 451
    hot flashes and, 605
    memory and, 587
    myths about, 46
    for pregnant women, 213–15
    premenstrual syndrome (PMS) and, 127
    resources, 657
    stress and, 325–28
    weight loss, 46–47

Differin (adapalene), 375
Dilatation and curettage (D&C), for fibroids, 130
Dilation, in labor, 242
Diphtheria, tetanus, and pertussis vaccine (DTP), 86
Doctors. *See* Health care providers; Physicians
Donor egg IVF, 186–87
Douching, as birth control method, 150
Doulas (labor assistants), 193
Dover, Jeffrey S., 550
Down syndrome, screening for, 204–5
D-penicillamine, 530
Drug abuse, 359–64. *See also* Substance abuse
  recreational (illegal) drugs, 362
  treatment for, 362–64
Drugs. *See also* Medications
  memory and, 587–88
  recreational, during pregnancy, 220
DTaP vaccine, 86
DTP (diphtheria, tetanus, and pertussis vaccine), 86
Dual energy X-ray absorptiometry (DEXA), 105–6, 464–66
Dual-photon absorptiometry, 105, 106
Dysmenorrhea (menstrual cramps), 118–19

E

Ear infections, vaccine for, 86
Eating disorders, 44, 57–66. *See also* Anorexia nervosa
  binge eating, 64–65
  bulimia nervosa, 62–64
  causes of, 58–59
  information sources on, 65–66
  mother-daughter connection and, 65
  resources, 658
  specialists in, 60
Eating Disorders Awareness and Prevention, 658
Eating habits. *See also* Eating disorders
  premenstrual syndrome (PMS) and, 127
EBV (Epstein-Barr virus), 513, 514
Echinacea, 173
Echocardiography, stress, 454
Ectopic pregnancy, 228–29
Educational Fund to End Handgun Violence, 675
Effacement, 242
EKG, 453
Electrocardiogram (ECG), 101
  frequency of, 105
Electrocoagulation/electrodesication, 166
Electroconvulsive treatment (ECT), 300–301
Electrolysis, 580–81
Embolization, fibroid, 133
Embryos, frozen, 187
Emergency Contraception Hotline, 660
Emergency rooms (ERs), 32
Encephalitis, Japanese, during pregnancy, 231
Endocrine diseases, 533–37
Endocrinologists, reproductive, 98–99
Endometrial biopsy
  for fibroids, 130
  as infertility test, 178
Endometrial cancer, 136–37, 425–27
Endometriosis, 134–39
  complications of, 136–37
  surgery for, 138–39
  symptoms of, 135–36
  tests for, 137
Environmental toxins, infertility and, 173
Epidurals, 238–39
Epilatories, 580
Epstein-Barr virus (EBV), 513, 514, 539
Estrace, 619
Estradiol, 618
17b-estradiol, 628–29
Estratest, 624

INDEX

Estrogen replacement (ERT), osteoporosis and, 477, 478
Estrogen replacement therapy, vaginal bleeding and, 122
Estrogen ring (Estring), 620–21, 628
Estrogens. *See also* Hormone replacement therapy (HRT)
  cancer and, 400
  depression and, 281
  in endometriosis treatment, 138
  low-dose, 622–23
  menstrual flow and, 119–20
  osteoporosis and, 474
  plant, 620
Estrone conjugate, 619–20
Evista (raloxifene), 407, 419, 474, 478–80, 621, 622
Exercise, 53–57. *See also* Physical activity
  after childbirth, 268, 269
  cholesterol and, 451
  consulting your doctor concerning, 55
  for depression, 306–7
  designing your own plan of, 53–55
  for mature women (40-64), 104
  for menstrual cramps, 119
  for older women, 56–57, 108
  osteoporosis and, 472–73
  during pregnancy, 216–17
  premenstrual syndrome (PMS) and, 127
  resources, 658–60
  stress and, 323–25
  women with school-age children and, 55
Eyelid lifts, 575
Eyes, of newborns, 265
Eye tests, 109

F

Face-lifts, 573–74
Facial hair, menopause and, 603
Fallopian tubes, sterilization and, 166
Family physicians (family practitioners), 191
Family planning, natural, 150, 151–52
  resources, 660
Family practitioners, choosing, 80–82
Famvir, 504
Fast food restaurants, 47–48
Fast foods, 95
Fat embolism, 74
Fatty acids, premenstrual syndrome (PMS) and, 127
Fecal occult blood test, 18, 101, 399
Federation of Feminist Women's Health Centers, 678
Female condoms, 155
Fertility. *See also* Infertility
Fertility Clinic Success Rate and Certification Act, 184
Fertility drugs, 180–81
Fertility specialists, finding, 174–78
Fertinex, 180
Fetal alcohol effect (FAE), 219
Fetal alcohol syndrome (FAS), 219, 353
Fiber, dietary, cardiovascular disease and, 451
Fibroid embolization, 133
Fibroids, 129–34
  menopause and, 596–97
  menstrual flow and, 119
  prevention of, 134
  symptoms of, 130
  treatment of, 130–33
Fifth disease, during pregnancy, 230
Fish, cholesterol and, 452
Flu, preventing, 486
Fluids, during pregnancy, 215, 217
Flu shots, 102, 106, 109, 487
  for children, 86–87
Folic acid, 48–49, 98
  depression and, 305–6
  during pregnancy, 215–16

Food Pyramid Guidelines, 50–51
Foods. *See* Diet; Nutrition
Fosamax (alendronate), 474, 475–76
Fraud, medical, 20
Frozen embryos, 187
Fruit acids, 560–67
FSH test, 616–17

G

Gamete intrafallopian transfer (GIFT), 186
Generalized anxiety disorder, 330, 333
Genetic diseases, resources on, 660
Genetic factors
  autoimmune diseases and, 523–24
  endometriosis and, 135
  premenstrual syndrome (PMS) and, 126
Genetic tests, for pregnant women, 202
Genital herpes, 502–4
  during pregnancy, 230
Genital warts, 500–502
  cervical cancer and, 428–29
German measles (rubella), during pregnancy, 230
GIFT (gamete intrafallopian transfer), 186
Ginkgo biloba, 173, 608
  for depression, 306
Ginseng, for hot flashes, 605
Girls. *See also* Children; Teenage girls
  body image of, 44
  vaginal bleeding in, 122
Glucose tolerance test, 536–37
GnRH (gonadotropin releasing hormone), 138
GnRH agonists (gonadotropin releasing hormone agonists), 131
Gonorrhea, 100, 504–5
  during pregnancy, 230
Gout, 52
Graves' disease, 534–35
Gray hair, 577–78

Group B strep, during pregnancy, 230–31
Gynecologists. *See also* Obstetrician/gynecologists
  choosing, 89

H

Hair, 575–82
  facial, menopause and, 603
  gray, 577–78
  loss, 576–77
  of newborns, 265
  removal of, 579–82
Hair dyes, 578–79
Hashimoto's thyroiditis, 534
Headaches
  menopause and, 601, 610
  resources, 660
Health care providers. *See also* Physicians; Specialists
  availability of, 6
  finding, 4–7
  partnership with, 5–7, 10–13
  specialists, 13–14
  unhappiness with, 13
Health Insurance Association of America, 664
Health maintenance organizations (HMOs), 22–32
  choosing, 24–25, 28
  disadvantages of, 23–24
  disclosure form (evidence of coverage) of, 26–27
  external review boards and, 32
  HMOs and, 23–24
  how to get the best care from, 27–29
  member satisfaction with, 26
  problems getting care from, 29–32
  questions to ask about, 25–26
  understanding coverage of, 26–27
Health Resource Center on Domestic Violence, 341
Healthy Weight Network, 677

INDEX

Heart, tests for assessing your, 453–55
Heart disease. *See* Cardiovascular disease
Heart palpitations, menopause and, 602
Hematologic autoimmune diseases, 542
Hepatitis A vaccine, 111
Hepatitis B, 505–7
   during pregnancy, 231
Hepatitis B vaccine, 87, 111
Herbal teas, for menstrual cramps, 119
Heredity, cancer and, 401
Herpes
   genital, 230, 502–4
   resources, 662
Herpes Home Page, 662
Herpes Resource Center, 662
Herpes simplex virus type I (HSV-I), 503
Herpes simplex virus type II (HSV-II), 503
Herpes Zone, 662
High blood pressure, 447–48
   smoking and, 346
HIV (human immunodeficiency virus), 508–10
   cervical cancer and, 429
   during pregnancy, 231
   substance abuse and, 361
Holter monitor, 453–54
Home births, 200
Homone replacement therapy (HRT), continuous, vaginal bleeding and, 122
Hormonal contraception. *See* Birth control (contraception), hormonal
Hormone replacement therapy (HRT), 618–43
   birth control pills as, 625–26
   cancer and, 400, 401
   deciding on, 632–34
   dosage regimens, 635–38
   heart attacks and, 631–32
   hormone pills, 626
   injections, 628
   low-dose estrogen, 622–23
   natural, 638–43
   osteoporosis and, 476–78
   progestins, 620–21
   pros and cons of, 629–32
   questions to ask about, 634–35
   SERMs (selective estrogen receptor modulators), 621–22
   side effects of, 635
   skin patch, 626–27
   stopping, 638
   testosterone, 623–25
   types of estrogen for, 619–20
   vaginal cream, 627–28
   vaginal rings (Estring), 620–21, 628
Hormones
   cancer and, 400–401
   depression and, 280–81
   male. *See also* Testosterone polycystic ovarian syndrome (PCOS) and, 144–45
   stress, 309–10
Hormone suppression, for endometriosis, 138
Hospice care programs, 36
Hospitals
   choosing, 34–36
   community, 34–36
   getting the care you need in, 36–37
   teaching, 35
Hot baths
   for menstrual cramps, 119
   premenstrual syndrome (PMS) and, 128
Hot flashes, 597–99, 604–6
Hot tubs, during pregnancy, 222
HPV (human papillomavirus), cervical cancer and, 428–30
HRT. *See* Hormone replacement therapy (HRT)
Human chorionic gonadotropin (hCG), 18, 189, 190, 204

Humanism, 288
Human papillomavirus (HPV), cervical cancer and, 428–30
Humegon, 180
Hypertension. *See* High blood pressure
Hypoglycemia, 88
Hysterectomy
 for endometriosis, 139
 for fibroids, 132–33
 resources, 662
Hysterectomy Educational Resources and Services Foundation (HERS), 662
Hysteroscopy, 132

I

IBD (inflammatory bowel disease), 537–38
Ibuprofen (Motrin or Nuprin)
 for menstrual cramps, 119
 during pregnancy, 221
Immune Deficiency Foundation, 647
Immunizations. *See* Vaccinations
Implants, contraceptive, 162–63
ImuLyme, 100
Incontinence, urinary, 21–22
 menopause and, 602–3
Infant car seats, 267
Infectious diseases, 485–517
 colds and flu, 486–88
 Lyme disease, 515–17
 mononucleosis, 513–15
 pelvic inflammatory disease (PID), 494–96
 resources, 662
 sexually transmitted diseases. *See* Sexually transmitted diseases
 toxic shock syndrome (TSS), 496–97
 tuberculosis, 510–13
 urinary tract infections, 488–91
 vaginal infections, 491–94

Infertility, 170–87. *See also* Assistive reproductive technology (ART)
 artificial insemination and, 181–84
 autoimmune diseases and, 542
 defined, 170
 endometriosis and, 136
 male factor, 171–72, 177
 non-physical factors and, 172–73
 resources, 663
 second opinion on, 179
 surgery to restore, 181
 unexplained, 179–80
Infertility tests, 174, 178–79
Inflammatory bowel disease (IBD), 537–38
Insider's Guide to HMOs, The (Steinberg), 29
Insomnia, menopause and, 599, 607
Insulin, polycystic ovarian syndrome (PCOS) and, 145
Insulin-dependent (type 1) diabetes mellitus (IDDM), 535–37
Insurance problems, resources on, 664
International Center for Research on Women, 678
International Childbirth Education Association, 233, 672
International Endometriosis Association, 136
International Society for Traumatic Stress Studies, 676
International Stress Management Association, 653
International Women's Health Coalition, 678
Internists, 99
Intrauterine devices (IUDs), 102, 118, 150, 158–59
Intrauterine growth restriction, 262–63

In vitro fertilization (IVF),
  185–86
  donor egg, 186–87
Iron, 48, 50, 98
  during pregnancy, 215
Irritability, menopause and,
  599–600, 607–8
Irritable bowel syndromes,
  resources on, 664
Isoflavones, 638, 640, 641
Isotretinoin (Accutane),
  376–77
Italian restaurants, 47
IUDs. *See* Intrauterine devices
IVF (in vitro fertilization),
  185–86
  donor egg, 186–87

J

Japanese encephalitis, during
  pregnancy, 231

K

Kava, 335
Kegel exercises, 610
Ketones, 537

L

Labor, 235–44
  beginning of, 240, 242
  common concerns about,
    235–37
  contractions, 243–44
    pushing, 251
  first stage of, 249–50
  induced, 247–48
  pain control during, 237
  pre-term, 224–25
  second stage of, 250–51
  signs of, 241–42
  stages of, 241, 249–52
  when to call the doctor,
    244–45
Labor assistants (doulas), 193
La Leche League
  International, 672
Laparoscopic surgery, for
  ovarian cysts, 143
Laparoscopy
  for endometriosis, 137, 139
  infertility test using, 178
  for ovarian problems, 141

Laser hair removal, 581–82
Laser resurfacing, 550–54
Laxatives, during
  pregnancy, 222
Lay midwives, 192
Libido, loss of, 602, 610
Lightening, 242
Light therapy, for seasonal
  affective disorder (SAD),
  279–80
Lignans, 638
Liposuction, 73–76
Listeriosis, during
  pregnancy, 232
Lithium, 299–300
Living will, 39–41
LPA (lysophosphatidic
  acid), 423
Lubricants, condoms and, 154
Lumpectomy, 415
Lung cancer, 346, 401
Lupron, 131
Lupus (systemic lupus
  erythematosus, or SLE),
  522, 523, 527–29
Lupus Foundation of
  America, 664
Lyme disease, 515–17, 664
  during pregnancy, 232
  vaccines against, 100–101,
    107, 110
Lyme Disease Information
  Resource, 665
Lyme Disease Network, 665
LYMErix, 100
Lysophosphatidic acid
  (LPA), 423

M

Magnesium, osteoporosis
  and, 471
Magnesium deficiency,
  premenstrual
  syndrome (PMS)
  and, 126
Male factor infertility, 171–72
Male hormones, polycystic
  ovarian syndrome
  (PCOS) and, 144–45
Male sterilization
  (vasectomy), 167
Malignant melanoma, 386–87

Mammograms, 101
  breast implants and, 68
  to detect cancers, 398, 409–11
    ultrasounds versus, 411
Managed care. *See* Health maintenance organizations (HMOs)
Mantoux test, 512
MAOIs (monoamine oxidase inhibitors), 297–99
Marijuana
  infertility and, 173
  during pregnancy, 218
Massage, for menstrual cramps, 119
Mastectomy, 406, 415, 416, 418
Mature women (40-64), 103–7. *See also* Menopause; Osteoporosis
  exercise for, 104
  vaccinations for, 106–7
Measles, mumps, rubella (MMR) vaccine, 87, 111
Medical tests. *See* Tests
Medications. *See also* Drugs
  abuse of, 361
  depression and, 283
  during pregnancy, 221–22
  questions to ask about, 19–20
  sun sensitivity and, 392–94
Meditation
  for depression, 305
  stress and, 320–21
Melanoma, malignant, 386–87
Melatonin, depression and, 279
Melpomene Institute for Women's Health Research, 659
Memory, improving, 588–89
Memory problems (memory loss)
  aging and, 582–89
  menopause and, 600–601, 608
Menopause, 104, 591–643
  breast changes and, 601
  coping with symptoms of, 604–11

depression and, 604
early (perimenopause), 96, 98
finding the right health care provider for, 613–16
"fuzzy thinking" and, 583–84
headaches and, 601, 610
heart palpitations and, 602
heavy bleeding and, 606
hormone replacement therapy and. *See* Hormone replacement therapy (HRT)
hormone tests and, 616–17
hot flashes and, 597–99, 604
insomnia and, 599, 607
irritability and mood swings and, 599–600
loss of sexual interest (libido) and, 602, 610
memory problems and, 600–601, 608
menstrual period changes and, 595–97
nutrition and, 49–50
onset of, 593–95
ovulation and, 591–93
resources on, 665–66
thinking and memory problems and, 600–601
urinary problems and, 602–3, 610–11
urinary tract infections and, 603
vaginal dryness and, 601, 608–10
Menstrual cramps (dysmenorrhea), 118–19
Menstrual problems, 115–23
  abnormal bleeding, 121–23
  absent periods (amenorrhea), 116–18
  heavy flow, 119–21
  painful periods (dysmenorrhea), 118–19
Menstruation
  menopause and, 595–97
  normal, 115–16
  nutrition and, 48
Mental health, resources on, 667–68

INDEX

Mental illness, substance abuse and, 345
Metamucil, 222
Metrodin, 180
Mexican restaurants, 47
Midwives
　certified nurse (CNMs), 192
　lay, 192
Mifepristone (RU-486), 169–70
Miscarriage, 258–59
Misoprostol (Cytotec), 248
Mitral valve prolapse, 440
Moisturizers, 569–71
　vaginal, 609
Moles, skin cancer distinguished from, 383
Monoamine oxidase inhibitors (MAOIs), 297–99
Mononucleosis, 513–15
Mood swings, menopause and, 599–600, 607–8
"Morning after" pill, 167–68
Mother-baby care, 198
Multiple sclerosis (MS), 531–32
Multivitamin supplements, 48, 108
　with iron, 50
　premenstrual syndrome (PMS) and, 127
Myasthenia gravis, 532–33
Mycoplasma, 488
Myomectomy, 132

N

Narcotics, during labor, 237
Narcotics Anonymous, 658
National Aging Information Center, 646
National AIDS Hotline, 647
National Alliance of Breast Cancer Organizations, 420, 655
National Arthritis and Musculoskeletal and Skin Diseases Information Clearinghouse, 653
National Association for Children of Alcoholics, 650
National Association of Anorexia Nervosa and Associated Disorders, 652
National Association of Insurance Commissioners, 31
National Association of People with AIDS, 648
National Cancer Institute, 655
National Center for Complementary and Alternative Medicine (NCCAM) Clearinghouse, 650–51
National Center for Education in Maternal and Child Health, 671
National Chronic Fatigue Syndrome Association, 654
National Clearinghouse for Alcohol and Drug Information, 648–49
National Clearinghouse on Child Abuse and Neglect Information, 655–56
National Coalition Against Domestic Violence, 341, 676
National Coalition Against Sexual Assault, 676
National Coalition for Promoting Physical Activity, 659
National Commission for the Certification of Acupuncturists, 351, 645
National Crime Prevention Council, 676
National Depressive and Manic Depressive Association, 656
National Diabetes Information Clearinghouse (NDIC), 657
National Digestive Diseases Information Clearinghouse, 664
National Domestic Violence hot line, 340

National Drug Information,
Treatment, and Referral
Line, 649
National Eating Disorders
Organization, 658
National Eating Disorders
Organization
(NEDO), 652
National Gay Task Force Crisis
Line, 648
National Headache
Foundation, 660
National Heart, Lung, and
Blood Institute
(NHLBI), 661
National Hypertension
Association, 661
National Institute of
Alcohol Abuse and
Alcoholism, 649
National Institute of Allergy
and Infectious
Diseases, 662
National Institute of Arthritis
and Musculoskeletal
and Skin Diseases,
654, 669
National Institute of Mental
Health (NIMH), 667–68
National Institute on Drug
Abuse, 649, 658
National Kidney and Urologic
Diseases Information
Clearinghouse, 675
National Maternal and Child
Health Clearinghouse,
671–72
National Medicare Issues
Hotline, 664
National Mental Health
Association, 667
National Organization for
Rare Diseases, 654
National Osteoporosis
Foundation, 669
National Osteoporosis
Foundation (NOF), 668
National Psoriasis
Foundation, 672
National Safety Council, 676
National Self-Help
Clearinghouse, 678
National Society of Genetic
Counselors, 660
National STD Hotline, 673
National Women's Health
Information Center, 678
National Women's Health
Network, 679
National Women's Health
Resource Center, 679
Natural Family Planning
(Couple-to-Couple
League), 660
Nausea, during labor, 243
Network for Size Esteem, 677
Neural tube defects, 203–4
Neural-tube defects, 215
Neuromuscular diseases,
531–33
Neurotransmitters,
premenstrual syndrome
(PMS) and, 126
Newborn girls, vaginal
bleeding in, 122
Newborns, 264–67
characteristics of, 270
feeding, 266
going home with, 267
holding, 265
Nicotine gum, 349–51
Nicotine patches, 349–50
Night sweating, 599
Norethindrone acetate, 620
North American Menopause
Society (NAMS), 99–100,
104, 666
North American Registry of
Midwives, 192
Nose job (rhinoplasty), 70–73
Novacet, 375
Nuclear scan (perfusion
imaging), 455
Nurse midwives, 6
certified (CNMs), 192
Nurse practitioners, 6
Nurseries, hospital, 198
Nutrition. *See also* Caloric
intake; Diet; *specific
nutrients*
after childbirth, 268
premenstrual syndrome
(PMS) and, 126
resources, 657

special needs of women, 48–50
teenagers and, 95–96
Nuts, cholesterol and, 452

O

Obesity, 51–53
  health risks of, 51–52
Obstetrician/gynecologists, 190
Occult blood test, 18
Office on Women's Health, 679
Office visits to health care providers
  first, 5, 6
  how to act during, 9–10
  preparing for, 8–9
Older women (over 65), 107–10. *See also* Aging
  exercise for, 56–57
  nutrition and, 50
  staying healthy, 110
Omega-3 fatty acids, 452
Oral contraceptives (birth control pills), 49, 102, 160–62. *See* Oral contraceptives
  cancer and, 400–401
  as hormone replacement therapy (HRT), 625–26
  menstrual cramps and, 119
  polycystic ovarian syndrome (PCOS) and, 146
  vaginal bleeding and, 122
Ortho Tri-Cyclen, 376
OsNET, 669
Osteoarthritis, 52
Osteoporosis, 97, 457–82
  bone density tests for, 104–6, 464–67
  causes of, 459–60
  diagnosis and monitoring of, 462–64
  prevention of, 480–82
  resources, 668–69
  risk factors for, 461–62
  symptoms of, 462
  treatment of, 467–80
    calcitonin, 480
    calcium intake, 468–69
    calcium supplements, 469–70
    drug treatments, 473–82
    exercise, 472–73
    future, 482–83
    hormone replacement therapy, 476–78
    magnesium, 471
    raloxifene (Evista), 478–80
    vitamin D, 470–71
Osteoporosis and Related Bone Diseases National Resource Center, 668
Ovarian cancer, 401, 420–25
  hereditary, 423–24
  mortality rate, 420
  risk factors, 421–23
  screening for, 423
  treatment of, 424–25
Ovarian cysts, 140–43. *See also* Polycystic ovarian syndrome (PCOS)
  treatment of, 142–43
Ovaries, problems of, 139–47
  cysts and tumors, 140–43
  infections, 140, 141
  polycystic ovarian syndrome (PCOS), 143–47
  polycystic ovary syndrome (PCOS), 140
Overeaters Anonymous, 676
Overweight. *See also* Obesity
  in older women (over 65), 108
Ovulation
  detection of, 171
  menopause and, 591–93
Ovulation predictor kit, in-home, 18–19
OWL (Older Women's League), 646
Oxytocin (Pitocin), 248

P

Panic attacks, 330
Panic disorder, 331–32
Pap smear, 88, 101
  cervical cancer and, 427, 429–30

Pap smear, (cont.)
  to detect cancers, 398
  for mature women
    (40 to 64), 105
  for older women
    (over 65), 109
  for pregnant women, 202
  for teenagers, 89–91
Paragard Copper T 380A, 158
Parathyroid hormone,
  osteoporosis and, 482
Parlodel, 180
Partnership with your health
  care provider, 5–7, 10–13
Patient(s), how to be a good,
  7–8
Patient's Bill of Rights, 37–38
Paxil, for premenstrual
  syndrome (PMS), 129
PCOS. See Polycystic ovarian
  syndrome
Pediatricians, choosing, 80–82
Pelvic exams, 101
  before childbirth, 247
  to detect cancers, 398
  sexually transmitted
    diseases (STDs) and, 498
  for teenagers, 91–94
Pelvic inflammatory disease
  (PID), 494–96
Pelvic training weights, 610–11
People's Plague Online, 674
Perfusion imaging (nuclear
  scan), 455
Pergonal, 180
Perimenopause, 96, 98
Perinatologists, 191
Phobias, 332–33
  treatment for, 335
Photosensitivity, 392–94
Physical abuse, 335–41
Physical activity.
  See also Exercise
  obesity and, 52–53
Physical examination. See also
  Tests; and specific
  procedures
  for teenagers, 87–88
Physician assistants, 6
Physicians. See also Health care
  providers; Specialists
  finding, 4–7, 99–100

Physicians Who Care, 32
PID (pelvic inflammatory
  disease), 494–96
Pill, the. See Oral
  contraceptives
Pinnell, Sheldon, 567
Pitocin (oxytocin), 248
Placenta previa, 227–28
Planned Parenthood, 92
Planned Parenthood
  Federation of
  America, 663
Plant estrogens, 620
Plastic surgery, 66–77. See also
  Skin (skin diseases),
  younger-looking
  breast surgery, cosmetic,
    66–70
  cost of common
    operations, 66
  finding a plastic surgeon,
    572–73
  liposuction, 73–76
  nose job (rhinoplasty),
    70–73
  resources, 669–70
  for skin conditions, 571–75
  tummy tucks (abdominal
    recontouring), 76–77
Plastic Surgery Network, 670
Pneumococcal (pneumonia)
  vaccine, 106, 109
Polio vaccines, 85–86
Polycystic ovarian syndrome
  (PCOS), 140, 143–47
  causes of, 144–45
  treatments for, 145–46
Postpartum depression,
  281–83
Poverty, substance abuse
  and, 345
Power Surge Reading Room,
  665–66
Preeclampsia, 225
Pregnancy, 189–233
  choosing health care
    providers, 190–96
  diet during, 213–15
  ectopic, 228–29
  electroconvulsive treatment
    (ECT) and, 301
  endometriosis and, 139

exercise during, 216
experience of, 207–13
    first trimester, 207–8
    second trimester, 208–10
    third trimester, 211–13
first prenatal visit, 200–201
fluids during, 215, 217
nutrition and, 48–49
problems during, 223–32
    abruptio placentae, 225–26
    bleeding, 226–27
    ectopic pregnancy, 228–29
    infections, 229–32
    placenta previa, 227–28
    preeclampsia, 225
    pre-term labor, 224–25
resources, 670–72
screening tests, 201–7
    alpha-fetoprotein (AFP) test, 203–4
    amniocentesis, 205–6
    basic tests, 201–2
    chorionic villus sampling (CVS), 206–7
    triple screening, 204–5
    ultrasound, 202–3
smoking and, 346
urinary tract infections during, 489
vitamin supplements during, 215–16
what to avoid during, 218–23
    alcohol, 218–19
    artificial sweeteners, 221
    caffeine, 220–21
    chemical exposure, 223
    hot tubs and saunas, 222
    medicines, 221–22
    recreational drugs, 220
    smoking, 220
    travel, 222–23
Pregnancy tests, 189–90
    home, 18

Premarin, 619
Premenopausal women, vaginal bleeding in, 122
Premenstrual syndrome (PMS), 123–29
    causes of, 125–26
    diagnosis of, 126–27
    easing symptoms of, 127
    medications for, 128–29
    menopause and, 611–13
    nutrition and, 48
    symptoms of, 124–25
Prenatal visit, first, 200–201
President's Council on Physical Fitness and Sports, 659–60
Progestasert Progesterone T., 158
Progesterone, 620
    in endometriosis treatment, 138
    menstrual flow and, 119–20
Progestins, 620–21
Project Inform HIV/AIDS Treatment Hotline, 647
Prolactin, infertility and, 172
Promensil, 453
Prostaglandins, 118
Provera, 620
Prozac, 294–95
    for premenstrual syndrome (PMS), 129
    for seasonal affective disorder (SAD), 280
Psoriasis, 538
    resources, 672
Psychoanalysis, for depression, 288
Psychotherapy, for anorexia nervosa, 62
Purging, bulimia nervosa and, 62–64
Pushing, during delivery, 251–52

Q

Quack cures, 20

R

Radiation therapy, for breast cancer, 415–17

Raloxifene (Evista), 407, 419, 474, 478–80, 621, 622
Read Natural Childbirth Foundation, 233
Relaxation. *See also* Meditation
  depression and, 305
  stress and, 319–20
Renova, 375, 377, 558–59
Reproductive endocrinologists, 98–99
Resolve, Inc., 176, 663
Resource Center on Child Custody and Protection, 341
Resources for Mid-Life and Older Women, 645
Restaurants, low-fat, healthy meals in, 47–48
Retin-A (tretinoin), 375, 377, 558–59, 568–69
  AHAs versus, 563
Retinol palmitate, 559
Rheumatoid arthritis, 529–30
Rhinoplasty (nose job), 70–73
"Rhythm" method of birth control, 152
Rooming in, 197–98
Rosacea, 378–81
RU-486 (mifepristone), 169–70
Rubella (German measles), during pregnancy, 230
Rupture of membranes, in labor, 242–43

S

Salad dressing, 451
Saline implant, 67
Salt, 48
Sarcoidosis, 540–41
Saunas, during pregnancy, 222
Scleroderma (systemic sclerosis), 530
Seasonal affective disorder (SAD), 278–80
Second opinion, on surgery, 21–22
Sedatives, during labor, 237
SERMs (selective estrogen receptor modulators), 474, 478, 482, 621, 622

Serotonin, 48
  depression and, 277–78
Serotonin reuptake inhibitors (SSRIs). *See* SSRIs
Sex
  menopause and loss of interest in, 602, 610
  resources, 672–73
Sexism, depression treatment and, 290
Sexuality Information and Education Council of the United States, 673
Sexually transmitted diseases (STDs), 100, 141
  chlamydia, 499–500
  condoms and, 154
  genital herpes, 502–4
  genital warts, 500–502
  gonorrhea, 504–5
  hepatitis B, 505–7
  HIV and AIDS, 508–10
  preventing, 497–510
  resources, 673
  syphilis, 507–8
  treatment outlook, 499
Shape Up America!, 676
Sidelines, 671
Sigmoidoscopy, 105, 109, 399
  flexible, 18
Size Acceptance Web Site, 677
Sjogren's syndrome (Sjogren's disease), 531
Skin (skin diseases), 367–96
  acne, 370–79
  autoimmune, 538–39
  cancer. *See* Skin cancer
  dry skin, 569–71
  of newborns, 264
  of older women (over 65), 108
  resources, 674
  rosacea, 378–81
  specialists in (dermatologists), 367–70
  younger-looking, 549–69
    AHA (alpha-hydroxy acid), 560–67
    botox injections, 555–56
    brow-lifts, 575

chemical peels, 557–58
collagen treatments, 554–55
combining skin products, 568–69
dermabrasion, 556
do-it-yourself peels (fruit acids), 560–67
eyelid-lifts, 575
face-lifts, 573–74
laser resurfacing, 550–54
plastic or cosmetic surgery, 571–75
vitamin A derivatives, 558–59
vitamin A-like products, 559–60
vitamin C, 567–68
of young women (20 to 39), 96–97
Skin cancer, 381–94
basal cell carcinoma, 383–85
checking for, 88
malignant melanoma, 386–87
moles distinguished from, 383
monthly check for, 381–83
quiz on, 387
squamous cell carcinoma, 385–86
sun safety and, 388
SLE (systemic lupus erythematosus), 522, 523, 527–29
Sleep. *See also* Insomnia
memory and, 587
premenstrual syndrome (PMS) and, 127
Sleep habits, of newborns, 270
Smoking, 345–51
cancer and, 401
health risks of, 346–47
heart disease and, 451
infertility and, 173
memory and, 587
pregnancy and, 220, 346
quitting, 347–51
stress and, 327

Social support. *See also* Support groups
cardiovascular disease and, 452
stress and, 329
Society for Assisted Reproductive Technology (SART), 184
Society for the Advancement of Women's Health Research, 679
Society for the Prevention of Human Infertility, 663
Soy foods (soy products)
cholesterol and, 452
hot flashes and, 606
osteoporosis and, 481–82
Specialists, 13–14. *See also specific types of specialists*
choosing, 80–82
eating disorders, 60
for young women (20 to 39), 98–99
Sperm, problems in producing, 171–72
Sperm banks, 181–84
Spermicide, 103, 153
Spinal block, 238–39
Sponge, birth control, 156–58
Sports bra, 53
Squamous cell carcinoma, 385–86
SSRIs (serotonin reuptake inhibitors), 294–96
for seasonal affective disorder (SAD), 280
St. John's wort (hypericum), 173
for depression, 302–4
for premenstrual syndrome (PMS), 129
Steinberg, Alan J., 29
Sterilization, surgical, 165–67
Stillbirth, 259–61
Stool screening, 101
frequency of, 105
StorkNet, 671
Strep, group B, during pregnancy, 230–31
Stress, 309–30
alcohol and, 327
benefits of, 329–30

Stress, (cont.)
  dealing with, 314–30
    anti-stress vitamins/herbs, 328–29
    breathing, 315–19
    diet and, 325–28
    exercise, 323–25
    meditation, 320–21
    relaxation, 319–20
    visualization, 321–23
  determining amount of, 311–14
  effects of, 310–11
  infertility and, 173
  memory and, 586
  resources, 652–53
  smoking and, 327
  substance abuse and, 345
Stress echocardiography, 454
Stress hormones, 309–10
Stress incontinence, 602
Stress test (treadmill), 311–13, 454
Stroke, 437–40
Substance abuse, 343–64
  alcohol. *See* Alcohol abuse (alcoholism)
  defined, 343–44
  infertility and, 172
  resources, 648–50, 658
  risk factors for, 344–45
  smoking. *See* Smoking
Substance Abuse and Mental Health Services Administration, 649
Substance and Alcohol Abuse Treatment Program, 649
Sulfur products, for acne, 375
Sunglasses, 392
Sun safety, 388–94
Sunscreen, 388–92
Supplements. *See* Multivitamin supplements; *and specific supplements*
Support groups. *See also* Social support
  alcoholism, 359
  breast cancer, 420
  depression, 304–5
  premenstrual syndrome (PMS), 128

Surgery, 20–22
  for breast cancer, 415–16
  for fibroids, 132
  for infertility, 181
  plastic. *See* Plastic surgery
  questions to ask about, 21
Sweating, night, 599
Synarel, 131
Syphilis, 507–8
  during pregnancy, 232
Systemic lupus erythematosus (SLE, or lupus), 522, 523, 527–29
Systemic sclerosis (scleroderma), 530

T

Tachycardia, 441–42
Take Off Pounds Sensibly (TOPS), 676
Tamoxifen, 407, 417–20, 426, 479, 621
Tans, indoor, 394–96
TB Resources, 675
TB Weekly, 675
Teaching hospitals, 35
Teenage girls, 87–96
  body image of, 44
  eating disorders in, 58
  gynecologists for, 89
  nutrition and, 95–96
  Pap smear for, 89–91
  pelvic exam for, 91–94
  physical exams for, 87–88
  vaccinations for, 87
Testosterone
  hormone replacement therapy (HRT) and, 623–25
  polycystic ovarian syndrome (PCOS) and, 144–45
Tests, 14–19. *See also specific tests*
  home, 16
    blood glucose, 17
    blood in stool, 18
    blood pressure, 17
    ovulation predictor kit, 18–19
    pregnancy, 18, 189–90
    urinalysis, 16

for mature women (40 to 64), 104–6
for older women (over 65), 108, 109
for ovarian cysts, 142
pregnancy, 189–90
for pregnant women, 201–7
refusing, 15
for young women (20-39), 100
Tetanus booster, 102, 107, 109
Tetanus/diphtheria (Td) booster, 87
Thyroid Foundation of America, 674
Thyroid tests, 109
Tissue backup, endometriosis and, 134–35
Toxic shock syndrome (TSS), 496–97
Toxoplasmosis, during pregnancy, 232
Tranquilizers, during labor, 237
Transitions for Health, 646
Travel, during pregnancy, 222–23
Tretinoin (Renova), 375, 377
Trichomoniasis, 494
Tri-Cyclen, 376
Tricyclic antidepressants, 295, 296–97
Triglycerides, 450
Triple screening, 204–5
TSS (toxic shock syndrome), 496–97
Tubal ligation, 166
Tuberculosis, 510–13
resources, 674
Tuberculosis (TB), testing for, 88
Tummy tucks (abdominal recontouring), 76–77
Tumors. *See also* Cancer
ovarian, 140
Tums, 49, 96, 222
Type 1 (insulin-dependent) diabetes mellitus (IDDM), 535–37

U

Ulcerative colitis, 538
Ultrafast CT scan, 454
Ultrasound
for ovarian problems, 141
for pregnant women, 202–3
Ultrasound densitometry, 465
United Soybean Board, 666
Urinalysis, 16
for teenagers, 88
Urinary incontinence, 21–22
menopause and, 602–3, 610–11
Urinary tract infections
menopause and, 603
preventing, 488–91
resources, 675
Urine tests, for osteoporosis, 466
Urologists, 21
Uterine fibroids. *See* Fibroids
UV Index, 388–89

V

Vaccinations (immunizations), 110–12
chicken pox, 83–85, 87, 111
for ear infections, 86
flu, 86–87, 102, 487
hepatitis A, 111
hepatitis B, 111
for infants, 83–85
for mature women (40-64), 106–7
measles, mumps, rubella (MMR), 87, 111
for older women, 108–10
pneumococcal (pneumonia), 106, 109
polio, 85–86
resources, 675
for teenagers, 87, 88
for young women (20-39), 100–102
Vaccine Adverse Event Reporting System, 675
Vaccines and Diseases News, 675
Vaginal bleeding, 121–23
during pregnancy, 226–27
Vaginal dryness, menopause and, 601, 608–10
Vaginal infections, 491–94
bacterial, infertility and, 173
Vaginal spermicide, 153

Vaginosis, bacterial, 493–94
Valium, 334
Valtrex, 504
Vasculitis syndromes, 541–42
Vasectomy (male
  sterilization), 167
Violent relationships, 335–41
  resources, 675
Visualization, stress and,
  321–23
Vitamin A
  cancer and, 399
  during pregnancy, 216
Vitamin A-like products,
  559–60
Vitamin B6
  depression and, 305
  premenstrual syndrome
    (PMS) and, 126
Vitamin C, 97
Vitamin C, skin and, 567–68
Vitamin D, 97
Vitamin D, osteoporosis and,
  470–71
Vitamin E, for hot flashes,
  605–6
Vitamin/mineral
  supplements. *See*
  Multivitamin
  supplements
  anti-stress, 328–29
  for depression, 305–6
  during pregnancy, 215–16
  prenatal, 216
Vitiligo, 539
Vulvovaginal candidiasis
  (VVC), 492–93
VVC (vulvovaginal
  candidiasis), 492–93

W

Weight, infertility and, 173
Weight Control Information
  Network, 677
Weight control resources,
  676–77
Weight gain
  in mature women
    (40 to 64), 97
  during pregnancy, 214
Weight loss diets (dieting), 46
  ineffectiveness of, 46–47
Wellspring for Women, 666
Withdrawal, as birth control
  method, 151
Women and AIDS Resource
  Network, 648
Women's Action Alliance, 646
Women's Health America
  Group, 679
Women's Health and Fertility
  Branch, 663
Women's Health Initiative, 680
Women's Helpline (now
  called the NYC Service
  Fund), 680

X

Xanax, 334
  for premenstrual syndrome
    (PMS), 128–29

Y

Yeast infections, 492–93
Young women (20 to 39),
  96–103

Z

ZIFT (zygote intrafallopian
  transfer), 186
Zinc oxide, 390
Zoloft, for premenstrual
  syndrome (PMS), 129
Zyderm, 554
Zygote intrafallopian transfer
  (ZIFT; tubal embryo
  transfer), 186
Zyplast, 554

The *Unofficial Guide*™ Reader Questionnaire

If you would like to express your opinion about women's health or this guide, please complete this questionnaire and mail it to:

The *Unofficial Guide*™ Reader Questionnaire
IDG Books Consumer Reference Group
1633 Broadway, floor 7
New York, NY 10019-6785

Gender: ___ M   ___ F

Age: ___ Under 30   ___ 31–40   ___ 41–50
___ Over 50

Education: ___ High school   ___ College
___ Graduate/Professional

What is your occupation?
_____

How did you hear about this guide?
___ Friend or relative
___ Newspaper, magazine, or Internet
___ Radio or TV
___ Recommended at bookstore
___ Recommended by librarian
___ Picked it up on my own
___ Familiar with the *Unofficial Guide*™ travel series

Did you go to the bookstore specifically for a book on women's health? Yes ___ No ___

Have you used any other *Unofficial Guides*™?
Yes ___ No ___

If Yes, which ones?
_____
_____
_____

What other book(s) on women's health have you purchased? _____
_____
_____

Was this book:
___ more helpful than other(s)
___ less helpful than other(s)

Do you think this book was worth its price?
Yes ___   No ___

Did this book cover all topics related to women's health adequately?
Yes ___   No ___

Please explain your answer:
_____
_____
_____

Were there any specific sections in this book that were of particular help to you?   Yes ___   No ___

Please explain your answer:
_____
_____
_____

On a scale of 1 to 10, with 10 being the best rating, how would you rate this guide? ___

What other titles would you like to see published in the *Unofficial Guide*™ series?
_____
_____

***Are Unofficial Guides*™ readily available in your area?**   Yes ___   No ___

Other comments:
_____
_____
_____
_____

Get the inside scoop...with the *Unofficial Guides*™!

Health and Fitness

The Unofficial Guide to Alternative Medicine
ISBN: 0-02-862526-9 Price: $15.95

The Unofficial Guide to Conquering Impotence
ISBN: 0-02-862870-5 Price: $15.95

The Unofficial Guide to Coping with Menopause
ISBN: 0-02-862694-x Price: $15.95

The Unofficial Guide to Cosmetic Surgery
ISBN: 0-02-862522-6 Price: $15.95

The Unofficial Guide to Dieting Safely
ISBN: 0-02-862521-8 Price: $15.95

The Unofficial Guide to Having a Baby
ISBN: 0-02-862695-8 Price: $15.95

The Unofficial Guide to Living with Diabetes
ISBN: 0-02-862919-1 Price: $15.95

The Unofficial Guide to Overcoming Arthritis
ISBN: 0-02-862714-8 Price: $15.95

The Unofficial Guide to Overcoming Infertility
ISBN: 0-02-862916-7 Price: $15.95

Career Planning

The Unofficial Guide to Acing the Interview
ISBN: 0-02-862924-8 Price: $15.95

The Unofficial Guide to Earning What You Deserve
ISBN: 0-02-862523-4 Price: $15.95

The Unofficial Guide to Hiring and Firing People
ISBN: 0-02-862523-4 Price: $15.95

Business and Personal Finance

The Unofficial Guide to Investing
ISBN: 0-02-862458-0 Price: $15.95

The Unofficial Guide to Investing in Mutual Funds
ISBN: 0-02-862920-5 Price: $15.95

The Unofficial Guide to Managing Your Personal Finances
ISBN: 0-02-862921-3 Price: $15.95

The Unofficial Guide to Starting a Small Business
ISBN: 0-02-862525-0 Price: $15.95

Home and Automotive

The Unofficial Guide to Buying a Home
ISBN: 0-02-862461-0 Price: $15.95

The Unofficial Guide to Buying or Leasing a Car
ISBN: 0-02-862524-2 Price: $15.95

The Unofficial Guide to Hiring Contractors
ISBN: 0-02-862460-2 Price: $15.95

Family and Relationships

The Unofficial Guide to Childcare
ISBN: 0-02-862457-2 Price: $15.95

The Unofficial Guide to Dating Again
ISBN: 0-02-862454-8 Price: $15.95

The Unofficial Guide to Divorce
ISBN: 0-02-862455-6 Price: $15.95

The Unofficial Guide to Eldercare
ISBN: 0-02-862456-4 Price: $15.95

The Unofficial Guide to Planning Your Wedding
ISBN: 0-02-862459-9 Price: $15.95

Hobbies and Recreation

The Unofficial Guide to Finding Rare Antiques
ISBN: 0-02-862922-1 Price: $15.95

The Unofficial Guide to Casino Gambling
ISBN: 0-02-862917-5 Price: $15.95

All books in the *Unofficial Guide*™ series are available at your local bookseller, or by calling 1-800-428-5331.